Weight Loss Kit
For Dummies®

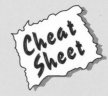

Cheat Sheet

Seven Health Problems Linked to Excess Weight

- Certain types of cancer
- Diabetes
- Gallbladder disease
- Heart disease
- High blood pressure
- High cholesterol
- Stroke

How Many Calories Do You Burn in 15 Minutes of Exercise?

- Aerobic dance: 171 calories
- Bicycling (12 mph): 142 calories
- Jumping rope (60 80 skips/minute): 143 calories
- Rowing machine: 104 calories
- Running (10-minute mile): 183 calories
- Walking (20-minute mile, flat ground): 60 calories
- Water aerobics: 70 calories

Seven Great Things About Regular Exercise

- It helps control obesity.
- It builds muscle.
- It makes bones stronger.
- It improves heart health.
- It lowers blood pressure.
- It lowers cholesterol.
- It reduces the risk of diabetes.

For Dummies™: Bestselling Book Series for Beginners

Weight Loss Kit For Dummies®

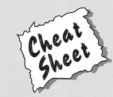

Cheat Sheet

Who's Fat?

Forget the weight charts. A better guide to healthy weight is BMI (body mass index), a number that describes your body's fat-to-lean-mass (muscle) composition.

- BMI below 18.5 is underweight.
- BMI of 18.5 to 24.9 is normal.
- BMI of 25 to 29.9 is Grade 1 obesity.
- BMI of 30 to 39.9 is Grade 2 obesity.
- BMI over 40 is Grade 3 obesity.

Four Fast Food Sandwiches Under 300 Calories

- McDonald's Hamburger (260 calories)
- Arby's Roast Chicken Deluxe Sandwich (276 calories)
- Pizza Hut Hand-Tossed Chicken Supreme Pizza (240 calories)
- Subway Veggie Delite (whole-wheat bread) (237 calories)

Three Ways to Identify a Fad Diet

- It claims you'll lose lots of weight very fast.
- It promotes "special" food or a very restricted diet.
- It says you can lose weight without exercising.

Avoid this diet!

Defining Food Label Terms for Fat Content

- Extra lean = (Meat, fish) less than 5 g fat
- Fat-free = Less than 0.5 g per serving
- Lean = (Meat, fish) less than 10 g fat & 0.5 g
- Light = 50 percent less than standard product
- Lowfat = 3 g or less per serving
- Reduced fat = 25 percent less than standard product

Counting Calories

- 1 gram protein = 4 calories
- 1 gram carbohydrate = 4 calories
- 1 gram fat = 9 calories
- 1 gram alcohol = 7 calories

Hungry Minds™

For Dummies™: Bestselling Book Series for Beginners

Praise for Weight Loss Kit For Dummies

"It's about time! Finally a weight loss book that's 100 percent fad-free! Carol Ann Rinzler speaks to the reader in a realistic, easily understood voice. I'd comfortably recommend this book to my patients."

— Bonnie Taub-Dix, M.A., R.D., C.D.N.,
Director, BTD Nutrition Consultants

"*Weight Loss Kit For Dummies* includes everything you need to get started and stay on a *successful* weight loss program — for first-timers and veteran dieters alike. And Carol's lighthearted conversational style weaves humor and scientific fact together so there's never a dull moment."

— Betty Ivie Goldblatt, R.D., M.P.H.,
Publisher, *Environmental Nutrition* newsletter

"Anyone who wants to lose weight should start with this simple, common sense guide. This is, by far, the best weight loss book around! Rinzler tells you what works, what doesn't work and why."

— Congresswoman Carolyn B. Maloney

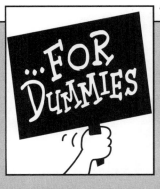
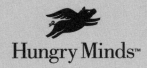

Weight Loss Kit
FOR
DUMMIES®

by Carol Ann Rinzler

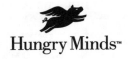

Hungry Minds™

HUNGRY MINDS, INC.

New York, NY ◆ Cleveland, OH ◆ Indianapolis, IN

Weight Loss Kit For Dummies®

Published by:
Hungry Minds, Inc.
909 Third Avenue
New York, NY 10022
www.hungryminds.com
www.dummies.com

Library of Congress Control Number: 00112173

ISBN: 0-7645-5334-8

Printed in the United States of America

10 9 8 7 6 5 4 3 2 1

1O/QV/QU/QR/IN

Distributed in the United States by Hungry Minds, Inc.

Distributed by CDG Books Canada Inc. for Canada; by Transworld Publishers Limited in the United Kingdom; by IDG Norge Books for Norway; by IDG Sweden Books for Sweden; by IDG Books Australia Publishing Corporation Pty. Ltd. for Australia and New Zealand; by TransQuest Publishers Pte Ltd. for Singapore, Malaysia, Thailand, Indonesia, and Hong Kong; by Gotop Information Inc. for Taiwan; by ICG Muse, Inc. for Japan; by Intersoft for South Africa; by Eyrolles for France; by International Thomson Publishing for Germany, Austria and Switzerland; by Distribuidora Cuspide for Argentina; by LR International for Brazil; by Galileo Libros for Chile; by Ediciones ZETA S.C.R. Ltda. for Peru; by WS Computer Publishing Corporation, Inc., for the Philippines; by Contemporanea de Ediciones for Venezuela; by Express Computer Distributors for the Caribbean and West Indies; by Micronesia Media Distributor, Inc. for Micronesia; by Chips Computadoras S.A. de C.V. for Mexico; by Editorial Norma de Panama S.A. for Panama; by American Bookshops for Finland.

For general information on Hungry Minds' products and services please contact our Customer Care department; within the U.S. at 800-762-2974, outside the U.S. at 317-572-3993 or fax 317-572-4002.

For sales inquiries and resellers information, including discounts, premium and bulk quantity sales and foreign language translations please contact our Customer Care department at 800-434-3422, fax 317-572-4002 or write to Hungry Minds, Inc., Attn: Customer Care department, 10475 Crosspoint Boulevard, Indianapolis, IN 46256.

For information on licensing foreign or domestic rights, please contact our Sub-Rights Customer Care department at 650-653-7098.

For information on using Hungry Minds' products and services in the classroom or for ordering examination copies, please contact our Educational Sales department at 800-434-2086 or fax 317-572-4005.

Please contact our Public Relations department at 212-884-5163 for press review copies or 212-884-5000 for author interviews and other publicity information or fax 212-884-5400.

For authorization to photocopy items for corporate, personal, or educational use, please contact Copyright Clearance Center, 222 Rosewood Drive, Danvers, MA 01923, or fax 978-750-4470.

Hungry Minds⁻ is a trademark of Hungry Minds, Inc.

About the Author

Carol Ann Rinzler is the author of *Nutrition For Dummies,* one of Amazon.com's ten best health books of 1999. A member of the National Association of Science Writers, she holds a master's degree from Columbia University. Carol's 20 books on nutrition, food, and health include *The New Complete Book of Herbs, Spices, and Condiments.* She lives in New York with her husband, wine writer Perry Luntz.

Dedication

To my husband, Perry Luntz, for more reasons than I could ever list, chief among them, his unfailing ability to see the good in every thing and every person.

Author's Acknowledgments

Oh, boy, do I have a long list of people to thank. Start with Stacy Collins, a woman who personifies the old-fashioned virtues such as honesty and practicality. Stacy brought the idea to me in the first place, so she's first in line for thanks. I want to thank my project editor Kelly Ewing (and Katie, too) as well as Suzanne Thomas who was with me on *Nutrition For Dummies* and had her fine hand in this book, too. And I have a special sense of gratitude to Carmen Krikorian. And, of course, my thanks go to Jennifer Young, Stacy Klein, and Nancee Reeves who (in order, of course), formatted the book, entered most of my changes, and coordinated the project through Production.

Wait! There's more. Joe D. Bartolomeo of Nutrisystems; Christine Bonney of Metropolitan Life Insurance Company; Jackie Havens and John Webster at the U.S. Department of Agriculture; Harold J. Holler of the American Dietetic Association; Maryann Gorman and Kathe Hooper of the American Society for Testing and Materials; Brenda Mack at the Federal Trade Commission; Richard E. Morris of the the National Academy of Sciences; Jean Bradley Rubel of Anorexia Nervosa and Related Eating Disorders (ANRED); and Gregg Szczesny of Tanita Corporation graciously answered questions and provided information we needed to complete this book. Yes, it's a cliche, but the truth is I could never have done it without them.

Finally, I am extraordinarily appreciative of Alfred Bushway, Mary Ellen Camire, Nancy Cohen, and Manfred Kroger, experts all who took the time to read and comment on the manuscript. If you find the *Weight Loss Kit For Dummies* reliable, it is these professionals who had a big hand in making it so.

Publisher's Acknowledgments

We're proud of this book; please send us your comments through our Online Registration Form located at www.dummies.com.

Some of the people who helped bring this book to market include the following:

Acquisitions, Editorial, and Media Development

Project Editor: Kelly Ewing

Acquisitions Editor: Stacy S. Collins

Acquisitions Coordinator: Stacy Klein

General Reviewers: Alfred Bushway, Mary Ellen Camire, Nancy Cohen, Manfred Kroger

Senior Permissions Editor: Carmen Krikorian

Media Development Specialist: Megan Decraene

Editorial Manager: Jennifer Ehrlich

Editorial Coordinator: Michelle Hacker

Media Development Manager: Laura Carpenter

Editorial Assistant: Jennifer Young

Cover Photos: Tony Stone, © James Darell

Production

Project Coordinator: Nancee Reeves

Layout and Graphics: Jackie Nicholas, Jacque Schneider, Jeremey Unger

Proofreaders: Angel Perez, Carl Pierce, Marianne Santy, York Production Services, Inc.

Indexer: York Production Services, Inc.

Special Help
Suzanne Thomas

General and Administrative

Hungry Minds, Inc.: John Kilcullen, CEO; Bill Barry, President and COO; John Ball, Executive VP, Operations & Administration; John Harris, CFO

Hungry Minds Consumer Reference Group

>   **Business:** Kathleen A. Welton, Vice President and Publisher; Kevin Thornton, Acquisitions Manager

>   **Cooking/Gardening:** Jennifer Feldman, Associate Vice President and Publisher

>   **Education/Reference:** Diane Graves Steele, Vice President and Publisher; Greg Tubach, Publishing Director

>   **Lifestyles:** Kathleen Nebenhaus, Vice President and Publisher; Tracy Boggier, Managing Editor

>   **Pets:** Dominique De Vito, Associate Vice President and Publisher; Tracy Boggier, Managing Editor

>   **Travel:** Michael Spring, Vice President and Publisher; Suzanne Jannetta, Editorial Director; Brice Gosnell, Managing Editor

Hungry Minds Consumer Editorial Services: Kathleen Nebenhaus, Vice President and Publisher; Kristin A. Cocks, Editorial Director; Cindy Kitchel, Editorial Director

Hungry Minds Consumer Production: Debbie Stailey, Production Director

◆

The publisher would like to give special thanks to Patrick J. McGovern, without whom this book would not have been possible.

◆

Contents at a Glance

Cartoons at a Glance

By Rich Tennant

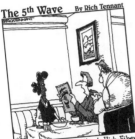

"I'll have the 'Healthy-Heart-High-Fiber-Lowfat-I'll-Just-Have-A-Bite-Of-My-Neighbors-Eggs-Benedict Breakfast.'"

page 147

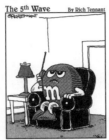

"My body type? I'm an 'M.' But I'd like to get down to an 'N,' maybe an 'H.'"

page 253

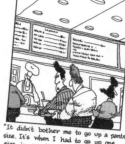

"It didn't bother me to go up a pants size. It's when I had to go up one size in camping tents that I began to worry."

page 5

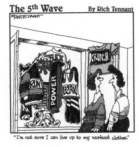

"I'm not sure I can live up to my workout clothes."

page 227

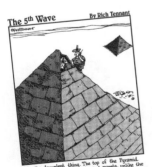

"It's the darnedest thing. The top of the Pyramid seems to be filled with fats and sweets, unlike the base, which contained mostly fresh vegetables, grains, and legumes."

page 43

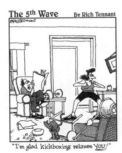

"I'm glad kickboxing relaxes _YOU!_"

page 197

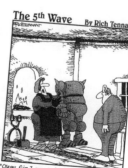

"Okay, Sir Loungealot, I was able to pound out another inch in the waist, but you're gonna have to start taking care of yourself or buy a new suit of armor."

page 275

Cartoon Information:
Fax: 978-546-7747
E-Mail: richtennant@the5thwave.com
World Wide Web: www.the5thwave.com

Table of Contents

Introduction

*J*ust as I started to write this introduction, some really important university whose name I cannot tell you because the newspaper clipping about the study has disappeared into the, um, clutter on my desk released a totally new study showing that most people are fed up to the eyeballs with diet advice.

No wonder. It seems that every morning you wake up to discover that (1) some food once absolutely Essential to Your Health has turned out to be Really Bad News, or (2) some food once considered Really Bad News has turned out to be absolutely Essential to Your Health, or (3) . . . well, who knows what (3) will turn out to be?

Not I. But I do know this: While specific foods go in and out of nutrition fashion as nutrition scientists continue to unpeel the Good-to-Eat Onion, some facts of healthy life never change. For example, no matter which foods are In and which are Out, when the skirt or pants that fit last summer don't close, it's time to lose weight.

This book aims to help you accomplish that goal.

What This Book Is About

Weight Loss Kit For Dummies does not insist that you control your weight by sticking to one particular diet. This book recognizes the fact that bodies differ. So do taste and food preferences. What works for me may not work for you or that guy over there in the next seat. As a result, this book is designed to give you the information you need to pick the weight loss program that works for you.

Some of the information here is totally basic stuff, like how to weigh yourself, a technique I bet you thought you mastered long ago. (I bet you haven't!) Other chapters provide tests you can use to determine whether a weight loss program is safe and effective and show you how to set reasonable long-term goals. There is a plethora of Web sites and 800-numbers giving access to even more info about weight loss possibilities. Plus another appendix introduces you to the world's greatest nutrient chart, the USDA Nutrient Data Base.

How This Book Is Organized

The following pages give you a brief but tasty summary of each of the 18 "regular" chapters, 4 Part of Tens chapters, and 3 Appendixes in the *Weight Loss Kit For Dummies*. These summaries make it easy to check out which chapter you want to dive into first. No need to start at Chapter 1 and read straight through to the end. You can start anywhere that tickles your fancy and go back and forth as your choose. What a pleasant way to discover how to change your body and change your life.

Part 1: Ready, Set, Lose!

Chapter 1 tells you why your weight is important to your health. Chapter 2 provides a plethora of tests you can use to answer the eternal question, "How do I know if I'm fat?" Chapter 3, a techie guide, tells you how to use a scale (not as easy as you think!).

Part 11: Choosing a Weight Loss Plan

Chapter 4 is the perfect intro to this section because it tells you what you need to know before you start to peel away the pounds. Chapter 5 explains why calories definitely do count. Chapter 6 lays out the intricacies of carbohydrate-based weight loss plans. Chapter 7 does the honors for low-carb, high protein plans. Chapter 8 evaluates the role of fats in weight control. And Chapter 9 is a mixed bag of unusual weight loss programs, some good, some (how shall I put this?) not so good.

Part 111: Strategic Food Choices

Part III begins with Chapter 10, which details nutrition essentials for people trying to lose weight. Chapter 11 is a guide to smart shopping for weight loss meals. Can you stick to your weight loss plan when you're dining out? Darn right you can — and Chapter 12 shows you how. Finally, for people who just can't cook or hate to count calories, there's Chapter 13, a list of products that you may use once a day in place of real food.

Part 1V: Other Ways to Lose Weight

Chapter 14 is serious stuff, a compendium of facts about weight loss drugs. Chapter 15, which describes surgery for weight reduction, is equally serious, although folks addicted to word play might just call it a cut above the rest. Ouch! Chapter 16 talks about gadgets and gimmicks, mostly ineffective.

Part V: Lifelong Weight Control

Once you take off the pounds, can you keep them off? The answer may depend on whether you use the techniques for behavior modification described in Chapter 17 or take up regular exercise such as the plans you find in Chapter 18.

Part VI: The Part of Tens

This is the part of the *Weight Loss Kit* that justifies *For Dummies*. Chapter 19 debunks ten weight loss myths. Chapter 20 identifies ten really good diet Web sites. Chapter 21 lists ten foods that help any weight loss plan succeed. Chapter 22 is pure pleasure: ten fast foods that won't bust your diet — or your waistline!

Part VII: Appendixes

Appendix A is the great nutrient chart I mention at the start of this Introduction, the USDA Nutrient Data Base. Appendix B is a reprise of all the Web sites and 800-numbers sprinkled through the book, plus a few more tossed in for good measure. Dial as needed! Appendix C is a guide to the CD-ROM packed in with this book. Click!

Icons Used in This Book

This little guy looks smart because he's pointing to clear, concise explanations of technical terms and processes.

The Official Word icon says, "Look here for scientific studies, statistics, definitions, and recommendations used to create standard nutrition policy."

Bull's-eye! This is information that you can use to improve your diet and health.

This is a watch-out-for-the-curves icon, alerting you to nutrition pitfalls, such as (oops!) leaving the skin on the chicken — turning a lowfat food into one that is high in fat and cholesterol.

Nutrition is full of stuff that "everybody knows." This masked marvel clues you in to the real facts when (as often happens) "everybody's" wrong!

This little icon points out all the great information you'll find on the handy CD located at the back of this book.

Part I
Ready, Set, Lose!

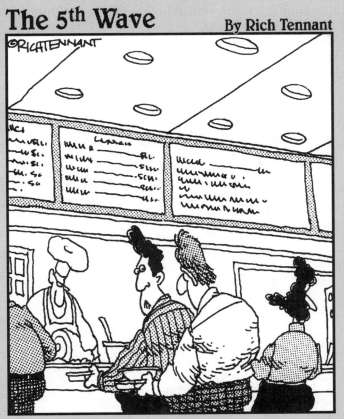

The 5th Wave   By Rich Tennant

"It didn't bother me to go up a pants size. It's when I had to go up one size in camping tents that I began to worry."

In this part . . .

Losing weight is hard work. You have to push yourself away from the table. You have to push yourself to avoid fat snacks. You have to push yourself to get moving, work out, stre-e-e-tch. So it helps to know that the result is worth the effort. This part tells how controlling your weight can improve your health and maybe even lengthen your life. Need I say more?

Chapter 1

Why Weight Matters

*I*f health professionals want you to hear one message about your weight, it is that how much you weigh may influence your quality of life and how long you live.

The important thing you should take from that sentence is the word *may*. There is more and more evidence each day that if your weight is higher than it should be, you are at risk of serious health problems. But, as you can find out later in this chapter, many people are exceptions to this rule.

As a result, the U.S. Departments of Agriculture/Health and Human Services Dietary Guidelines for American 2000 no longer ask you to decide whether you are overweight. Instead, the Guidelines have come up with a small but significant difference. Now their advice is to decide whether you are at a "healthy weight" — which is why you need this book.

Your Weight and Your Health

Skirt doesn't close?

Pants a bit snug?

Well, I know what *you* were doing last year: brunching and lunching and munching up a storm. Now you're toting around some extra pounds, and you want to get rid of them. Fast.

Join the crowd. According to data from the National Health and Nutrition Survey, the number of obese adults has risen from 13 percent in 1960 to 22.5 percent today. As a result, the *Journal of the American Medical Association* says two out of every three adults in this country are trying to lose weight. The *American Journal of Public Health* breaks that down by gender to report that 45 percent of women and 25 percent of men are on a reducing diet. Yipes.

The collective failure to slice off the pounds probably has less to do with lack of will power than with the stubborn refusal to accept the boring truth. Unfortunately, the only way to lose weight and keep it off is to follow a sensible weight loss diet to produce a trimmer, healthier, probably happier you and stay that way through a life-long pattern of healthful eating and regular exercise.

What? You thought there was another way? Sorry about that.

But the news isn't all bump — ooops! make that "work" — and grind. Notice that the earlier paragraph talks about a "trimmer" you, not necessarily a skinny you. Healthy bodies come in different sizes and shapes. The trick (as you can discover in Chapter 2) is to find your best weight and then hold onto it for dear life.

And I mean that literally because, as this chapter discusses, being overweight may mean taking on unnecessary health risks.

Many people want to lose weight to look better. Others want to gain weight for the same reason. But maintaining a healthy weight is more than a question of looking good. It's also about feeling good.

Years and years of studies comparing death rates with adult weight have demonstrated that people with excess poundage are at higher risk of weight-related health condition such as

- Heart disease
- High cholesterol
- High blood pressure
- Stroke
- Diabetes
- Certain types of cancer
- Gallbladder disease
- Osteoarthritis and gout (a form of arthritis)
- Sleep apnea (frequent awakening at night due to respiratory problems)
- Problem pregnancy
- Urine leakage caused by weak pelvic muscles

On the other hand, these same studies (or similar ones) show that weighing less than your optimal weight may also be risky. Surprised? You shouldn't be. People may be thin for a variety of reasons, some of them health-related. For example:

✔ Some skinny people eat like the proverbial horses, but are genetically programmed to have small bodies or burn up energy (food) so fast that they stay thin no matter what they eat.

✔ Some people are thin because food is not a major source of pleasure in their lives, so if they are very busy, they may just plain forget to eat enough.

✔ Some people are very thin because they have a medical condition, such as cancer or AIDS, which robs them of their appetite or prevents them from absorbing the nutrients in food.

✔ Some people are very thin because they have an eating disorder that leads them to diet obsessively. (More about that in Chapter 2.)

Clearly, the last two reasons, both potentially fatal situations, are more dangerous than the first and second reasons. Nonetheless, anyone who is very thin has a higher risk of

✔ Osteoporosis due to small, lightweight bones

✔ Frequent chilling due to a lack of fat padding to insulate his or her body in cold weather

✔ Respiratory illness including tuberculosis

✔ Infertility

✔ Digestive disorders

Finally, both people who are very fat and those who are very thin have this in common: Even if they are healthy, they are at higher risk of psychological problems such as depression because they do not fit the norm. Whether the norm is really normal for them, of course, is another question entirely, which is discussed in "Fat but Fit" later on in this chapter.

Judging Your Own Risk of Weight-Related Illness

Given the list of things that can go wrong if you're above your healthy weight, you may be convinced that extra pounds are an inevitable early death sentence. They aren't. Real people and their real differences keep sneaking in to mess up the predictions.

For example:

- ✔ No matter what the weight charts say, real people tend to gain weight as they grow older — and manage to stay healthy, anyway.

- ✔ Age may influence the effect of weight. For example, the value of standards such as the body mass index (BMI) described in Chapter 2 in predicting weight-related health risks may depend on how old you are. In your 30s, a lower BMI is clearly linked to better health. In your 70s or older, no convincing evidence indicates that it makes a difference. In between, from age 30 to age 74, the relationship between BMI and health is, well, in between — more important early on, less important later in life.

Americans may be crazy over weight, but the truth is that many large people, some of them obese, live long, happy, healthy lives.

Possibilities, possibilities

The wonderful thing about individual human beings is that they really are individuals, each one a unique bundle of genes and possibilities. Trying to make these unique individual fit into strict, predictable categories is like trying to map the stars in the skies. It works, but only up to a point.

In other words, you can't avoid the evidence of lots of studies showing that — common wisdom aside — some fat people are healthy.

How come? Well:

- ✔ Maybe overweight people have a higher overall death rate not because they weigh more but because they exercise less. If that's true, those who work out can reduce the risk associated with obesity. To see this with your very own eyes, slide your eyes over to "Fat but Fit: Exceptions that Prove the Rule," which describes a humdinger of a study showing that fit fat men (can you say that five times fast?) have a lower death rate than fit thin men.

- ✔ Maybe overweight people have a higher overall death rate because they eat lots of "bad" foods (such as foods high in saturated fat), which increase their risk of cardiovascular disease. If that's true, those who eat healthy will be — how else to say it — healthier.

- ✔ Maybe overweight people have a higher overall death rate because many of them carry a genetic predisposition to a serious disease such as diabetes, which is clearly more common among fat people than among lean ones. If that's true, you would have to ask whether losing 20 pounds will really lower their risk of disease to the level of a person who is natu-rally 20 pounds lighter. In some cases, the answer is definitely in the affirmative. For example, losing as little as five or ten pounds may bring a person's blood pressure down from "dangerous" to "safe." In other cases, though, weight loss may not be a final answer. In several studies, the data show that people who successfully lost weight actually had a higher rate of death. (!!!) Why? Alas, no explanation was given.

But enough about them. What about you? What do these conflicting numbers say about your own personal risk of weight-related illness and death?

One way to find out is to check with your doctor. Is your blood pressure normal? Are your cholesterol numbers okay? Can you climb those stairs without puffing? No guarantees, but these signs suggest you're healthy.

Coloring the leaves on your family tree

Another way to see where you fit in the weight/health continuum is to see what your genes have to say about your weight and health by filling in a chart of your own. I call it The Family Fat Tree.

Click onto your CD-ROM for Figure 1-1: Your Family Fat Tree. Print the table and fill in the blanks. If you have a lot of relatives, you may want to print several copies of the table. In addition to your parents and siblings, you'll want to complete this table for all grandparents, aunts, and uncles. Don't forget to complete the table for yourself, too.

When you're completing this chart, keep in mind that reasonable guesses are fine. For example, if you don't know a relative's exact weight, you can just say, "fat," "thin," or "average." At the end, you should have a pretty good picture of what your genes have to say about your weight. More important, you can see at a glance whether your near and dear have a history of weight-related problems such as diabetes or high blood pressure that may lead to *premature death* (loosely pegged as younger than 50 to 55 years for a man and younger than 60 to 65 years for a woman).

Once you've filled in your Family Fat Tree, look it over carefully to check out the status of your large relatives. If you've got several family members who appear to weigh more than they should by current standards, but who still refuse to keel over early in life, that's good. But does that mean you don't have to worry about those nasty weight charts and standards?

What an interesting question!

The answer is, I don't know. Unfortunately, neither does anyone else. The best guess is that people with weight-related problems should lose weight. For those without problems, the answer is . . . well, no answer right now. But these rules always work:

  ✔ Don't smoke.

  ✔ Watch your diet.

  ✔ Exercise.

  ✔ Check with your doctor.

Relax. Do the best you can to control your weight. Get a life you can enjoy. And live it. After all, who's to say you're not the exception that proves the rule?

Figure 1-1: Your Family Fat Tree			
Grandmother Grandfather		Grandmother Grandfather	
Name: _____ _____		Name: _____ _____	
Weight: _____ _____		Weight: _____ _____	
Body frame: _____ _____		Body frame: _____ _____	
Cause of death: _____ _____		Cause of death: _____ _____	
Age at death: _____ _____		Age at death: _____ _____	
Aunts & Uncles		Aunts & Uncles	
Name: _____ _____		Name: _____ _____	
Weight: _____ _____		Weight: _____ _____	
Body frame: _____ _____		Body frame: _____ _____	
Cause of death: _____ _____		Cause of death: _____ _____	
Age at death: _____ _____		Age at death: _____ _____	
Mother Father			
Name: _____ _____			
Weight: _____ _____			
Body frame: _____ _____			
Cause of death: _____ _____			
Age at death: _____ _____			
Sisters & Brothers		YOU	
Name: _____ _____		Name: _____	
Weight: _____ _____		Weight: _____	
Body frame: _____ _____		Body frame: _____	
Cause of death: _____ _____		_____	
Age at death: _____ _____		_____	

Figure 1-1:
Your Family
Fat Tree.

Fat but Fit: Exceptions that Prove the Rule

Imagine a world in which you can't find clothes in your size or a seat that fits. Where comedians and commercials poke fun at people who look like you. Where you know you're not going to get the job for which you're qualified because the personnel person thinks you're undisciplined. Imagine having no way to change any of this.

Well, if you weigh a lot more than the rest of the people you know, you don't have to use your imagination. You live these situations first hand, every day.

If you are large but healthy, should you have to lose weight to fit in? No way, says the National Association to Advance Fat Acceptance (NAAFA). The group, which calls what fat people experience *size discrimination,* is zealous about protecting the rights of large people. In the past few years, the organization has waged letter writing campaigns and rallies to protest skinny airline seats, job discrimination, and offensive advertising, while representing large Americans at scientific conferences, seeking to switch the agenda from "finding ways to make fat people thin to ways to make fat people healthy." NAAFA also serves as a national clearinghouse for lawyers and others challenging size discrimination. In May 2000, they participated in a campaign that won a ruling from the San Francisco Board of Supervisors making it illegal to discriminate against anyone based on size (a category that protects very thin people, too). Similar measures have been in place in other parts of California, as well as in Michigan and Washington, D.C.

Are you tempted to giggle here? Would you still feel like laughing if we were talking about "religion" or "race" instead of "size"? Worth thinking about, isn't it?

Here's another sentence worth thinking about. In fact, you may want to read it v-e-r-y s-l-o-w-l-y: Yes, obesity-related health problems may increase your risk of early death, but simply being overweight doesn't. As I say, you may want to read that slowly.

I bet you've always thought that being fat guarantees your having high blood pressure, high cholesterol, and other nasties that can lead to early death. Well, as they sing in Porgy and Bess, it ain't necessarily so. Lots of people who tip the scale at more than their recommended weight have perfectly normal blood pressure and low cholesterol to boot. More important, they may be fit as fiddles, meaning that they meet all the criteria for aerobic health and can do the following without running out of breath:

- Climb stairs.
- Carry packages, maybe even up stairs.
- Run short distances (or walk a treadmill for short periods of time).

Being fit is not only a useful tool for taking weight off and keeping it off, it's also a crucial variable in determining the risk of early death among people who are overweight. And you can bet I have the numbers to back up my statement.

Around 1989, researchers at the Cooper Institute for Aerobic Research in Dallas, Texas, began a study designed to keep tabs on a group of 25,000 men to see who was more likely to die first: Thin men, medium-size men, or fat men. The men who joined the study were given a physical exam and a stress test (treadmill) to establish a baseline for individual fitness and health.

Overall, the heavier men had higher blood pressure and higher cholesterol and were less fit than their slimmer counterparts. But here's the kicker. In 1997, when the Cooper scientists totaled up the numbers, they discovered that, yes, the annual death rate was higher among severely overweight men than among men of average weight. But the equation was different among fit overweight men. As you can see by running your finger down the columns in Table 1-1, when the number of deaths per year per 10,000 men is linked to fitness, the death rate for very fit overweight men is lower — yes, *lower* — than the death rate for very fit average weight men.

Table 1-1	Weight, Fitness, and Death: Number of Deaths per Year per 10,000 Men		
	Very Fit	*Sort of Fit*	*Not Fit*
Average-weight men	20	28.6	52
Moderately overweight men	19.7	29.8	49.1
Very overweight men	18	18	62.1

Source: Adapted from Cooper Institute for Aerobics.

While you're mulling that one over, you can find out more about NAAFA by clicking onto www.naafa.org. Or, you can read more about weight and size discrimination by clicking onto the aptly named Council on Size & Weight Discrimination home page at www.cswd.org.

I haven't found a similar Web site for the naturally (healthy) skinny. Nonetheless, I am sure that that any woman who wears pants to hide her skinny legs or any man who buys really bulky sweaters to hide a concave chest considers her/his situation equally painful. If you know of an appropriate Web site, send it to me at the address at the beginning of this book, and I'll include it in any future editions of the *Weight Loss Kit For Dummies*.

Weight and Kids

According to a 27-country World Health Organization survey of children ages 11, 13, and 15, American kids

- ✔ Eat more candy and fries than their counterparts in Northern Ireland, Scotland, Israel, and England.

- ✔ Exercise less than kids in Austria, Germany, and the Slovak Republic — yes, the Slovak Republic.

- ✔ Are in the top three student groups when it comes to slurping up soda every day.

The inevitable result is a generation of butterballs at higher risk of weight-related illness, such as diabetes and heart disease. According to the American Heart Association (AHA), by age 12, as many as seven of every ten American children has fatty deposits in their arteries. This statistic leads AHA to recommend testing cholesterol levels in any kids older than 2 who have a family history of coronary artery disease in parents or grandparents younger than 55. In addition, as you can see in Table 1-2, there are now cholesterol guidelines for children.

Table 1-2	Cholesterol Guidelines for Children and Adolescents (Ages 2 to 19)	
	Total Cholesterol (mg/dL)	*LDL Cholesterol mg/dL*
Acceptable	<170	<110
Borderline	170–199	110–129
High	200 or higher	130 or higher

Source: American Heart Association.

Overweight children are at a higher risk of lifelong obesity. An overweight 6-month old has a 14 percent risk of becoming an overweight adult. For an overweight 7-year-old, it's 41 percent. For an adolescent, the risk is 80 percent.

But here's the problem. Exactly what constitutes overweight for children is still open to interpretation. New growth charts have figures similar to the Body Mass Index measurement for adults (yes, Chapter 2, again), but taking these measurements is more complex for children whose height changes as they grow. And, like adults, children may weigh more and have higher BMIs because they are muscular rather than fat.

So what's the solution? Should chubby children be on weight loss diets? Not without the advice of a physician, say experts at the Centers for Disease Control and Prevention and co-author of the American Academy of Pediatrics *Guide to Your Child's Nutrition.* For one thing, overweight is sometimes in the eye of the beholder. For another, children with modest weight problems don't need a weight loss diet as much as their parents need to pay attention to what their kids eat and how much they exercise.

To maintain a healthful weight with good nutrition, the American Academy of Pediatrics now recommends that children older than 2 adopt a diet that mirrors their parents' — with no more than 30 percent of calories from fat, 10 percent or less from saturated fats, and less than 300 mg cholesterol a day.

Or parents could just turn off the TV. As the American Dietetic Association notes, food ads aimed at children generally do not reflect healthful eating patterns. Hey, after watching six gazillion ads for super chocobars, who wants to eat a carrot?

A Bonus for Those Who Want to Read It for Themselves

Some people just have to see it all in person. That's why there are Web sites, more Web sites, and still more Web sites. To check on why healthy weight matters, the click-on address is your CD-ROM, where you will find the American Dietetic Association's most recent statement on weight management.

Go for it!

Chapter 2

How to Tell Who's Fat

*B*efore you start a weight loss program, you need to find out whether you just feel fat or actually need to lose weight for health reasons. To help you decide, this chapter describes several methods that health professionals use to measure body weight and to predict your risk of weight-related health problems

You can read this chapter in parts, or you can just plunge right in and barrel through to the end. For energy, you may want to have a (nutritional) snack at hand. So wash that apple, shine that pear, slice it up, and go!

The Bulging American Body

Boy, are Americans chubby! Everybody says so. The American Society of Bariatric Physicians, a professional group of doctors specializing in obesity treatment, reveals that 58 million Americans — 26 million men and 32 million women — are overweight. And the National Health and Nutrition Survey shows that the number of obese adults is up from 13 percent in 1960 to 22.5 percent in 1999.

The average American adult weighs 8 pounds more today than he or she did 16 years ago, and the *Journal of the American Medical Association* says two out of every three adults are trying to lose weight. But in a country obsessed with being young and skinny, how do you know that all these people are fat rather than, say, naturally chunky? It's all in the numbers.

Pounds of charts

For years, the standard definitions of obesity have included weight charts. To decide who's carrying too many pounds, doctors usually compare a person's weight with what's written on the weight chart: If you weigh 20 to 40 percent more than the chart says you should, you're mildly obese. If you weigh 40 to 100 percent more than the chart says you should, you're moderately obese. If your weight is more than double the weight on the chart, you're severely obese.

This interpretation sounds sensible, but here's the catch. The standard or healthy weights for adult Americans shown on the earliest charts are weights most adult Americans cannot achieve without severely restricting what they eat — or being born again with a different body. Take a look and see what I mean.

Weight charts #1: The MetLife classics

In 1959, the Metropolitan Life Insurance Company (MetLife) published the first set of standard weight charts. The weights were drawn from insurance statistics showing what the healthiest, longest-living people weighed — with clothes and 1-inch heels on. The problem with this is that people with insurance back then constituted a narrow class of all human beings, so who's to say their stats predict anything for the rest of us?

In fact, my favorite nutrition textbook, *Understanding Normal and Clinical Nutrition* by three savvy ladies named Eleanor Noss Whitney, Corinne Balog Cataldo, and Sharon Rady Rolfes, quotes one physician as saying that with new methods of gauging healthy weight, we should consign weight tables to the "medical museum."

Table 2-1 and Table 2-2 show the MetLife weight charts for men and women. Note that the charts indicate different weight ranges for people with small, medium, or large frames. The frame size refers to bone structure. People with small frames typically have narrow wrists, ankles, and shoulders. People with large frames typically have large wrists and ankles and broad shoulders. People with medium frames have, well, medium wrists, ankles, and shoulders. When it comes to the actual measurements for "small," "medium" and "large," though, your guess is as good as mine. Maybe better. My editor, Kelly Ewing, says she's heard a general rule about putting your hand around your wrist and if your third and middle finger easily overlap, you're small frame; if they just touch, you have a medium frame; and if they don't touch, you have a large frame. Of course, she admits, how large a hand you have may skew the test!

Table 2-1	Height & Weight Table for Women*		
Height (Feet and Inches)	**Small Frame**	**Medium Frame**	**Large Frame**
4'10"	102–111	109–111	118–131
4'11	103–113	111–123	120–134
5'0"	104–115	113–126	122–137
5'1"	106–118	115–129	125–140
5'2"	108–121	118–132	128–143
5'3"	111–124	121–135	131–147
5'4"	114–127	124–138	134–151
5'5"	117–130	127–141	137–155
5'6"	120–133	130–144	140–159
5'7"	123–136	133–147	143–163
5'8"	126–139	136–150	146–167
5'9"	129–142	139–153	149–170
5'10"	132–145	142–156	152–173
5'11"	135–148	145–159	155–176
6'0"	138–151	148–162	158–179

*Weights at age 25–59 based on lowest mortality. Weight in pounds according to frame (in indoor clothing weighing 3 pounds; shoes with 1-inch heels). Copyright 1996, 1999. Metropolitan Life Insurance Company, New York, New York. All Rights Reserved.

Table 2-2	Height & Weight Table for Men*		
Height (Feet and Inches)	**Small Frame**	**Medium Frame**	**Large Frame**
5'2"	128–134	131–141	138–150
5'3"	130–136	133–143	140–153
5'4"	132–138	135–145	142–156
5'5"	134–140	137–148	144–160
5'6"	136–142	139–151	146–164
5'7"	138–145	142–154	149–168

(continued)

Table 2-2 *(continued)*

Height (Feet and Inches)	Small Frame	Medium Frame	Large Frame
5'8"	140–148	145–157	153–172
5'9"	142–151	148–160	155–176
5'10"	144–154	151–163	158–180
5'11"	146–157	154–166	161–184
6'0"	149–160	157–170	164–188
6'1"	152–164	160–174	168–192
6'2"	155–168	164–178	172–197
6'3"	158–172	167–182	176–202
6'4"	162–176	171–187	181–207

Weights at age 25–59 based on lowest mortality. Weight in pounds according to frame (in indoor clothing weighing 3 pounds; shoes with 1-inch heels). Copyright 1996, 1999. Metropolitan Life Insurance Company, New York, New York. All Rights Reserved.

Weight charts #2: Dietary Guidelines advice

The second standard set of American weight charts was created for the U.S. Department of Agriculture/Health and Human Services Dietary Guidelines for Americans. The weight ranges on the charts appearing in the 1990 edition of the guidelines listed more forgiving weight ranges for adults than those in the skinny MetLife charts.

And, because most people do gain some weight as they get older, the charts sensibly divided the weights into two broad categories, one for people age 19 to 34, the other for people age 35 and older. This not only recognizes reality but also science.

Table 2-3 shows the weight charts for adult men and women from the 1990 edition of the Dietary Guidelines for Americans. If you have a small frame and proportionately more fat tissue than muscle tissue (muscle is heavier than fat), you are likely to weigh in at the low end. If you have a large frame and proportionately more muscle than fat, you are likely to weigh in at the high end. As a general (but by no means invariable) rule, women who have smaller frames and less muscle weigh less than men of the same height and age.

In healthy adults, acceptable levels of body fat increase with age. Men should have 18 to 25 percent body fat, and women should have 25 to 30 percent body fat. The lower number is for young men and women; the higher number is for older men and women.

Table 2-3	Guidelines for Weight for Men and Women	
	Weight (Pounds)	
Height	**Age 19 to 34**	**Age 35 and Older**
5′	97–128	108–138
5′1″	101–132	111–143
5′2″	104–137	115–148
5′3″	107–141	122–157
5′4″	111–146	122–157
5′5″	114–150	126–152
5′6″	118–155	130–167
5′7″	121–160	134–172
5′8″	125–164	138–178
5′9″	129–169	142–183
5′10″	132–174	146–188
5′11″	136–179	151–194
6′	140–184	155–199
6′1″	144–189	159–205
6′2″	148–195	164–210
6′3″	152–200	168–216
6′4″	156–205	173–222
6′5″	160–211	177–228
6′6″	164–216	182–234

Source: Nutrition and Your Health: Dietary Guidelines for Americans, 3rd ed. (Washington, D.C.: U.S. Department of Agriculture, U.S. Department of Health and Human Services, 1990).

Weight charts #3: Stricter standards

Well, wouldn't you know it? Having created such user-friendly weight charts in 1990, the folks at USDA/HHS immediately felt guilty, so guilty that they changed their minds in later editions of the guidelines. The Dietary Guidelines for Americans published in 2000 does not include the table with higher weight allowances for older people. In other words, the "healthy" weights for everyone, young or old, are the ones listed in the column for 19- to 35-year-olds in the 1990 guidelines.

Reading that sentence may lead you to wonder if the people who design weight charts live in some parallel universe where everyone is skinny regardless of gender, age, or family history.

Many health professionals have had the same concern. Until recently, *overweight* meant that a person carried more pounds than the weight chart said he or she should. But modern obesity research has come up with a new wrinkle: defining who's fat by taking into consideration body composition (fat tissue versus lean tissue, or muscle) along with body weight.

The method is called *Body Mass Index (BMI)*. Emphasizing body fat content has led to a whole new philosophy of weight measurement called *body fat testing,* which is the topic of the next section.

The Body Mass Index

In 1990, the National Heart, Lung, and Blood Institute published a new set of "fat rules," the first federal guidelines on how to identify, evaluate, and treat people with excess poundage. These rules, which apply to men and women age 19 to 70, are special because they introduce a new measurement called *Body Mass Index,* or BMI. BMI is a number — such as 24 — which symbolizes the relationship between height and weight as a means for predicting your risk of weight-related illnesses such as diabetes, high blood pressure, heart disease, stroke, gallbladder disease, and arthritic pain.

The World Health Organization uses these standards for interpreting BMI:

- A BMI below 18.5 is underweight.
- A BMI of 18.5 to 24.9 is "normal."
- A BMI of 25 to 29.9 is "Grade 1 obesity." Translation: You're moderately overweight.
- A BMI of 30 to 39.9 is "Grade 2 obesity." Translation: You're severely overweight.
- A BMI over 40 is "Grade 3 obesity." Translation: You're massively overweight.

When to worry

If your BMI is higher than you'd like (see Table 2-4), don't panic. If you're an athlete, for example, muscle tissue weighs more than fat tissue, so heavily muscled bodies may pack on more pounds than the weight chart says is okay. So if you're very muscular, like Arnold Schwarzenegger, you might have a higher BMI but still not be fat.

The virtue of the BMI is that it gives health professionals — and you, too — an idea of what treatment is appropriate. With a BMI below 29.9, you know you're not a candidate for really risky treatment like weight loss surgery. With a BMI higher than 30, you need to consider more stringent options.

The exception to the preceding rule is having other weight-related health problems. Regardless of your BMI, your risks of weight-related health problems increase if you have the following existing health conditions:

- High blood pressure
- High levels of LDL ("bad") cholesterol
- Low levels of HDL ("good") cholesterol
- High levels of triglycerides (a kind of fat in your blood)
- A family history of premature heart disease (close relatives who suffered heart attacks before age 60)

Your risk is also higher if you are not physically active or if you are a smoker.

Table 2-4 lists the health-risk level of various BMIs.

Table 2-4	Your BMI and Your Health Risks	
BMI	*Health Risk*	*BMI+Existing Health Risks*
<25	Very low	Low
25–26.9	Low	Moderate
27–29.9	Moderate	High
30–34.9	High	Very high
35–39.9	Very high	Extremely high
>40	Extremely high	Extremely high

The man who invented the average man

Lambert Adolphe Jacques Quetelet (1795–1874) was a Belgian mathematician, astronomer, statistician, and sociologist who invented the concept of the "middle man" *(homme moyen),* the average Joe who stands at the center of any bell curve.

Quetelet's main concern was predicting criminal behavior. To this end, he hoped to develop statistical patterns based on a person's deviation from

average (normal) social behavior that could be used to predict his actions including moral (good) and criminal (bad) behavior. While this idea provoked many lively discussions among 19th century social scientists, it never really worked as a crime-fighting tool, but became extremely useful in estimating health risks. One good example: the BMI, which explains your weight in relation to a statistically average person.

The BMI is not a reliable guide for

✔ Women who are pregnant or nursing

✔ People who are very tall or very short

✔ Professional athletes or weight trainers with well-developed muscle tissue

What's my BMI?

The equation used to calculate your BMI is called the *Quetelet Index,* named after the 19th century Belgian mathematician and astronomer who invented the concept of "the average man." (See "The man who invented the average man" sidebar, later in this chapter.) The equation is W/H^2, which originally meant weight (in kilograms) divided by height (in meters) squared.

Forget the kilograms and meters. You can do this in pounds and inches. All you have to do is add one more step. The new equation looks like this:

```
W/H² x 705
```

Plug your personal numbers into the BMI equation. For example, if you are 5'3" and weigh 138 pounds, the equation for your BMI looks like this:

```
BMI = W/H² x 705 = (138 pounds/63 x 63 inches) x 705 =
          (138/3969) x 705 = 24.5 BMI
```

Or you could just run your finger down Table 2-5, also on your CD-ROM, which does the math for men and women from 4'11" to 6'4"starting with a weight of 91 pounds.

Table 2-5

Body Mass Index

Height (inches)	Body Weight (Pounds)																
	19	20	21	22	23	24	25	26	27	28	29	30	31	32	33	34	35
58	91	96	100	105	110	115	119	124	129	134	138	143	148	153	158	162	167
59	94	99	104	109	114	119	124	128	133	138	143	148	153	158	163	168	173
60	97	102	107	112	118	123	128	133	138	143	148	153	158	163	168	174	179
61	100	106	111	116	122	127	132	137	143	148	153	158	164	169	175	180	185
62	104	109	115	120	126	131	136	142	147	153	158	164	169	175	180	186	191
63	107	113	118	124	130	135	141	146	152	158	163	169	175	180	186	191	197
64	110	116	122	128	134	140	145	151	157	163	169	174	180	186	192	197	204
65	114	120	126	132	138	144	150	156	162	168	174	180	186	192	198	204	210
66	118	124	130	136	142	148	155	161	167	173	179	185	192	198	204	210	216
67	121	127	134	140	146	153	159	166	172	178	185	191	198	204	211	217	223
68	125	131	138	144	151	158	164	171	177	184	190	197	203	210	216	223	230
69	128	135	142	149	155	162	169	176	182	189	196	203	209	216	223	230	236
70	132	139	146	153	160	167	174	181	188	195	202	209	216	222	229	236	243
71	136	143	150	157	165	172	179	186	193	200	208	215	222	229	236	243	250
72	140	147	154	162	169	177	184	191	199	206	213	221	228	235	242	250	258
73	144	151	159	166	174	182	189	197	204	212	219	227	235	242	250	257	265
74	148	155	163	171	179	186	194	202	210	218	225	233	241	249	256	264	272
75	152	160	168	176	184	192	200	208	216	224	232	240	248	256	264	272	279
76	156	164	172	180	189	197	205	213	221	230	238	246	254	263	271	279	287

Source: The National Heart, Lung, and Blood Institute.

Other Ways to Measure Body Fat

Depressed by weight charts? Not sure about BMI? Have I got some body-fat tests for you!

- ✔ Pinching your skin together and measuring the fat fold
- ✔ Measuring the circumference of your arm midway between elbow and shoulder
- ✔ Calculating your hip-to-waist ratio
- ✔ Seeing how much water you displace when dunked in a tank
- ✔ Measuring your body's ability to resist an electrical current

Each of these methods is an estimate. The more body fat you have, the less reliable the tests will be. Sorry about that.

Pinch an inch

Most of the fat in your body lies just beneath the surface of your skin. This fatty tissue is an insulator that holds body heat in, keeping you warm in winter (nice) but making you uncomfortably hot in the summer (not nice).

How much fat do you have? The easy way to find out is to pinch your skin together at a place where it's sort of loose, such as the back of your arm right above your elbow. You can do this with your fingers; professionals use medical pincers. Either way, the scientific name for the skin and fat you pinch is a fat fold. Measuring the width of the fat fold tells you where you stand in relation to other people: less fat than most, an average amount of fat, more fat than most. For example, five percent of all women age 25 to 35 — the skinny ones — have a fat fold of about 18 millimeters. At the other end of the scale, five percent of all women have a fat fold of 37 millimeters. The ones in the middle — the average — have a fat fold in the middle, as shown in Table 2-6.

Table 2-6 shows the size of the fat fold for average adult men and women. Scientists measure fat folds in millimeters. But because most Americans prefer inches, I've translated these numbers to inches. (FYI: 25 millimeters is just about equal to one inch.)

The female fat fold is always larger than the male fat fold because women have proportionately more body fat, while men have proportionately more muscle tissue. Check out Chapter 5 to see how this affects daily calorie allowances for men and women.

Table 2-6	Pinch Test Results
Age	**Average Fat Fold for Men**
25–34	12 mm = .48 in = ½ in
35–44	12 mm = .48 in = ½ in
45–54	12 mm = .48 in = ½ in
55–64	11 mm = .44 in = ½ in
Age	**Average Fat Fold for Women**
25–34	21 mm = .84 in = ⅘ in
35–44	23 mm = .92 in = 9/10 in
45–54	25 mm = 1 in
55–64	25 mm = 1 in

Source: Adapted from A.R. Frisancho, "New Norms of Upper Limb Fat and Muscle Areas for the Assessment of Nutritional Status," American Journal of Clinical Nutrition (1981): 2540-2645.

Make a muscle

Another guide to how much fat padding you are carrying is the circumference (the measurement around) of your arm midway between your elbow and your shoulder, right at the bulge you create when you make a muscle. To measure the circumference, your health professional wraps a nonstretch tape measure around your arm and reads the result in centimeters (10 millimeters = 1 centimeter). To convert centimeters (cm) to inches, you multiply the number in centimeters by 0.39.

Table 2-7 shows the average upper arm circumference for adult men and women, again handily translated to inches. Notice that Table 2-7 is the reverse of Table 2-6, gender-wise. Men have proportionately more muscle, so they have larger average upper arm measurements. But you knew that, right?

Table 2-7	How Big Is Your Muscle?
Age	**Average Upper Arm Circumference for Men**
25–34	27.9 cm = 10.8 in
35–44	28.6 cm = 11.2 in

(continued)

Table 2-7 (continued)

Age	Average Upper Arm Circumference for Men
45–54	28.1 cm = 10.9 in
55–64	27.8 cm = 10.8 in

Age	Average Upper Arm Circumference for Women
25–34	21.2 cm = 8.2 in
35–44	21.8 cm = 8.5 in
45–54	22.0 cm = 8.6 in
55–64	22.5 cm = 8.8 in

Source: Adapted from A.R. Frisancho, "New Norms of Upper Limb Fat and Muscle Areas for the Assessment of Nutritional Status," American Journal of Clinical Nutrition (1981): 2540-2645.

Hip, hip, hooray!

Or maybe not. As everyone who has even a passing interest in weight and health must know by now:

- An apple-shape body with fat around the middle predicts a higher risk of heart disease.
- A pear-shape body with fat around the hips predicts a lower risk of heart disease.

You can find out what shape your body is just by looking in the mirror. But, hey, why take the easy way when there's an honest-to-goodness scientific test available?

Forget the mirror. Instead, get out your tape measure.

1. **Run the tape just above the navel.**

2. **Write down the results (in inches).**

3. **Run the tape around the widest part of your hips.**

4. **Write down the results (in inches).**

5. **Divide the measurement of your waist by the measurement of your hips: Waist (29 inches)/Hips (39 inches) = 0.74.**

That's your *waist/hip ratio,* a number you can use to predict your risk of weight-related health problems. Women whose waist/hip ratio is higher than 0.8 and men whose waist/hip ratio is higher than .95 are at higher risk of weight-related health problems.

Dunkin' people

When you put a solid body, such as your own, into a tub of water, some water is pushed aside (displaced). Fatty tissue weighs less than muscle, so a body with more fat than muscle displaces less water than a body with more muscle than fat. Serious obesity researchers invest tons of money in large, bulky tubs and scales that can lower you into the water, measure how much water was displaced, and then lift you out again. Then they spend hours doing the really complicated math that tells them how much body fat you have. Frankly, I'd rather pinch my upper arm.

Shocking! Just shocking!

Come back. I was just kidding. But, yes, I'm talking electricity here — a painless amount of current used for a method of body fat measurement called *bioelectrical impedance.*

Your body (and mine, and everyone else's) is full of fluids packed with *electrolytes,* ions that conduct the electrical impulses that send messages back and forth among your cells. More fluid is in muscle tissue than in fat tissue, so a body with more muscle than fat is less resistant to an outside electrical current.

To test your body's resistance to electrical current (impedance), a researcher places electrodes on your wrists and ankles and zaps a harmless low intensity electrical current through. Then, he or she figures out how resistant your tissues were to the current.

The final number indicates how much body fat you have.

Understanding What the Numbers Mean

Given the complex ways to measure weight and where you fit in, you might reasonably assume that these methods provide a reliable guide to who's healthy and who's not.

Surprise. They don't. As anyone can plainly see, some fat people are healthy; others aren't. But that observation also applies to skinny people, not to mention those in-betweeners often labeled "average."

The problem is that variables, little things like eating habits, fitness, genetics, and attitude, exercise their own influence on health. For more on these subjects, check out the genetic angle in Chapter 1. Turn to Chapter 18 to see how fitness affects longevity. And flip through the various chapters on specific weight loss plans to read how what you eat may (or may not) help you live a longer, healthier life.

After you're done, you may want to just toss out your scale and forget about weight altogether. Do me a favor: Wait until you've read Chapter 3, which tells you how scales work. It starts on the very next page.

Chapter 3

How to Tell If You're Losing Weight

*Q*uestion: When you're on a weight loss program, how can you be sure that you're losing weight? Answer: Read this chapter. Okay, okay, so that's sort of a smart-alecky answer, but it's true. This chapter tells you all about scales and two other tests of weight loss, not to mention showing you how to set up a reasonable weight-tracking schedule.

Measuring Weight Loss

You can tell whether you're losing weight in three basic ways:

- ✔ The clothing test
- ✔ The waistband test
- ✔ The bathroom scale

Each one has its good and bad points.

The Clothing Test

Every woman I know has had this experience. Although she usually wears, say, a size 12, when she's trying on clothes while shopping, she gets a pleasant surprise when one size 10 skirt is a perfect fit. Then, horrors! Another skirt, in another style, is too small in a size 14. Has this girl lost weight? Or has she gained weight? Probably neither.

Men's clothing sizes are pretty much a standard affair, all cut to the same measurements no matter whose name is on the label. If a man's shirt is marked "15-35, tapered body," for example, you can pretty much bet it has a 15-inch neck, a 35-inch sleeve, and a body that slims down as it approaches the waist.

You can't say that about women's clothes. Female clothing sizes are incredibly elastic. One manufacturer or designer's size 10 can easily be equivalent to another's size 12 or even a third designer's size 8. What a mess!

Measuring women's sizes

In 1972, the U.S. Department of Commerce (DOC) National Bureau of Standards attempted to bring some order to the chaos in women's clothing by drawing up a table of 49 Body Measurements for the Sizing of Women's Patterns and Apparel for junior, junior petite, junior tall, misses, misses petite, and misses tall. The table also included an estimate of what a woman fitting each size might weigh.

Unfortunately, as DOC carefully noted in its intro to this multipage document, "The adoption and use of a Voluntary Product Standard is completely voluntary." Well, duh. The unfortunate result is that the sizing standards did not become standard, and women's clothing continued on its merry way, up and down, down and up, around and about, according to the whims of individual manufacturers.

Eventually, the DOC standards (which weren't standard) were withdrawn and replaced with a new set of voluntary standards, 39 measurements created by the American Society for Testing and Materials (ASTM). The new nonstandard standards are based on body measurements submitted by clothing manufacturers and retailers and from surveys of real human beings conducted by the U.S. Army and the U.S. Navy. The measurements are available in centimeters as well as inches, to make them more useful to marketers who sell their clothes overseas where metric is the rule. Unlike the old DOC standards, the new ones from ASTM do not include weight.

Both the DOC and ASTM standards are based on specific body stats — the measurement of your chest, your waist, your hips, and so on. The definition of each measurement is careful and precise. No one could accuse these guys of pulling any punches. For example, according to ASTM,

- The bust measurement is the "circumference horizontally around the body under the arms, across the nipples, and parallel to the floor."

- The waist measurement is the "circumference horizontally around the body at waist level."

- The hip measurement is the "maximum hip circumference of the body at the hip level and parallel to the floor."

It sounds a bit techie, but at least the words are familiar. But what about your "armscye"? Or your "sitting spread girth," which sounded not quite ladylike to me until I read the definition, which explains that it is the width around your legs when you are sitting down? Who knew? To clear up any confusion in terms, get out your tape measure, call a friend to help with the places you can't reach, and scan Table 3-1, a list of terms adapted from both the DOC and ASTM definitions for women's measurements (for example, bust, waist, hip, and so on). Keep in mind that not all terms appear on both the DOC and ASTM charts.

Table 3-1	What the Words Mean
Measurement	**Definition**
Bust	Around the fullest part of the bust, when wearing a bra
Waist	Around the natural waistline, ½ inch below your lowest rib
High hip	About 3 inches below your waist, around the rounded part of your middle commonly called your "tummy"
Hip	About two inches below your high hip, where your hip bones stick out
Sitting spread	Around both legs at the widest bottom when you are sitting down
Neck base	Around the lowest point where your neck meets your body
Armscye	A circle down from your shoulder to your armpit, under your armpit, and back up again
Upper arm	Around the widest part of your arm just below the armscye
Elbow	Around your elbow
Wrist	Around the bony part of your wrist
Thigh, max	Around the upper part of your thigh, closest to your body
Thigh, mid	Around the upper leg, halfway up from your knee
Knee	Around your knee
Calf	Around the widest part of your leg between knee and ankle
Ankle	Around the bony part of your ankle
Vertical trunk	Down from your right shoulder, midway between your neck and your arm, through your legs, and back up over your breast to your shoulder

(continued)

Table 3-1 *(continued)*

Measurement	Definition
Total crotch	Down from your center front waist, through your legs, and back up to your center back waist

Sources: Adapted from U.S. Department of Commerce, National Bureau of Standards, Voluntary Product Standard PS-70, Body Measurements for the Sizing of Women's Patterns and Apparel (Washington, D.C.: Government Printing Office, nd) and the Annual Book of ASTM Standards, copyright American Society for Testing and Materials, 100 Barr Harbor Drive, West Conshohocken, PA 19428.

So what size are you anyway?

With voluntary standards, who knows what size you are? Table 3-2 shows the DOC girth measurements (measurements taken by running a measuring tape around something) for women's clothing in inches. Table 3-3 shows the same ASTM measurements, again in inches. Bookmark this page, look carefully at the two tables, and then come right back to this spot.

You're reading, you're reading, you're reading, you're reading, you're done.

Okay. Did you see something interesting? No? Look again. Look carefully at the measurements for size 12 on the DOC charts and size 8 on the ASTM list. Good for you: You caught the fact that sizes have changed. Radically. A woman who requires a size 12 under the 1972 DOC standards can fit neatly into a size 8 on the ASTM charts, without trimming back even a miniscule fraction of an inch. In fact, her new size 8 waist is 27 inches around, an entire inch larger than her earlier size 12 middle. How's that for painless slimming?

The serious point, of course, is that in the real world, women's clothing size may not be a reliable test of weight loss. The possible exception is a consistent downward trend in sizes of clothes made by a single manufacturer. If you used to wear Designer Smith's clothes in size 14s and size 16s, and now you're fitting comfortably into Designer Smith's size 8s and 10s, that's pretty good proof your weight loss program's working.

Table 3-2	Body Measurements for the Sizing of Women's Patterns and Apparel						
Size	*6*	*8*	*10*	*12*	*14*	*16*	*18*
Bust	31½	32½	33½	35	36½	38	40
Waist	22½	23½	24½	26	27½	29	31
Hip	33½	34½	35½	37	38½	40	42

Size	*6*	*8*	*10*	*12*	*14*	*16*	*18*
Mid neck	13⅛	13⅜	13⅝	14	14⅜	14¾	15¼
Armscye	13⅞	14¼	14⅝	15¼	15⅞	16½	17¼
Abdominal extension	29⅝	30⅝	31⅝	33⅛	34⅝	36⅛	38⅛
Sitting spread	33½	34½	35½	37	38½	40	42
Thigh, maximum	18¾	19½	20¼	21¼	22¼	23¼	24½
Thigh, mid	17	17½	18	18¾	19½	20¼	21¼
Knee	12	12⅜	12¾	13¼	13¾	14¼	14¾
Calf	11½	11⅞	12¼	12¾	13¼	13¾	14¼
Ankle	8⅛	8⅜	8⅝	8⅞	9⅛	9⅜	9⅝
Upper arm	9⅝	9⅞	10⅛	10½	10⅞	11¼	11⅞
Elbow	9¼	9⅜	9½	9¾	10	10¼	10⅝
Wrist	5¼	5⅜	5½	5⅝	5¾	5⅞	6
Vertical Trunk	55½	57	58½	60	61½	63	64½

Source: U.S. Department of Commerce, National Bureau of Standards, Voluntary Product Standard PS-70, Body Measurements for the Sizing of Women's Patterns and Apparel (Washington, D.C.: Government Printing Office, nd).

Table 3-3 Standard Table of Body Measurements for Adult Female Misses Figure Type, Sizes 2–20

Size	*6*	*8*	*10*	*12*	*14*	*16*	*18*
Bust	34	35	36	37½	39	40½	44½
Waist	26	27	28	29½	31	32½	34½
Hip	33½	34½	35½	37	38½	40	42
Mid neck	13½	13¾	14	14⅜	14¾	15⅛	15⅝
Neck base	14	14¼	14½	14⅞	15¼	15⅝	16⅛
Armscye	15	15⅜	15¾	16⅜	17	17⅝	18⅜
Upper arm	10½	10¾	11	11⅜	11¾	12⅛	12¾
Elbow	9 ⅝	9¾	9 ⅞	10⅛	10⅜	10⅝	11

(continued)

Table 3-3 *(continued)*

Size	6	8	10	12	14	16	18
Wrist	5$\frac{7}{8}$	6	6$\frac{1}{8}$	6$\frac{1}{4}$	6$\frac{3}{8}$	6$\frac{1}{2}$	6$\frac{5}{8}$
Thigh, max	21	21$\frac{3}{4}$	22$\frac{1}{2}$	23$\frac{1}{2}$	24$\frac{1}{2}$	25$\frac{1}{2}$	26$\frac{3}{4}$
Thigh, mid	19$\frac{1}{4}$	19$\frac{3}{4}$	20$\frac{1}{4}$	21	21$\frac{3}{4}$	22$\frac{1}{2}$	23$\frac{1}{2}$
Knee	13$\frac{3}{4}$	14$\frac{1}{8}$	14$\frac{1}{2}$	15	15$\frac{1}{2}$	16	16$\frac{1}{2}$
Calf	13$\frac{1}{4}$	13$\frac{5}{8}$	14	14$\frac{1}{2}$	15	15$\frac{1}{2}$	16
Ankle	8$\frac{7}{8}$	9$\frac{1}{8}$	9$\frac{3}{8}$	9$\frac{5}{8}$	9$\frac{7}{8}$	10$\frac{1}{8}$	10$\frac{3}{8}$
Vertical Trunk	59	60$\frac{1}{2}$	62	63$\frac{1}{2}$	65	66$\frac{1}{2}$	68
Total crotch	26$\frac{1}{2}$	27$\frac{1}{4}$	28	28$\frac{3}{4}$	29$\frac{1}{2}$	30$\frac{1}{4}$	31

Reprinted with permission, from the Annual Book of ASTM Standards, copyright American Society for Testing and Materials, 100 Barr Harbor Drive, West Conshokocken, PA 19428.

Traveling sizes

You probably have a pretty good idea what size you are in the United States. But suppose that you're shopping in Great Britain or Western Europe, and you see a totally strange set of numbers on the clothing labels. What to do? Just read down Tables 3-4 through 3-9, which show equivalent sizes for women's and men's clothing sold in the United States, Great Britain, and Western Europe. These tables make it easy as pie (hey, easy on that pie!) to find out where you fit. Or, more appropriately, what fits you.

Table 3-4 — International Clothing Sizes for Women — Dresses, Coats, Jackets, Skirts, and Pants

Country	Sizes						
United States	6	8	10	12	14	16	18
Great Britain	8	10	12	14	16	18	20
Western Europe	38	40	42	44	46	48	50

Table 3-5	International Clothing Sizes for Women — Blouses, Sweaters, and T-Shirts						
Country	*Sizes*						
United States	32	34	36	38	40	42	44
Great Britain	34	36	38	40	42	44	46
Western Europe	40	42	44	46	48	50	52

Table 3-6	International Clothing Sizes for Women — Shoes and Boots						
Country	*Sizes*						
United States	4	5	6	7	8	9	10
Great Britain	2.5	3.5	4.5	5.5	6.5	8.5	9.5
Western Europe	35	36	37	38	39	40	41

Table 3-7	International Clothing Sizes for Men — Suits, Jackets, Coats, Pants, and Sweaters						
Country	*Sizes*						
United States	34	36	38	40	42	44	46
Great Britain	34	36	38	40	42	44	46
Western Europe	44	46	48	50	52	54	56

Table 3-8	International Clothing Sizes for Men — Shirts				
Country	*Sizes*				
United States	14	15	16	17	18
Great Britain	14	15	16	17	18
Western Europe	36	38	41	43	45

Table 3-9	International Clothing Sizes for Men — Shoes and Boots						
Country	*Sizes*						
United States	7.5	8.5	9.5	10.5	11.5	12.5	13.5
Great Britain	7	8	9	10	11	12	13
Western Europe	40	41	42	43	44	45	46

The Waistband Test

Does the skirt or pants that once pinched around the waist and sort of hugged your bottom feel just a tad more comfortable? Congrats. That's positive proof you're losing weight. For some people, the waistband test is quite enough. When old clothes fit again, or are so loose that new ones seem in order, these folks know they've met their weight loss goal.

But if you need hard evidence, it's not enough. That's why scales where invented.

The Scale

A scale is an instrument that measures weight. In principle, all scales are see-saws, with you at one end and the scale's weight-sensing device at the other. The point where the see-saw balances is your weight.

- ✔ **Spring scales:** The earliest scales really were balancing acts, with weights piled on one side and wheat, coal, or you on the other. When the scale balanced, bingo! There's your weight. Then, "Bam!", as TV's Emeril Legasse might say, the invention of the spring scale kicked things up a notch. The spring scale is still a simple mechanical device. You step on, the metal inside the scale stretches, and where it stops is your weight. Your basic bathroom scale (no flashing lights) is a spring scale. So is the scale in your doctor's office.

The familiar basic square-ish white enamel box with mechanical levers inside usually accommodates someone weighing up to 300 pounds or maybe 320. It has a spinning dial that stops like a slot machine at your weight. Ready for bi-focals? Get the *big* dial scale. Big feet? Get the longer model. Just make sure that this scale (and any other scale you buy) has a nonskid bottom. Nothing ruins your day like slipping off a scale and hitting your chin on a wet bathroom floor.

Your doctor's scale — no, not the scaled-down home version, but the authentic old-fashioned standing model with the ruler on top to measure your height — is the one you want if accuracy is your thing. On the Internet or in a medical supply store, it is priced at about $300.

✔ **Electronic scales:** The electronic scale, also known as the *digital strain gauge scale,* is still a see-saw, but in place of metal springs it has an electronic device called a *load cell.* When you step on an electronic scale, the load cell analyzes the strain your body is exerting on the scale and translates that into a number that is displayed in bright red on an LED (light emitting diode) in the display window at the top of the scale. The numbers — in bright red — are ½ inch to 1½ inches high, depending on make and model.

Some electronic scales are powered with *lithium batteries,* special long-lasting thingees meant to last "a lifetime" — the scale's lifetime, that is, not yours. Color me suspicious, but did you notice the tag never says how long a lifetime is? Besides, who wants to give up that heart-stopping moment of panic when the battery runs down, your weight goes haywire, and you burn, oh, at least five calories jumping off the darned thing.

Earth to Captain Kirk! Your scale is waiting, solar-powered, of course. Electronic scales with solar power soak up energy from light. No window in the bathroom, you say? No problem. The solar cell will absorb energy from plain old electric light bulbs. Forget the Starship Enterprise: Think of this scale as a puppy you have to feed and water each day.

✔ **Body fat monitor:** The body fat monitor looks like a scale, but it doesn't count your pounds. Instead, this high-tech device uses a gee-whiz process called *bioeletrical impedance* to measure your body composition — the amount of fatty tissue versus the amount of muscle tissue. For more on body fat monitors, thumb back to Chapter 2.

Choosing the perfect scale

A perfect scale is

✔ Convenient to use

✔ Priced within reason

✔ Accurate to a fault

A real scale for your bathroom is

✔ Convenient to use

✔ Priced within reason

✔ Sort of accurate

The trick is to consider your home scale a guide to what you weigh, not an absolute guarantee. In tests conducted by Consumer Watch in 1999, various bathroom scales produced results from 0.5 to 4 pounds off the tester's real weight. Scales that give you your weight within 0.5 to 1 pound are considered okay.

So how do you get the more accurate models? According to the technical support team at Tanita Corporation of America in Arlington Heights, Illinois, a higher price usually translates into better accuracy for both spring scales and electronic scales. In my heart of hearts, I know they're right, but honesty (and a tight wallet) compels me to point out that while weighing myself on the Old Reliable, no-name $5 bargain tucked under my bed gives me a number 2 pounds lower than the weight on my doctor's scale, the 2-pound difference never varies. In other words, my tacky little scale is wrong, but consistent. Hey, it works for me.

When to weigh yourself

Whether you step on the scale at home or at the gym or in your doctor's office, numbers going down mean that you're losing weight. The real question is, how often should you check to find out whether you are losing?

Most weight loss programs suggest holding yourself to once a week, at the same time, on the same day, say, Monday morning at 8 a.m. Their reasoning is sound, of course. Any number of variables, such as rainy weather — falling *barometric pressure,* a measure of the pressure the earth's atmosphere exerts against your body (and everything else on earth), which allows you to balloon out a bit — or one day's dietary riot (I don't care how dedicated you are, nobody can resist chocolate cake all the time) can bubble your weight up a bit from day to day. So if you weigh in every single day, you may not see a steady downward progress, and that can be discouraging.

Well, sure. They're right. Except . . . making a really detailed chart and keeping a running daily total works wonders for obsessive, compulsive, picky perfectionists like me. Yes, the numbers bounce, but if you stick to your weight loss program, after a week or so, the trend will be clearly downward. Besides, filling in the chart uses up some energy (calories, see Chapter 5), doesn't it?

Oh, boy, is this chart ever simple Simon time. Table 3-10, on your CD-ROM, shows you a record of a full month of tracking your weight. Just print it and fill it in with your daily weight in the Weight column. In the Comments column, put, well, comments, such as "ate ice cream last night," or "had a sandwich with just one slice of bread," or (if you're a female type) "my period's due," or any other happening you think might affect your weight. By the end of the month, not only will you have a record of your weight loss, you just might also have a pattern showing how your daily life affects your ability to lose weight. Remember: One or two days' small gain or a few days' at the same weight is totally normal.

Table 3-10	Tracking Your Weight	
Date	*Weight*	*Comments*
March 1	135	Started my new eating plan
March 2		
March 3		
March 4		
March 5		
March 6		
March 7		
March 8		
March 9		
March 10		
March 11		
March 12		
March 13		
March 14		
March 15		
March 16		
March 17		
March 18		
March 19		
March 20		
March 21		
March 22		
March 23		
March 24		
March 25		
March 26		
March 27		

(continued)

Table 3-10 *(continued)*		
Date	*Weight*	*Comments*
March 28		
March 29		
March 30		
March 31		

How to use a scale

Believe it or not, there's a right way and a wrong way to weigh yourself. The following steps walk you through the correct procedure.

1. Take off all your clothes.

Yes, I know some weight charts in Chapter 2 list weight with clothes, but who are we kidding? What we want here is the lowest consistent weight. And that's buck-nekkid, kids.

2. Put the scale on a hard, flat surface.

No carpet, please. Carpet bounces, making the springs or load cell rrrrrrr-ock.

3. On a spring scale, adjust the dial so that the indicator sits at zero. With an electronic scale, just wait until it says zero.

4. Step on and off the scale. If the indicator does not return to zero, repeat Step 2 and try again.

5. Now step on the scale with your feet squarely planted on each side so that your weight is evenly divided.

6. Read your weight.

What? You forgot to put on your glasses? No, no, no— don't bend down to try to read the dial. Step off the scale, put on your glasses, and step back on. Oh, wait, did you check to see that the dial returned to zero when you stepped off? If it didn't, readjust it. If it did, step on and read your weight.

There, that was easy, wasn't it?

Part II
Choosing a Weight Loss Plan

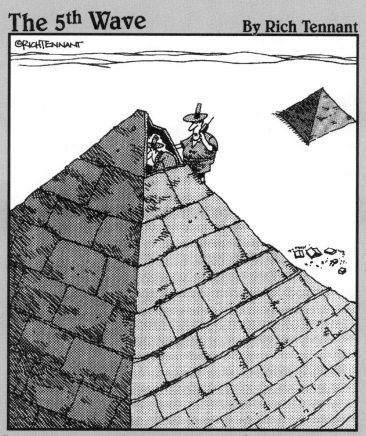

The 5th Wave   By Rich Tennant

@RICHTENNANT

"It's the darnedest thing. The top of the Pyramid seems to be filled with fats and sweets, unlike the base, which contained mostly fresh vegetables, grains, and legumes."

In this part . . .

Deciding to lose weight is just the first step toward a slimmer, trimmer you. Picking a weight loss program is a really Big Step. How to evaluate the claims of conflicting weight loss plans? This part tells you how to separate the reasonable healthful stratagems from the unproven or nutritionally deficient alternatives. What a good idea!

Chapter 4

Healthful Rules for Healthy Weight Loss Programs

*T*he fact that you are reading this book means you're serious about weight control. And you probably want to get to the main event *right now*. But you stopped at this chapter because you know in your heart that before you plunge into a new meal plan, it makes sense to sit back, take a deep breath, and spend a minute — okay, maybe ten minutes — learning The Rules. No, no, *not* those rules for finding a romantic partner (although many people want to lose weight to make themselves more attractive so that they can get around to The Rules).

But that set of guidelines is for another day, maybe even a whole other book such as *Dating For Dummies* (Hungry Minds, Inc.) by Dr. Joy Browne. The rules I plan to list here are designed to enable to you recognize a healthful diet while avoiding the nasty fad diets that promise miracles but often end up keeping you from meeting your long-term weight control goals. If you need a nice low-cal beverage or treat (I won't even mention how good a piece of fruit would be) to get you through this chapter, now's the time to get it. Hurry back.

Five Rules of the Game

Like riding a bicycle, playing tennis, or singing at the Met, successful weight loss takes practice. Sometimes a lot of practice. Nobody's born knowing exactly what to eat to lose weight, but learning the ropes makes it easier to pick a better way to go. In other words, to win at weight loss, you have to know the rules. Translation: You have to know when you're ready to lose weight, and once you've decided that, you have to know how to distinguish a healthful program from the merely okay or the truly awful.

The five rules listed here are a good guide.

Rule #1: Be sure you actually need to lose weight

Your assignment, if you choose to accept it, is to be certain that you really do need to lose weight. Chapter 2 lays out guidelines you can use to assess your own weight realistically: too high, too low (!), or just right. These guidelines can help you avoid the pitfall of trying to lose weight for the wrong reason, such as an eating disorder that makes you feel fatter than your really are (more about that in Chapter 2, too).

On the other hand, if you really are a couple of pounds on the wrong side of the scale (you can find out how to weigh yourself in Chapter 3), and your doctor agrees that losing weight will improve your health, proceed to Rule #2.

Rule #2: Don't start a weight loss program until you're ready

I mean really, really ready. Trying to lose weight is like trying to give up smoking. I know how hard that is because when I finally threw away the butts, my habit had reached three, count 'em three, packs a day. My hair smelled, my clothes smelled, I couldn't sleep, and I couldn't corral enough breath to walk a city block. In fact, I took so many taxis that my boyfriend, now my husband, called me "The Princess."

Giving up cigarettes wasn't easy. After several missed attempts, I started it one hour at a time. Then I pushed for half a day. Then I made it through a day. Each time I raised the bar I told myself that I would make it through this period of time and then decide whether to continue. When I hit six months without lighting up, I said, "Hey, I'll go for a year and then make a final decision." I made the year, and never looked back. Sometimes I still miss an after-dinner smoke, and sometimes I follow smokers down the street just for the fragrant aroma. But I'm not smoking, and let me tell you, now that cigarettes are $3.50 a pack, I am pleased as punch not to be burning up $73.50 every week.

But enough about me. My point is that I know how you feel, and I sympathize. You've tried to lose weight before, and either didn't make it or gained back everything you lost. So how do know if you're ready this time? Glad you asked, because I have this teensy little multiple choice five-question quiz, which you can find in Table 4-1 on your CD-ROM. Yes, it's baby simple, and yes, I know you'll get the idea right off the bat, but humor me: Try it anyway.

Table 4-1	Are You Ready to Lose Weight?

I want to lose weight because . . .

(a) My boyfriend/girlfriend/parents say I'll look better.

(b) My doctor says it will improve my health.

(c) I think losing weight will improve my health. And I'll look better.

I am willing to try to lose weight right now because . . .

(a) I've lost my job, and dieting will keep me occupied.

(b) I broke up with my boyfriend/girlfriend, and dieting will take my mind off my broken heart.

(c) Things are pretty good, so I figure I have the energy to change my eating habits.

My goal is to lose . . .

(a) Ten pounds the first week.

(b) Ten pounds the first month.

(c) Ten pounds.

My diet is . . .

(a) Oranges three time a day; after all, they're high in fiber and vitamin C.

(b) All fruit; nobody can live on just one food, not even oranges.

(c) Fruit, veggies, grains, dairy foods, meat, fish, and poultry — only in measured portions, smaller than I usually eat.

After I lose weight . . .

(a) My whole life will change.

(b) I'll never eat ice cream again.

(c) I'll continue an active, nutritious lifestyle.

Okey-dokey, you're right. The correct answer to every question is (c). Why? Because it describes a decision based on what you want to do and what you can do, not on someone else's opinion or on unrealistic assumptions about weight. Lose ten pounds in a week? Wave bye-bye to all your problems? Never eat ice cream again? Give me — and yourself — a break!

Rule #3: Pick a diet that provides all the essential nutrients

If you're not sure exactly how much of which vitamins and minerals you need each day, stick a book mark in this page and flip ahead to Chapter 10. For your daily requirements of calories, protein, fats, and carbohydrates, keep the bookmark in place while you skim through Chapter 5, Chapter 6, Chapter 7, and Chapter 8. When you come back to this page, you should have a good idea of what you need to consume each day and how to count up totals to make sure that the diet you're thinking of using meets the test.

The corollary to Rule #3 — call it Rule #3A — is that a healthful diet, even one designed to take off pounds, provides a variety of different foods. I don't care how much you love, say, broccoli. Even though the vegetable is packed with with anticancer carotenoid pigments, plus vitamin A, vitamin C, the B vitamin folate, carbs, and dietary fiber, man (and woman) cannot live by green florets alone.

Variety in food is important to weight loss. Food is meant to be enjoyed, even diet food. When your weight loss diet is interesting and tastes good, sticking to it is less of a chore. Besides, human beings are omnivores, which means they have digestive tracts equipped to handle foods from plants and foods from animals. While vegetarianism may certainly be a healthful choice, maybe even a moral one for folks who do not want to consume animals, human bodies have the ability to metabolize and use all kinds of food: meat, dairy, grains, fruits, and veggies. Who are you to contradict Mother Nature by eating only one food?

Rule #4: Choose a diet with sensible goals

Obesity has become such an important health issue that oodles of reputable organizations, such as the American Heart Association, the American Diabetes Association, the American Dietetic Association, not to mention all the relevant government agencies, are ready and willing to offer sensible weight loss advice. The funny thing is that all of them offer pretty much the same prescription: Eat less, eat a variety of foods, get the nutrients you need, step up your exercise, and take the time you need to lose pounds safely.

This advice is boring, no doubt about that. But it's a darn sight better than testimonials on the order of "My sister's boyfriend's cousin Ethel tried this, and I heard she lost ten pounds overnight." If I believed it, I would say, "Good for Ethel." But you and I both know the story's nonsense. Boring or not, the simple truth is that like the tortoise in Aesop's tale whose slow but steady pace left the jumpy hare in the dust, slow but steady weight loss is a sure winner over the long haul. Which takes you gracefully to Rule #5.

Rule #5: Pick a diet you can live with forever

If the thought of sticking with your weight loss program triggers pure panic — what? asparagus and toast every day for the next 40 years? — you have a pretty good clue that you have picked the wrong diet. However, if your reaction is, "Yeah, I guess I could learn to live with more veggies, more fruits, and fewer coconut cream cupcakes so long as I can have a McBurger (see Chapter 22) or a fat-free frozen yogurt once in a while," that suggests you're on the right track. Remember, true weight control is a lifestyle change, and a healthy lifestyle can (and should) be a pleasurable lifelong commitment.

How to Recognize a Fad Diet

Of all the words written about weight loss, *fad diet* are the two that stir the greatest ire in a nutritionist's heart. Say the words slowly. Let them roll around on your tongue. You can practically hear the sound of distant thunder as the Nutrition Establishment rises as one to proclaim: Bah, humbug!

Fad diets come and go, which is why they are called fads. But experts say all fad diets have several traits in common:

- ✔ They claim you can lose lots of weight really, really fast.
- ✔ They promote "special" foods or a severely restricted diet.
- ✔ They claim you can lose weight without exercising.
- ✔ They quote sources nobody knows or use before-and-after pictures and anecdotes or testimonials.
- ✔ They have no long-term scientific back-up.

Before you bite, check out the following worms in these too-good-to-be-true diet apples.

Promises, promises

If a diet claim sounds too good to be true, it probably is. The perfect example is a diet that promises to take off 30 pounds in 30 days, a formula chosen presumably because some months do have 30 days, and the numbers sound good together.

According to the American Society of Bariatric Physicians, a group of doctors specializing in weight control, it is an impossibility because:

- ✔ You need to cut your calorie intake by 3,500 to lose one pound.

- ✔ To lose 30 pounds in 30 days, you need to cut out 105,000 calories (30 lbs x 3,500 calories = 105,000 calories).

- ✔ A person who consumes 2,800 calories a day — more than most American women — takes in only 84,000 calories in 30 days.

- ✔ If this person stopped eating entirely, she would still have to get rid of another 21,000 calories to reach 105,000 — the number equivalent to 30 pounds.

Anyone here think that will happen?

On the other hand, a slow but steady loss of five pounds in that 30-day means cutting back just 17,500 calories (5 lbs x 3,500 calories = 17,500 calories). Divide 17,500 by 30, and you come up with 580 calories a day, a reduction most serious weight loss programs can handle.

So the next time someone says he's knows how to lose 30 pounds in 30 days, tell him to take a hike. The exercise will do him good.

Funny food plans

A second hallmark of a fad diet is its reliance on strange food plans based on

- ✔ "Fat burning" foods such as grapefruit, a perennial favorite.

- ✔ Unusual meals such as fruit alone or grains alone or meat alone . . . whatever.

- ✔ Special products, such as costly liquid or powdered food substitutes available only from the people pushing the diet.

I hate to be the one to break this to you, but no one food will rev up your metabolism to burn fat. In addition, your body is perfectly equipped to handle all kinds of food at one meal. Restricting your food intake to one food or one type of food will not only bore you silly after a while, it will also cheat your body of essential nutrients. Imagine going on a diet to lose weight and ending up with a vitamin deficiency disease. Or, here's a surprise: A weight loss diet for people who need to lose weight but are not morbidly obese should have at least 1,200 calories, sometimes more. A diet with fewer calories may be hazardous to your health because it eventually forces your starving body to nibble on its own muscles, a situation fraught with potentially fatal consequences, as you can read in Chapter 9.

In the late 1970s, liquid protein diet products made from *collagen* (connective tissue), an inferior source of protein, were touted as a quick solution to obesity. Unfortunately, for at least 60 people the solution was — ugh! — death. The liquid protein diets contained no added nutrients, so they were deficient in essential vitamins and minerals, including minerals such as potassium that keep your heart muscle pumping. Without enough nutrients, the 60 unfortunate liquid protein consumers suffered fatal heart failure, leading to the government taking the diet products off the market. As a result of this disaster, the government now monitors the nutritional content of meals substitutes. For more about high-protein diets and the different kinds of protein your body needs, see Chapter 7. For the moment, the lesson is, there's no such thing as a free lunch.

As for "special," "high potency," or "high energy" liquids, powders, and other potions, they will certainly enrich your diet guru, but their value as a diet aid is questionable. One exception is the Very Low Calorie Diet described in Chapter 5. A second exception is the group of meal substitute products in Chapter 13. The first is serious medicine for people who are morbidly obese, meaning their weight is life-threatening; the second is convenience food for folks who need one meal in a hurry. Neither claims to be miraculous.

No hard work, no hard body

This book has a whole chapter (Chapter 18) on the virtues of exercise, so I won't waste your time by repeating the arguments in favor of movement here. The only thing you need to know to judge a weight loss program is that losing weight and keeping it off takes more than the brainpower required to identify a healthful diet. True, you need to exercise your intelligence, but you also need to exercise your muscles. The old song says, "Every little movement has a meaning all its own." The new tune tells you, "Every movement uses calories." The more you move, the easier it is to use up calories and melt away the pounds.

Who says so?

Finally, fad diets came naked, without the requisite recommendations from reputable health organizations such as the American Dietetic Association or the American Heart Association or an arm of the National Institutes of Health. Instead, a fad diet:

- Bases its advice on the results of one study, often a dubious one (65 overweight pet rats or five middle-aged men lost weight after three months on a diet of nothing but fresh apricots and peaches).

- Comes with endorsements from people who may be well meaning but have no real expertise (the rats' owners or the mother of one of those men).

> ✔ Contradicts the generally accepted advice of health and nutrition professionals (rats and people need nutrients other than those supplied by apricots and peaches).

Fad versus fit

No matter how you slice the food, healthful weight loss programs require time and effort to melt away the excess pounds. Fad diets are so appealing because they promise maximum results with minimum investment (other than the dollars you may be asked to cough up for those miracle products).

To find out whether a weight loss plan you've chosen is a sensible investment or a (boo!) fad diet, click onto your CD-ROM and fill in the blanks on Table 4-2. A "Yes" answer to each statement means you're really smart, diet-wise. Lots of "No" answers? Tsk. Tsk. Time to choose another diet.

Table 4-2	Fad versus Fit: Does Your Weight Loss Plan Measure Up?		
My Diet		*Yes*	*No*
Has a variety of foods			
Provides at least 1,200 calories a day for a woman/1,400 calories a day for a man			
Provides RDA amounts of essential nutrients			
Does not ask me to buy "special" products			
Has an exercise plan			
Comes with endorsements from reputable sources			
Is approved by my doctor			

When Dieting Is a Disease

If *For Dummies* books came with color graphics, you would see a bright red flag next to the following sentence: Before you decide to lose weight, be sure you're not already too thin.

Fashion mags and fashion gurus continue to push the image of a flat-chested, flat-hipped, flat-thighed female body that has more in common with a teenage girl or boy's than a grown-up woman's. As a result, "beauty" remains an impossible dream for millions of women, young and old, who can never achieve this streamlined body.

For an unfortunate minority, the impossible dream escalates to a psychological illness called an eating disorder. People with eating disorders do not eat enough or they eat too much. This may sound like old hat to you — doesn't everyone go through days of dieting or days of eating too much? — but an eating disorder is nothing like your cutting calories for three weeks so that you can fit into last year's dress this New Year's or (conversely) diving into a hot fudge sundae once in a while.

The difference between normal dieting and normal indulgence versus an eating disorder is that the former are normal behavior; the latter are not. An eating disorder is a serious emotional illness in which some people persistently consume extraordinarily large amounts of food to relieve anxiety, using food not as a source of physical sustenance, but as a tool for coping with emotional distress. Others do just the opposite. When anxious, they stop eating, or they force their bodies to reject the food they've eaten. Either way, their behavior is abnormal.

The three most common forms of eating disorder are

- ✔ Anorexia nervosa
- ✔ Bulimia nervosa
- ✔ Binge-eating disorder

Some lesser-known, less-common forms of eating disorder are

- ✔ Muscle dysmorphia
- ✔ Night-eating syndrome
- ✔ Pica

As you can see in Table 4-3, current statistics on the incidence of eating disorders show them to be more common among women than among men. However, it is well to keep in mind the fact that boys are less likely than girls to seek help for eating disorders, so these figures are generally regarded only as estimates. As a side note, pica is most common among pregnant women.

Table 4-3	Female-to-Male Ratio of Eating Disorders
Eating Disorder	*Female-to-Male Ratio*
Anorexia nervosa	5:1
Binge eating	1:1
Bulimia nervosa	9:1
Muscle dysmorphia	1:1
Night-eating syndrome	N/A
Pica	N/A

Source: Anorexia Nervosa and Related Eating Disorders, Inc. (www.anred.com).

Anorexia nervosa

Anorexia nervosa, a.k.a. voluntary starvation, is classically defined by one important symptom: Although they may be literally "skin and bones," when people suffering from this illness look in the mirror, they see a fat person. Treating the disease means reversing this distorted body image, an arduous task.

Anorexia is overwhelmingly a disease of wealth and privilege, virtually unknown in places where food is hard to come by. The most frequent victims of anorexia nervosa are the young and the well-to-do. The illness appears to be anywhere from six to nine times more common among young women than among young men. These figures are suspect because anorexia is so commonly characterized as a young women's problem that young men may be unwilling to admit to suffering from it; the same is likely to be true for bulimia.

Whatever its cause, the refusal to eat has real physical consequences, including

- Low body temperature and a constant sense of chill.
- Low blood pressure leading to dizziness or faintness.
- Loss of minerals, raising the risk of osteoporosis.
- Irregular heartbeat and an increased risk of sudden death.

Bulimia nervosa

Bulimia nervosa (voluntary vomiting) also occurs chiefly among the young and also seems to be more common among women than among men. Like people with anorexia, people suffering from bulimia have a distorted body image that makes them feel fat when they're not. But unlike anorexia sufferers, people with bulimia do eat. The problem is that they refuse to keep the food they eat in their bodies. In an effort to get rid of the food, they may use laxatives, but their most characteristic stratagem is to induce vomiting after meals by retiring to the bathroom and simply sticking their fingers into their throats or by taking *emetics* (drugs that cause vomiting).

Either way, danger looms. The intestinal tract is not designed for repeated stuffing followed by repeated vomiting. Forcing yourself to regurgitate the acidic contents of your stomach may

- ✔ Irritate or tear the lining of the esophagus (throat).
- ✔ Erode the enamel on your teeth, one sure sign of bulimia.
- ✔ Cause dehydration, damaging your kidneys.
- ✔ Cause a loss of minerals such as potassium required for the transmission of impulses between cells, leading to irregular heartbeat and, in extreme cases, sudden death.

Binge-eating disorder

Binge-eating disorder is a term used to describe periodic bouts of gorging. A person who is bingeing may consume astoundingly large amounts of food at one sitting: a whole chicken, several pints of ice cream, a loaf of bread, and so on.

Theoretically, pushing this much food into your stomach can dilate the stomach to the point of rupture. Realistically, if a bingeing person does not purge herself/himself afterward, either by vomiting or using large amounts of laxatives, overeating will produce obesity. (No, no, no — not all people who are overweight are binge eaters. See Chapter 2.)

Muscle dysmorphia

Muscle dysmorphia is pretty much the mirror image of anorexia nervosa, a condition that causes people to see themselves as small and thin (rather than big and fat) even when they are perfectly normal size. Eating more is one way to increase body size; another is obsessive exercising, which becomes the focus of the person's life, crowding out all other activities. (See Chapter 18, which explains the role of exercise in maintaining a healthy weight.)

Night-eating syndrome

Night-eating syndrome leads people to cram most of the calorie consumption in the hours after their evening meal. The question is not whether you have a slice of cake before you go to bed. It's whether you have three. Or four. Or more. People with night-eating syndrome may actually eat more than half of all the food they consume all day in late night "snacks," "meals," "noshes" — whatever. All that food at an odd hour tends to add up to — what else? — weight gain. In fact, statistics suggest that up to 27 percent of the Americans who are more than 100 pounds overweight eat this way — no, again, not everyone who's overweight has late night eating syndrome.

Pica

Pica gets its name from the Latin word for magpie, a bird famous for eating virtually anything it can get its beak on. In human beings, pica is an intense craving for nonfood items. The best known example may be a craving for clay or dirt or laundry starch during pregnancy. Some people say that pica may reflect the body's need for minerals lacking in the normal diet. On the other hand, regardless of nutritional value of the diet, eating clay or dirt or starch while pregnant is an old folk tradition in some parts of the world such as Africa and the Southeastern United States. These substances are not poisonous, but lots of starch can cause intestinal blockage. And eating nonfood can reduce consumption of nutritious food.

How to Recognize and Treat Eating Disorders

Eating disorders are serious medical problems that require serious medical attention. Although people with eating disorders have difficult problems to overcome, with treatment:

- ✔ About 60 percent recover.
- ✔ About 20 percent make a partial recovery.
- ✔ About 2 to 3 percent die (without treatment, that number may be as high as 20 percent).

Recognizing an eating disorder

Because so many people diet to improve their health or their looks, it is important to differentiate between a sensible weight loss diet and one that puts your health at risk. Table 4-4 gives you some guidelines culled from the advice of various reputable experts. Once you know the differences between these two patterns of weight loss, run your finger over to Table 4-5, which shows the warning signs for anorexia, bulimia, and binge eating.

Table 4-4	Patterns of Dieting	
Characteristic	*Healthful*	*Hazardous*
Rate of weight loss	Slow but steady	Very fast
Total weight loss	Within reasonable limits as outlined in standard weight charts (see Chapter 2)	Dramatic
Nutritional value of diet	Sufficient amounts of all essential nutrients	Deficient in essential nutrients
Daily calorie consumption	Within reasonable limits (see Chapter 5)	Extremely low
Food choices	Wide variety	Very limited, sometimes as few as one or two foods
Portion size	Reasonable (see Chapter 6)	Miniscule (sometimes as small as one lettuce leaf or five peas or one spoon full)

Source: American Anorexia Bulimia Association, Inc. (www.aabainc.org) and Anorexia Nervosa and Related Eating Disorders, Inc. (www.anred.com).

Table 4-5	Warning Signs of Eating Disorders
Eating Disorder	*Warning Signs*
Anorexia nervosa	Preoccupation with body weight
	Significant, fast weight loss
	Unrealistic body image
	Intense fear of weight gain
	Hair loss, very dry skin
	Failure to menstruate and growth of body hair (women) due to hormonal imbalance
	Irregular heartbeat
	Shortness of breath
	Weakness, fatigue
	Constipation
	Depression/anxiety/hyperactivity

(continued)

Table 4-5 (continued)

Eating Disorder	Warning Signs
Bulimia nervosa	Preoccupation with body weight
	Significant weight loss
	Unrealistic body image
	Binge eating
	Unexplained use of laxatives or diuretics
	Using the bathroom frequently after meals (vomiting)
	Unusual damage to dental enamel due to frequent vomiting
	Sore throat, vomiting blood
	Constipation, indigestion
	Weakness, fatigue
Binge eating disorder	Episodes of binge eating
	Eating when not hungry
	Inability to stop eating when full
	Weight fluctuations
	Weight gain
	Depression/anxiety

Source: American Anorexia Bulimia Association, Inc. (www.aabainc.org).

Are you at risk for an eating disorder?

If you spend a lot of time trying new diets in an attempt to lose weight, by now you may be wondering if you have an eating disorder.

Probably not: The simple fact that you have bought and are reading a moderate book designed to help you lose weight safely is a good clue to the fact that you have a reasonable approach to weight loss and weight control.

For those who want to be sure, the Anorexia Nervosa and Related Eating Disorders, Inc. (ANRED) Web site offers a simple multiquestion self test. The more "yes" answers you give, the higher your risk for sliding off the rails, diet-wise. To take the test, click onto www.anred.com.

Treating an eating disorder

Treating people with eating disorders means treating not only their extreme weight loss and potentially life-threatening physical problems but also their emotional upset. If you or someone you know experiences any of the signs of an eating disorder, the safest course is to seek immediate medical advice.

For more information, you may want to contact the organizations listed in Table 4-6. You can find a longer list of resources at the American Anorexia Bulimia Association Web site.

Table 4-6	Help for People with Eating Disorders	
Organization	*Web Site*	*Telephone*
American Anorexia Bulimia Association	www.aabainc.org	
Anorexia Nervosa & Related Eating Disorders (ANRED)	www.anred.com	
Eating Disorder Referral & Information Center	www.edreferralcom	(858) 792-7463
1-800-Therapist Network	www.1-800-therapist.com	(800) 843-7274

Chapter 5

Calories Count

*R*educing body fat by cutting calories is plain vanilla weight control, the basic principle on which most successful weight loss programs are built. You can call a diet lowfat, high-carb, high-protein, vegetarian, fruitarian, or whatever, but if you look closely, what you see is likely to be plain old calorie cutting dressed up in fancy clothes.

This chapter is a good introduction to all the other chapters dealing with specific diet regimens. The information here includes a definition of calories, a guide to how your body uses them, an estimate of how many you need each day, and some suggestions on how to create your own low-calorie diet. Because counting calories means working with numbers, you find a fair amount of math in the middle of the chapter. Not to worry — each step is spelled out in baby-simple detail.

What a Calorie Is

Machines burn fuel such as gasoline or kerosene to get the energy (heat) they need to move. Living things — dogs, cats, bacteria, you, and I — burn *(metabolize)* food to produce the energy (heat) needed to get up and about. Nutritionists measure the energy you get from food in units called — surprise! — *calories*.

When you increase your energy (calorie) intake, you gain weight. When you decrease your energy (calorie) intake, you lose weight. A controlled calorie diet — sometimes called a low-calorie diet — should lower your calorie consumption enough to make you spend more energy in work than you take in from food. To be healthful, this diet should provide a variety of foods and all the nutrients you need while lowering energy (calorie) intake just enough to take off about a pound a week.

Counting the calories in food

In science-speak, 1 calorie is the amount of energy (heat) it takes to raise the temperature of 1 gram of water 1 degree on the Centigrade scale at sea level.

To find out how many calories are in a serving of food, nutrition scientists burn the food in a *calorimeter,* a special box with two chambers, one inside the other.

First, they weigh out a standard 100-gram serving of, say, cooked dried beans. They put the beans on a dish. They put the dish into the inner chamber of the calorimeter (see figure). They fill this chamber with oxygen and then seal it. Then they fill the outer chamber with water and ignite the oxygen inside the inner chamber (inside the chamber filled with water . . . stick with me here) with an electric spark. As the beans burn, somebody carefully records the temperature of the water in the outside chamber. If the temperature of the water goes up 1 degree, the beans have 1 calorie. Two degrees, 2 calories, and so on. When you check out the Web site for the USDA Nutrient Database (see Chapter 22) and find that 100 grams of cooked black beans has 132 calories, you know that metabolizing the beans produces 132 calories worth of heat, energy your body can use for work.

By the way, did you notice the size of the standard serving? Not ½ cup or 3 tablespoons or a can of beans, but 100 grams. That's no accident. The United States and Burma are the only two countries in the world that do not use the metric system of grams and meters as primary units of measurement. In 1975, President Gerald Ford signed a bill that required Americans to convert

gradually to metric. But ordinary Americans said, "No, thank you," so they have never fully switched from the U.S. Conventional System with its ounces and inches.

Worldwide, however, science uses metrics. As a result, while you and I think of food in terms of common servings such as one fresh apple, or one chicken breast, or a slice of whole wheat bread, nutrition scientists often think of a standard food portion, measured as 100 grams, a more precise amount roughly equivalent to 3.5 ounces.

All modern nutrition data tables begin with the nutrients for a 100-gram serving of any particular food. The USDA Nutrient Database also lists several real-life portions, such as ½ cup cooked beans. The values listed on Nutrition Facts food labels at the supermarket may show both the metric equivalent (58 g) and the real serving ("one English muffin").

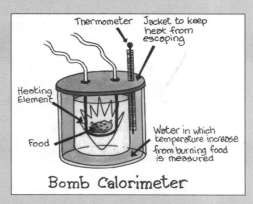

Bomb Calorimeter

Some low-calorie diets are gimmicky, like the I'm-so-bored-I-can't-eat-diet built around a single food such as a grapefruit diet or a diet based on cabbage soup. Or a low-calorie diet, such as the Scarsdale diet (which bills itself as low-carb, but is also low-cal) may simply feature meals so lacking in taste appeal that nobody wants to eat them. (For more on low-carb diets, see Chapter 6.) Cutting calories this way does take off weight, but after a few days your taste buds will rebel, demanding something that tastes good. When you give in, you gain weight.

Another way to cut calories is to serve measured portions. Two good examples are the prepared servings sold by programs such as Weight Watchers or Jenny Craig (more about that in Chapter 17). Or you can create your own version of measured portions by using the Food Guide Pyramid created by the U.S. Departments of Agriculture (USDA) and Health and Human Services (HHS). For more on using the Food Guide Pyramid, see Chapter 6.

A diet based on measured servings is a gimmick, but a good one because it provides

- ✔ A variety of foods
- ✔ Plenty of nutrients
- ✔ No need to cook, thus reducing temptation time in the kitchen — or really big servings of otherwise diet-friendly food

Using commercial products has a downside in that it does not show you how to assemble your own meals, but using the Food Guide Pyramid is a super way to learn.

A diet based on measured portions works because it serves up fewer calories than you ordinarily eat but enough calories to keep your body healthy. How many calories is that? I thought you'd never ask.

How Many Calories Does a Healthy Body Need?

Your body needs energy (calories) to do two kinds of daily work, involuntary work and voluntary work.

Involuntary work comprises the essential chores your body does even when you are just lying there doing absolutely nothing:

- ✔ Breathing
- ✔ Pumping blood
- ✔ Digesting food
- ✔ Absorbing nutrients

> ✔ Building new cells and tissues
>
> ✔ Producing biochemical compounds such as enzymes

and . . . well, you get the picture.

On average, a resting man uses more energy (cal . . . oh, heck, by now you know the terms are synonyms) than a resting woman of the same weight and height because he has proportionately more muscle tissue than she does. Muscle is active; it works (moves) and burns calories. Fat is passive; it stores energy and insulates the body and its internal organs, but it doesn't use up as many calories as muscle. (Did I mention women have proportionately more fat?)

The precise number of calories/energy you need to accomplish these essential jobs is called *resting energy expenditure (REE),* also known as *basal metabolic rate (BMR).* You can find out how to determine your own REE, or BMR, in the next section.

Voluntary work is the work you do when you are up and going about your daily business: walking, running, driving, cooking, thinking (yes, thinking uses energy, although not as much as you think it might).

Adding up your own REE

Before you start this section, take a deep breath and repeat after me: I am not afraid of math. This section contains lots of math, but it's done step by simple step. Trust me, you will sail through like a pro.

Okay. Your REE accounts for a whopping 79 percent of all the energy (remember: calories) you need each day. The National Research Council, the arm of the National Academy of Sciences in Washington, which sets RDAs and other nutritional guidelines, has created a set of age- and gender-related equations you can use to calculate how many calories that is. All you have to do is plug in the right numbers.

Unless you can multiply multidigit numbers in your head, you'll need your calculator for this exercise. Get it. Got it? Good.

1. **Convert your weight in pounds (lbs) to kilograms (kg).**

   One kilogram = 2.2 pounds, so divide your weight in pounds by 2.2 to find your weight in kilograms. Example: 130 lbs divided by 2.2 = 59 kg.

2. **Pick the appropriate equation from Table 5-1 (for males) or Table 5-2 (for females).**

Table 5-1	Male REE Equations
Age	*REE Equation*
0–3 years	(60.9 x weight) – 54
3–10 years	(22.7 x weight) + 495
10–18 years	(17.5 x weight) + 651
18–30 years	(15.3 x weight) + 679
30–60 years	(11.6 x weight) + 879
>60 years	(13.5 x weight) + 487

Source: Adapted with permission from The National Research Council, Recommended Dietary Allowances (Washington, D.C.: National Academy Press, 1989).

Table 5-2	Female REE Equations
Age	*REE Equation*
0–3 years	(61.0 x weight) – 51
3–10 years	(22.5 x weight) + 499
10–18 years	(12.2 x weight) + 746
18–30 years	(14.7 x weight) + 496
30–60 years	(8.7 x weight) + 829
>60 years	(10.5 x weight) + 596

Source: Adapted with permission from The National Research Council, Recommended Dietary Allowances (Washington, D.C.: National Academy Press, 1989).

3. Plug in the numbers.

Math tip: Numbers grouped together in parentheses represent one unit. For example, $(2 \times 6) + 4$ means, "Multiply 2×6 and then add 4."

Okay, now I'll do some REEs for you. (Note to the very picky: We are rounding off numbers to avoid pesky decimals.)

Example #1: You are a 30-year-old woman who weighs 130 pounds.

1. Convert your weight in pounds to kilograms: 130 lbs/2.2 = 59 kg.

2. Pick the appropriate REE equation: $(8.7 \times 59) + 829$.

3. **Do the math: $8.7 \times 59 = 513$ and then $513 + 879 = 1,392$.**

   Your REE is 1,392 calories a day.

Example #2: You are a 30-year-old man who weighs 130 pounds.

1. **Convert your weight in pounds to kilograms: 130 lbs/2.2 = 59 kg.**
2. **Pick the appropriate REE equation $(11.6 \times 59) + 879$.**
3. **Do the math: $11.6 \times 59 = 684$ and then $684 + 879 = 1,563$.**

   Your REE is 1,563 calories a day.

Do you see the interesting difference? Two people, same weight, same age. But one (the male) uses about 12 percent more calories to run his body at rest. Aha! It's his active muscle tissue, working even when he's at rest. (By the way, children and adolescents have relatively high REEs because they are building new tissue at a fast clip every day. An adult's REE goes up temporarily when he or she is recuperating from an injury such as a torn muscle or a broken bone temporarily and busily making new tissue.)

But what about when he (and she) is actually working? Good question.

Finding out your total daily calorie requirements

The REE represents a big chunk of your calorie requirements, but it's not the whole story. Every day you also do voluntary work — walking, running, vacuuming the floor — and that takes energy, too. You can calculate your total daily calorie requirement — calories for involuntary plus voluntary work — in one of two ways.

Use an REE multiple

The simplest way to figure out how many calories your body needs each day is to multiply your REE by a standard number the National Research Council calls, with admirable directness, an *REE multiple*.

Tables 5-3 and 5-4 show REE multiples for adolescent and adult men and women.

Table 5-3	Male REE Multiples
Age	*REE Multiple*
11–14 years	1.70
15–18 years	1.67
19–24 years	1.67
25–50 years	1.60
>51years	1.50

Source: Adapted with permission from The National Research Council, Recommended Dietary Allowances (Washington, D.C.: National Academy Press, 1989).

Table 5-4	Female REE Multiples
Age	*REE Multiple*
11–14 years	1.67
15–18 years	1.60
19–24 years	1.60
25–50 years	1.55
>51 years	1.50

Source: Adapted with permission from The National Research Council, Recommended Dietary Allowances (Washington, D.C.: National Academy Press, 1989).

Now I'll use the REE multiples to find out how many calories the 30-year-old man and woman actually need each day to do their work. Ladies first:

Example #1: The recommended daily calorie allowance for a 30-year-old, 130-pound woman with an REE of 1,392 is 2,158 calories. 1,392 (REE) × 1.55 (REE multiple) = 2,158.

Example #2: The recommended daily calorie allowance for a 30-year-old, 130-pound man with an REE of 1,563 is 2,422 calories. 1,563 (REE) × 1.60 (REE multiple) = 2,500.

Once again, he's got the calorie advantage. His larger body with its bulkier muscles requires 342 calories more a day than her lighter, fatter frame. Bummer.

Skip the math

If you were a nutrition scientist working in a lab with lots of machines to measure every teensy little bit of work your body does, you could calculate your calorie requirements precisely.

But you're not. So you can't.

Luckily, the National Research Council has done all the pesky math for you. The numbers in Tables 5-5 and 5-6 are recommended daily energy allowances (read: calories) for people of average height and weight doing an average day's average amount of work. If the average Joe and Jane stick to the number of calories listed here, they should just keep truckin' along, neither gaining nor losing weight.

Do I really have to say that if non-average you may need more (or less) energy for your non-average day? Check out Chapter 18 for details on the amount of energy (calories) you use doing various kinds of exercise and work. Or thumb through *Fitness For Dummies* (Hungry Minds, Inc.) by Suzanne Schlosberg and Liz Neporent. Or check with your weight loss professional for a more personal calorie count.

Table 5-5	Recommended Daily Calorie Allowances for Males		
Age (Years)	*Weight*	*Height (Ft/In)*	*Calories*
11–14	99 lbs/45 kg	5'2"	2,500
15–18	145 lbs/66 kg	5'9"	3,000
19–24	160 lbs/72 kg	5'10"	2,900
25–50	174 lbs/79 kg	5'10"	2,900
>51	170 lbs/77 kg	5'8"	2,300

Source: Adapted with permission from The National Research Council, Recommended Dietary Allowances (Washington, D.C.:National Academy Press, 1989).

Table 5-6	Recommended Calorie Allowances for Females		
Age (Years)	*Weight*	*Height (Ft/In)*	*Calories*
11–14	101 lbs/46 kg	5'2"	2,200
15–18	120 lbs/55 kg	5'4"	2,200
19–24	128 lbs/58 kg	5'5"	2,200

Age	Weight	Height (Ft/In)	Calories
25–50	138 lbs/63 kg	5'4"	2,200
>51 years	143 lbs/65 kg	5'3"	1,900

Source: Adapted with permission from The National Research Council, Recommended Dietary Allowances (Washington, D.C.:National Academy Press, 1989).

Building a Sensible Controlled-Calorie Weight Loss Program

The magic number for controlling weight by counting calories is 3,500, the amount of calories it takes to add or subtract one pound of body fat.

✔ If you cut your daily calorie consumption by 3,500 calories over a period of time, you will lose one pound. For example, a person who goes down from 2,000 calories a day to 1,700 and continues to do the same amount of physical work will lose one pound in just about 11 days.

✔ If you increase your daily calorie consumption by 3,500 calories over a period of time, you will gain one pound. For example, a person who goes up from 1,700 to 2,000 calories a day, without increasing the amount of work he does, will be one pound heavier 11 days later.

Caution! Nutrition wisdom says that you must consume at least 10 calories per pound of body weight per day to lose weight without doing harm to your body. For example, a woman who weighs 137 pounds and wants to lose weight safely must get at least 1,370 calories a day. The lower limit for safe calorie cutting is 1,200 calories a day. This figure is not one pulled out of the air. On a diet providing less than 1,200 calories, it is virtually impossible to get the nutrients your body needs. Besides, 1,200 calories is adequate for a person who weighs 120 pounds, a weight at which most adults are already v-e-r-y slim and unlikely to need to lose weight.

Counting your personal calories

To decide how many calories you want to eliminate each day in order to lose one pound, you must start by knowing how many calories you are currently consuming.

Every nutrition person worth his weight in vitamins knows that folks are likely to underestimate their calorie intake. The only way to be sure what you're eating is to keep a list.

For a chart that you can use to list your daily food (and calorie) intake, click onto your CD-ROM for Counting Your Personal Calories, my version of the National Heart, Lung, and Blood Institute's own diagram. You can also go to the National Heart, Lung, and Blood Institute Web site at

www.nhlbi.nih.gov/health/public/heart/obesity/lose_wt/diaryint.html

Print a copy of the chart. Cross out the section labeled "activity" (we're just doing food and calories here) and write in "Snacks." Then use the chart as a daily record to see how many calories you're actually consuming (see Table 5-7).

Wait! Don't forget to include beverages and extras, such as seasonings, on your daily food chart!

Then print four more copies and try cutting back 250 calories a day for four weeks. At the end of this period, if you're doing the same amount of physical work you did before, you should be two pounds lighter. Good luck!

Table 5-7	Counting Your Personal Calories		
Day	*Meal*	*Food/Portion Size*	*Calories*
Day 1	Breakfast		
	Lunch		
	Dinner		
	Snacks		
Day 2	Breakfast		
	Lunch		
	Dinner		
	Snacks		
Day 3	Breakfast		
	Lunch		
	Dinner		
	Snacks		
Day 4	Breakfast		
	Lunch		
	Dinner		

Age	Weight	Height (Ft/In)	Calories
	Snacks		
Day 5	Breakfast		
	Lunch		
	Dinner		
	Snacks		
Day 6	Breakfast		
	Lunch		
	Dinner		
	Snacks		
Day 7	Breakfast		
	Lunch		
	Dinner		
	Snacks		

Creating your own lower-calorie eating plan

Once you know how many calories you're taking in each day, you can easily figure out how many you have to eliminate to add up to 3,500 in a specific period of time. For example, if you regularly consume about 2,000 calories a day, cutting back to around 1,500 calories, a net reduction of about 500 calories a day, will take off one pound in one week ($550 \times 7 = 3,500$).

Here's the good news: If that sounds too drastic, take heart. Cutting back just 300 calories a day will take off one pound in about 11 days ($11 \times 300 = 3300$. Close enough).

Here's the even-better news: When you're counting calories, even very little things mean a lot. Most people start a new weight loss diet with big expectations, promising to eat nothing but lettuce leaves (oh, sure) or no more than 1,000 calories a day (ditto), so that they can take off the pounds so fast their friends will turn green with envy. In real life, this kind of weight loss plan usually lasts about a day and a half, at which point you reward yourself for a strenuous 36 hours by wolfing down pastrami on rye or a bagel with an extra schmear.

The better way is the Little Things Theory of Dieting, a name I invented to explain how you can maintain slow but steady weight loss by cutting calories in amounts so small that you won't even notice they're gone. Once again, you're dealing with the magic 3,500 — the amount of calories you have to drop to melt away one pound of body fat.

This time, though, instead of thinking in the hundreds or calories, think in terms of ones or tens and make your weight loss program a one-year plan. To drop ten pounds in one year, you have to lose 35,000 calories ($10 \times 3,500$). The Little Things Theory of Dieting says

- ✔ One teaspoon of sugar is worth 16 calories. If you put sugar in your coffee and if you drink three cups a day, that's 48 calories. Switching to a no-cal sugar substitute saves 48 calories a day. Multiply that by 365, and you save — can you believe this? — 17,520 calories a year. At 3,500 calories a pound, that's 5 pounds less of you just by giving up 3 teaspoons of sugar a day.

- ✔ One slice of bread is worth 90 calories. Make your lunch time sandwich with one slice of bread rather than the customary two, and you save 90 calories a day or 32,850 calories a year for a net loss of 9 — count 'em, 9 — pounds of body fat.

- ✔ One 12-ounce can of regular soda a day equals 150 calories. One 12-ounce can of diet soda equals 0 calories. Switching to the diet brand saves 54,750 calories a year and peels off 15 pounds.

I could go on and on like this, but do I really have to? You get the idea: When you're trying to cut calories, little things can mean a lot. You won't turn skinny overnight, but if you keep it up, you will lose steadily without feeling deprived — and without depriving your body of the nutrients it needs. Not a bad definition of a healthful diet.

Table 5-8 shows you how to cut calories from a typical American diet. This is just an example: It lists three meals a day, but no snacks. But nobody says you can't juggle the food around, using one slice of bread from breakfast as an afternoon munchie with the apple from lunch or increase your exercise time (check out Chapter 18). Enjoy.

Table 5-8	Cutting 500 Calories the Easy Way	
Meal/Item	*Regular Serving (Amount, Calories)*	*Lower-Calorie Serving (Amount, Calories)*
Breakfast		
Orange juice	6 oz (67 cal)	6 oz (67 cal)
Whole-wheat toast	2 slices (140 cal)	1 slice (70 cal)
Jelly	2 T (30 cal)	1 T (15 cal)

Meal/Item	Regular Serving (Amount, Calories)	Lower-Calorie Serving (Amount, Calories)
Breakfast		
Cereal	1 cup (207 cal)	1 cup (207 cal)
Milk (skim)	1 cup (85 cal)	1 cup (85 cal)
Breakfast		
Coffee	1 cup (5 cal)	1 cup (5 cal)
Total	*551 calories*	*466 calories*
Lunch		
Whole-wheat bread	2 slices (140 cal)	2 slices (140 cal)
Roast beef	3 oz (90 cal)	2 oz (60 cal)
Lettuce	1 leaf (1 cal)	1 leaf (1 cal)
Tomato	3 slices (10 cal)	3 slices (10 cal)
Mayonnaise	1 T, regular (99 cal)	1 T, lowfat (36 cal)
Apple pie/apple	1 slice (374 cal)	2.5" fresh apple (81 cal)
Cola, diet	12 oz (0–4 cal)	12 oz (0–4 cal)
Total	*718 calories*	*541 calories*
Dinner		
Salmon, baked	6 oz (310 cal)	3 oz (155 cal)
Baked potato, with skin	Medium (229 cal)	Medium (229 cal)
Margarine, regular	1 pat (36 cal)	No margarine (0 cal)
Green beans, cooked	1/2 cup (22 cal)	1/2 cup (22 cal)
Carrots, cooked	1/2 cup (35 cal)	1/2 cup (35 cal)
Dinner roll	Medium (80 cal)	Medium (80 cal)
Margarine	1 pat (36 cal)	No margarine (0 cal)
Iced tea	12 ounces (0 cal)	12 ounces (0 cal)
Total	*748 calories*	*521 calories*
Day's total	*2,000 calories*	*1,511 calories*

Well, that sounds fine. But wait! There are two traps waiting. Can you see what they are? First, calcium. Second, the Food Guide Pyramid. If you scrutinize the "regular" diet and the "slim down" version, you'll see that neither one provides all the calcium recommended by the RDA, and neither one has all the servings recommended by the Food Guide Pyramid. These are not unusual problems. And the solutions are easy. For the calcium, just add two 8-ounce cups of skim milk per day. If that does not give you all the calcium you need, ask your doctor about the virtue of calcium supplements. As for servings, check out the Food Guide Pyramid yourself and adjust your diet as required. What this little exercise should show you is that both "typical" diets and "weight loss" diets can be less than perfect. So check them out. Every time.

Is that easy, or what?

The very low-calorie diet

The very low-calorie diet (VLCD) is a 400- to 800-calorie prepared liquid formula containing twice the RDA for protein, a little carbohydrate, little or no fat, and vitamin and minerals supplements that provide sufficient amounts of all the essential nutrients.

VLCDs are so low in calories that your body reacts to them as a kind of mini-fast (see Chapter 11 for the skinny on true fasting). First, realizing how few calories it is taking in, your body begins to draw on the energy stored in fat deposits, producing real weight loss. Continued calorie deprivation, however, can lead to potentially serious adverse effects such as:

- Dry skin, hair loss, body odor
- Fatigue, insomnia,
- Gastric upset
- Slowdown of the intestinal tract
- Dehydration
- Breathing difficulties
- Irregular heartbeat
- Sudden death
- Higher cholesterol

As a result, the medically supervised VLCD is recommended only as a relatively short-term first step to life-long weight control for:

- People who must lose more than 100 pounds
- People with a BMI higher than 30
- People with a BMI 27 to 30 who have weight-related health problems such as diabetes or high blood pressure

The VLCD regimen is not recommended for:

- Women who are pregnant
- Women who are breast-feeding
- Children or adolescents
- Older people who may have medical conditions or be using medication that makes it difficult to tolerate the side effects of severe calorie cutting

Caution! A medically supervised VLCD is not the same as liquids or products sold over-the-counter to be used in place of one or two meals a day (more about these products in Chapter 13). While home VLCDs were once popular, a series of serious problems, including sudden death, quickly reduced demand. VLCDs require medical supervision; they are not a do-it-yourself weight loss plan.

Chapter 6

Playing with Carbs

*W*eight loss mavens love high-carb foods, such as fruits, veggies, and grains, because they are low in calories, but high in essential nutrients. You and I love carbs because their low-cal bulk can fill the tummy without filling out the hips.

This chapter, therefore, gives you the skinny on carbs. It explains why carbs are important to your body, evaluates various high-carb meal plans, and shows you how to build your very own tasty, nutritious, and totally painless carb-based weight loss plan that not only lowers your risk of heart disease, high blood pressure, and diabetes, but also helps you take off those extra pounds.

The Joy of Carbs

Carbohydrates — sugars, starch, dietary fiber — are compounds produced when plants are exposed to light. The process by which plants make carbs is called *photosynthesis,* from the Greek words for light *(photo),* together *(syn),* and place *(thesis).* As a result, most plant foods — fruits, vegetables, grains, nuts, and seeds — have seven things in common. They are

↳ High in carbohydrates

↳ Chock-full of vitamins and minerals

↳ Rich in *phytochemicals,* the newly identified plant compounds such as the deep yellow pigment beta carotene, which seems to protect against chronic illnesses, like heart disease and cancer

↳ Low in calories

- Low in fat, including the saturated fats that clog your arteries
- Cholesterol-free
- Full of fiber and bulk (meaning they fill you up so you have less room for high-fat, high-calorie indulgences)

It's no surprise to hear that high-carb meals are the mainstay of the basic everyday healthy diet recommended by the following authoritative organizations, medical-based weight loss plans, and pop weight loss programs:

- The U.S. Departments of Agriculture and Health and Human Services Dietary Guidelines for Americans 2000
- The American Heart Association
- The American Diabetes Association
- The Pritikin diet
- The Ornish diet
- Eater's Choice
- Eat to Win
- Susan Powter (author of *Stop the Insanity*)
- Dr. Bob Arnot's Revolutionary Weight Control Program

I know you're raring to find out how high-carb foods help you slim down. But take a minute or two to read in the next section about how your body uses carbs. The nutritional and physiological info will help you understand carbs' role in weight loss. On the other hand, if you really can't wait, who am I to stand in your way? You have my permission to skip past the next section and go straight to the weight loss plans.

How Your Body Uses Carbohydrates

Your organs, systems, and cells run on *glucose*, a sugar molecule you burn to produce the energy you need. You get this necessary glucose from carbohydrates, which are composed of units (molecules) of sugar.

As soon as you eat high-carb foods, you digest — separate — the compound into its sugar units. As you can see from the "Classifying carbohydrates" sidebar, some of these sugar units are plain glucose. Others are compounds such as sucrose, which can be broken apart quickly into more glucose.

Insulin — an enzyme secreted by your pancreas — moves the glucose into your cells. If you need the glucose for instant energy, your body burns it right away. If you have enough glucose for your immediate needs, the extra supply on hand is converted to glycogen ("animal starch") and tucked away as stored energy in your liver and muscle cells, which can accommodate about 400 grams (14 ounces) of glycogen.

One gram of carbohydrates has 4 calories, so a quick multiplication (4 × 400) shows that you can store approximately 1,600 calories of energy as glycogen. If you take in more carbs than you can store as glycogen or glucose, the rest becomes — ugh! — stored fat. But that's not going to happen after you read this chapter and find out how to use carbs in a weight loss program, right? Right!

In addition to giving you energy, carbs also do the following for your body:

- ✔ Regulate the amount of sugar circulating in your blood.
- ✔ Protect your muscles.
- ✔ Influence your mood.

Carbs and blood sugar

Healthy people produce enough insulin to process all the sugars from the carbs they consume. Folks with certain metabolic problems such as diabetes do not produce enough insulin to carry all the glucose into their body cells. As a result, the glucose continues to circulate in their blood stream until it is excreted through the kidneys. (One way to check for diabetes is to test the level of sugar in urine.)

Other people can't digest carbohydrates because they lack the specific enzymes they need to break the bonds that hold a carbohydrate's sugar units together. The best known example is *lactose intolerance,* an inability to digest the sugar in milk. Nearly three-quarters of all adults (other than those from northwest Europe) are deficient in *lactase,* the enzyme that splits lactose (milk sugar) into glucose and galactose. The undigested lactose provides a rich banquet for intestinal bacteria, which chomp away on it and excrete, um, gas, which makes people with this particular problem, um, gassy.

Some recent weight loss programs such as Sugar Busters! base their dietary recommendations on the assumption that eating carbs provokes your body to release lots of insulin, which makes you hungrier, which makes you eat more, which makes you (what else?) gain weight. As a result, these diets pass up carbs for proteins. You can read more about these diets in Chapter 7.

Healthy people can cope with high-carb diets. But if you have a metabolic disorder (you know who you are), you should seek your physician's advice in setting up a diet — don't merely rely on a pop diet book, not even this one.

Carbs and your muscles

Chapter 7 explains how carbs protect your muscles and how a carb-deficient diet can cause your body to burn its own protein tissues (muscles) for energy. A diet that provides sufficient amounts of carbohydrates keeps your body from "eating" its own muscles, so a diet with enough carbs is sometimes labeled "protein sparing." A medically supervised fast in a hospital setting spares protein, too, because it provides . . . well, why not just check out Chapter 10?

Carbs and your mood

Yes, indeed, milk and cookies will make you feel mellow. So will pasta. Or a sweet roll. Forget what you've heard about sugar pepping you up. All carbs, including sugar, are super calmer-downers.

Your emotional responses arise from the transmission of impulses between nerve cells in your brain. To transmit impulses, these cells require chemicals called neurotransmitters (*neuro* = nerve) to be present in the liquid surrounding the cells.

The neurotransmitters (dopamine, norepinephrine, and serotonin) are made from tyrosine and tryptophan, amino acids (components of proteins) found abundantly in protein foods. Tyrosine is the most important ingredient in dopamine and norepinephrine, the "alertness" neurotransmitters. (This explains why a high-protein meal makes you feel alert and peppy.) Tryptophan is the most important ingredient in serotonin, the "calming" neurotransmitter.

All amino acids get to your brain eventually, but tyrosine usually zips up there way ahead of tryptophan. But when you eat carbs, which provide glucose, your pancreas releases that old reliable insulin, which — in addition to pushing glucose into body cells — keeps tyrosine circulating in your blood. As a result, tryptophan can slide into your brain to increase your production of serotonin. And voilà! After a meal of starchy high-glucose pasta, you're calmer. Or, some people complain, too mellow to clinch a deal at lunch.

How many carbohydrates does it take to make this happen? According to Judith Wurtman, a scientist at the Massachusetts Institute of Technology who (with her husband, Richard Wurtman) practically pioneered the study of food and mood, one ounce of sugar plus two ounces of protein food are enough to groove your mood. And maybe increase the odds of your sticking to your weight loss plan.

Classifying carbohydrates

All carbohydrates are made of units (molecules) of sugar. But not all carbs are sweet, because *sugar* refers to a specific chemical structure, not a flavor. What makes some carbs sweet and other carbs starchy is the number and type of sugar units they contain.

Nutrition For Dummies (written by me and published by Hungry Minds, Inc.) includes the chemical structure of various carbs, so I could tell you to run out and buy the book right now, or just to take the book off your shelf if you already have it. But, heck, it's easier to include a quick set of facts and definitions right here — rewritten, of course, so that you don't experience déjà vu in case you've already gone through *Nutrition For Dummies*.

> Fact #1: The word *carbohydrates* comes from *carbon* (carbo-) and *water* (hydr-).

> Fact #2: All carbs are made of units of sugar.

> Fact #3: Depending on how many sugar units a carbohydrate has or how the units are attached to one another, a carbohydrate is either *simple* or *complex*.

A simple carbohydrate has only one or two units of sugar. A carb with one sugar unit is a *monosaccharide* (*mono* = one; *saccharide* = sugar). Examples of monosaccharides are *fructose* (fruit sugar), *glucose* (blood sugar — the sugar produced when you digest carbs), and *galactose* (the sugar produced when you digest lactose, milk sugar).

A carb with two sugar units is a *double sugar,* also known as *disaccharide* (*di* = two). The most familiar disaccharide is *sucrose* (table sugar), which is composed of one unit of fructose and one unit of glucose.

Complex carbohydrates, sometimes labeled *polysaccharides* (*poly* = many), have more than two units of sugar. (Technically speaking, *oligosaccharides* are generally those with 3 to 10 sugar units and poly those greater than 10.)

A *trisaccharide* (*tri* = three) has three sugar units. One example of a trisaccharide is *raffinose,* a complex carb in potatoes, beans, and beets that has one unit each of galactose, glucose, and fructose. A *tetrasaccharide* (*tetra* = four) has four sugar units. *Stachyose,* a tetrasacharride in veggies, has one fructose unit, one glucose unit, and two galactose units. A plain old polysaccharide has lots of sugar units. *Starch,* a complex carbohydrate in potatoes, pasta, and rice, is definitely a polysaccharide with multiple units of glucose.

Dietary fiber is a special kind of carb. The word *dietary* is stuck in front of *fiber* to make sure that you understand that this fiber, from food, is different from the natural and synthetic fibers such as silk, cotton, wool, or nylon that you find in fabrics.

Like starch, dietary fiber is a polysaccharide. But you don't have the enzymes needed to break dietary fiber into its separate sugar units, so eating dietary fiber doesn't give you any energy (calories) or nutrients. Some diet gurus think this makes fiber a bonus in a weight loss meal plans. More about that later in this chapter.

Comparing High-Carb Meal Plans

High-carb diets come in four sizes: Moderate, strict, popular, and for-athletes-only. The following sections detail the differences among these regimens.

Moderate high-carb plans

The Recommended Dietary Allowances (RDAs) published periodically by the National Academy of Sciences Food and Nutrition Board establishes RDAs for nutrients including calories, protein, fats, carbohydrates, vitamins, and minerals. In 1989, the 10th edition of the Recommended Dietary Allowances suggested reducing the amount of fat in your daily diet to less than 30 percent of your daily calories, with a subsequent increase in the amount of calories from complex carbohydrates.

These sensible suggestions form the basis for the USDA/HHS Food Guide Pyramid, as well as the USDA/HHS Dietary Guidelines 2000, which includes three specific recommendations on carbs and dietary fat:

  ✔ Choose a variety of grains daily, especially whole grains.

  ✔ Choose a variety of fruit and vegetables daily.

  ✔ Choose a diet that is low in saturated fat and cholesterol and moderate in total fat.

The American Heart Association Step I and Step II diets, promoted in conjunction with the National Cholesterol Education Program, echo this nutritional wisdom, as does the American Diabetes Association's exchange plan, which has its very own Food Guide Pyramid, similar to the USDA/HHS Food Guide Pyramid.

Figure 6-1 shows how high-carb food can form the basis of a healthful diet. Table 6-1 shows the recommended servings of different foods from the USDA/HHS Food Guide Pyramid. The ranges shown represent the different number of servings allowed for people consuming a different number of calories per day. The number at the lower end is for people consuming 1,500 calories per day; the higher end, for those consuming as many as 2,800 calories per day.

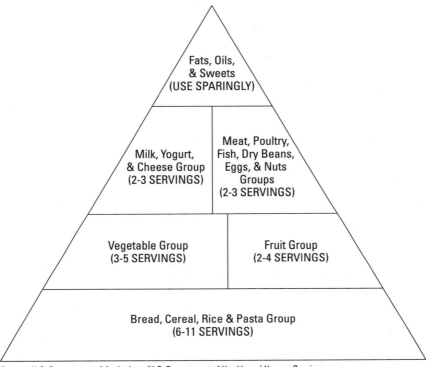

Figure 6-1:
The Food
Guide
Pyramid.

Source: U.S. Department of Agriculture/U.S. Department of Health and Human Services

Table 6-1	Counting Servings: Daily Choices Based on the Food Guide Pyramid 2000
Food Group	**Number of Servings**
Bread group	6 – 11
Fruit group	2 – 4
Vegetable group	3 – 5
Milk group	2 – 3
Meat group	5 ounces – 7 ounces

Source: Dietary Guidelines for Americans 2000, U.S. Departments of Agriculture & Health and Human Services, Home and Garden Bulletin 232 (Washington, D.C.: Government Printing Office, 2000).

Strictly speaking, neither the Food Guide Pyramid, the American Heart Association Step I and Step II Diets, nor the American Diabetes Association plans are weight loss programs. Their primary goal is to provide a nutritious meal plan that

✔ Provides a variety of food choices

✔ Provides sufficient amounts of all essential nutrients

✔ Reduces the risk of heart disease by controlling fat and cholesterol intake

✔ Reduces the risk of other chronic conditions such as high blood pressure and diabetes

But a funny thing happens on the way to better health. When you go on a high-carb diet that reduces the number of calories you get from fat, you lose weight.

Amazing, ain't it?

Strict high-carb plans

The special characteristics of a moderate carb-based diet are that it derives up to 30 percent of its calories from fat and up to 20 percent of its calories from protein. No such luxury exists for people on strict high-carb plans such as the Pritikin diet or the Ornish diet.

The Pritikin diet

The Pritikin diet, created in 1980 by Nathan Pritikin, is a plant-based regimen that serves up

✔ Frequent small meals

✔ Lots of plant foods

✔ Lots of whole grains

✔ Lots of fresh fruits and vegetables

✔ Very small amounts of unsalted nuts and seeds (for unsaturated fatty acids)

✔ A little seafood, the preferred choice for animal protein because it contains heart healthy omega-3 fatty acids

✔ A little skin-free poultry (limited to 3–4 ounces a day)

The "preferred foods" on the Pritikin diet are high-fiber, high-carb plant stuff such as whole grains, salads, beans, potatoes, corn, peas, and fruit. These "preferred" foods are considered both satisfying and filling. To enable you to switch from more commonly preferred foods — ice cream, chocolate cake, potato chips, burgers, and colas — the Pritikin people maintain a soup-to-nuts organization complete with live-in retreat centers, cookbooks, and Web sites that stress good messages, such as a cup of broccoli is lower in calories and higher in the nutrients you need than a cup of high-fat nuts.

Like the Food Guide Pyramid, the American Heart Association Step I and Step II diets, and the American Diabetes Association diet, the Pritikin diet is not a weight loss plan per se. But if you stick with Pritikin, which gets only 10 to 15 percent of its calories from fat, you will lose weight. Oh boy, will you lose weight! Table 6-2 shows why.

Table 6-2	Sample 1-Day Pritikin Meal Plan
Food Group	*Breakfast*
Grain	Oatmeal, barley, or cold cereal
Fruit	Raisins plus grapefruit or banana
Dairy	Skim milk or soy milk plus nonfat yogurt or cottage cheese
Food Group	*Snack*
Vegetables	Fresh vegetables plus salsa plus vegetable soup
Food Group	*Lunch*
Vegetables	Salads plus steamed vegetables
Grains	Vegetable pizza
Fruit	Fresh
Food Group	*Snack*
Vegetables	Soup or salad
Food Group	*Dinner*
Vegetables	Salads, cooked vegetables
Meat, fish, poultry	One serving
Fruits	Poached or fresh

Source: www.pritikin.com/samplemenus.html.

The Ornish diet

Compared to the Ornish regimen, Pritikin is a dietary orgy. After all, Pritikin allows you to get up to 15 percent of your calories from fat. Ornish draws the line at 10 percent. The Ornish diet, outlined in several books, including *Eat More, Weigh Less,* is serious vegetarian — fruits, vegetables, whole grains, and legumes (peas and beans) — with no animal foods except nonfat milk products and egg whites. Ornish dieters get fat from one full serving of tofu a day, plus omega-3 oil (flaxseed or flaxseed oil). Yes, you can have a little salt, a little sugar, a little alcohol, but no coffee, thank you. And you have to take a multivitamin: up to 20,000 IU beta carotene (mostly from foods); 1,000 to 3,000 mg vitamin C; 100 to 400 IU vitamin E; and 400 to 2,000 mcg folate.

Good news, bad news

The Pritikin and Ornish diets are designed to stop or even reverse the forma-tion of plaque, the gunky fat stuff that can block your arteries and trigger heart attack. Several studies have shown the meal plans work. In one study, for example, patients on the Ornish diet lowered their total cholesterol an average 24 percent and lowered their LDL cholesterol (the "bad" particles that carry cholesterol into arteries) by 37 percent, while plaque already in the arteries seemed to melt away. In other words, staying with the Pritikin and Ornish diets appears to make people less likely to experience "cardiac events." And once again, the weight goes down.

But here's the rub. While Pritikin is a restrictive diet, it allows some animal-based foods, which makes it easier (if not easy) for people to follow. But when Dr. Ornish first introduced his diet, critics complained that it was

- ✔ Too restrictive in its food choices
- ✔ Likely to reduce levels of HDLs (the "good" cholesterol) along with levels of LDLs (the "bad" cholesterol)
- ✔ Linked to higher levels of triglycerides, another kind of fat in the blood
- ✔ Lacking in some essential fatty acids, including the heart protective omega-3 fatty acids found primarily in fish that swim in cold water (the oils keep the fish's liquids liquid so the little fella doesn't turn into a fish-shaped ice cube)

Today, the Ornish diet has been revised to include omega-3s, but the food list is still so restrictive that the American Heart Association considers the diet too difficult for most people to follow. On the other hand, if you're a Bad Heart Baby whose father had a heart attack before age 50 (mother, before age 60), or if you've had very high cholesterol that doesn't respond to the moder-ate AHA diet, you may want to ask your doctor about Pritikin and Ornish along with the regulation exercise and medications.

Popular high-carb weight loss plans

Some high-carb diets seem a tad over the limit on fiber. Susan Powter's regi-men, first described in a book called *Stop the Insanity,* is an example of a diet some experts suggest may give you more fiber than you need at the expense of some other nutrients.

Powter gets good marks for encouraging exercise, but her diet frowns on any food that derives more than 30 percent of its calories from fat. The Real Rule, as promoted by the Dietary Guidelines for Americans 2000 and the American Heart Association, is that no more than 30 percent of your total daily calories — meaning all the calories you consume in one 24-hour period — should come from fat. That means that you can utterly pig out on a food with 40 percent or even 50 percent of its calories from fat, as long as you keep your daily total of calories from fat at the 30 percent mark.

The other drawback to a very high-fiber diet is, well, very high fiber. According to the U.S. Department of Agriculture, the average American woman gets about 12 grams of fiber a day from food; the average American man, about 17 grams. That's well below the current recommendations of 20 to 30 grams a day thought to confer the benefits of fiber without causing fiber-related "unpleasantries."

If you exceed the 20- to 30-gram recommendation, your body may rebel, issuing an unmistakable protest in the form of intestinal gas or diarrhea. In extreme cases, if you load up on dietary fiber but fail to drink sufficient amounts of liquids to swish the fiber you eat through your intestines, you can end up with an intestinal obstruction. Not a pleasant prospect.

The point? If you choose to increase your consumption of dietary fiber, keep it within reasonable boundaries and step up gradually, a little bit more every day. That way, you are less likely to experience intestinal distress. Which foods are good sources of dietary fiber? Table 6-3 shows the amount of all types of dietary fiber — insoluble plus soluble — in a 100-gram (3.5 ounce) serving of specific foods. (Nutritionists like to measure things in terms of 100-gram portions because that lets them compare foods at a glance.)

Table 6-3	Getting Fiber from Food
Food	*Amount of Fiber in 1 Gram (3.5 ounce) Serving*
Bread	
Bagel	2.1
Bran bread	8.5
Pita bread	
White	1.6
White bread	1.9
Whole wheat	7.4

(continued)

Table 6-3 *(continued)*

Food	Amount of Fiber in 1 Gram (3.5 ounce) Serving
Cereals	
Bran cereal	35.3
Bran flakes	18.8
Corn flakes	2.0
Oatmeal	10.6
Wheat flakes	9.0
Grains	
Barley, pearled, (minus its outer covering) raw	15.6
Cornmeal, degermed	5.2
Cornmeal, whole grain	11.0
Oat bran, raw	6.6
Rice, raw	
Rice, brown	3.5
Rice, white	1.0 – 2.8
Rice, wild	5.2
Wheat bran	15.0
Fruits	
Apple, with skin	2.8
Apricots, dried	7.8
Figs, dried	9.3
Kiwi	3.4
Pear, raw	2.6
Prunes, stewed	6.6
Raisins	5.3

Food	Amount of Fiber in 1 Gram (3.5 ounce) Serving
Vegetables	
Beans	
Baked (vegetarian)	7.7
Broccoli, raw	2.8
Brussels sprouts, cooked	2.6
Cabbage, white, raw	2.4
Cauliflower, raw	2.4
Chickpeas (canned)	5.4
Corn, sweet, cooked	3.7
Lima, cooked	7.2
Peas with edible pods, raw	2.6
Potatoes, white, baked, w/skin	5.5
Sweet potato, cooked	3.0
Tomatoes, raw	1.3
Other	
Corn chips, toasted	4.4
Nuts	
Almonds, oil-roasted	11.2
Coconut, raw	9.0
Hazelnuts, oil-roasted	6.4
Peanuts, dry-roasted	8.0
Pistachios	10.8
Tahini	9.3
Tofu	1.2

Source: Provisional Table on the Dietary Fiber Content of Selected Foods (Washington, D.C.: U.S. Department of Agriculture, 1988).

To find the amount of dietary fiber in your own serving, divide the gram total by 3.5 and multiply the result by the number of ounces in your portion. For example, if you're having 1 ounce of cereal, the customary serving of ready-to-eat breakfast cereals, divide the gram total of dietary fiber by 3.5, and then

Fiber FAQs

Does dietary fiber provide energy? No. Dietary fiber is a complex carbohydrate (really several varieties of complex carbohydrates), but it is not a source of energy for human beings. Because human digestive enzymes cannot break the bonds that hold its sugar units together, it adds no calories to your diet and cannot be converted to glucose.

Okay, no energy. So is dietary fiber a source of vitamins and minerals?

Sorry, no, again. Ruminants (animals such as cows that "chew the cud") do have digestive enzymes that allow them to get at the nutrients in the insoluble fibers cellulose, hemicellulose, pectins, and gums. But even these animals cannot drag nutrients out of lignin, an insoluble fiber in plant stems and leaves and the predominant fiber in wood. In fact, the U.S. Department of Agriculture specifically prohibits the use of wood or sawdust in animal feed.

Does a high-fiber diet reduce the risk of colon cancer?

For more than 30 years, nutrition studies and experts said yes. Then, whammo! In January 2001, the respected Nurses Health Study at Harvard, Brigham, and Women's Hospital, and Dana Farber Cancer Institute in Boston released new data showing no relationship — zip, zero, zilch — between dietary fiber and the risk of colon cancer. Among the 88,757 women in the 16-year study, the incidence of colon cancer was the same whether the women ate lots of fiber or practically none. In fact, some women who ate lots of fruit and veggies were actually at higher risk.

Where's the fiber in foods? There is fiber in all plant foods — fruits, vegetables, and grains. There is absolutely no fiber in foods from animals: Meat, fish, poultry, milk, milk products, and eggs.

What are the two kinds of fiber? Foods have two kinds of dietary fiber, soluble fiber and insoluble fiber, classified by whether they dissolve in water. Soluble dietary fiber — pectins, beta-glucans, gums — dissolves. Insoluble dietary fiber — cellulose, hemicellulose, lignin — does not.

Which fiber is in what food? Most foods with fiber have both soluble fiber and insoluble fiber, although balance may tilt one way one or the other. For example, the predominant fiber in an apple is pectin (a soluble fiber), but there is also some cellulose, hemicellulose, and lignin in the apple peel.

To get the soluble dietary fiber you need, look for:

- Pectin in fruits

- Beta-glucans in oats and barley

- Gums in beans, cereals, and seeds

To get the insoluble dietary fiber you need, look for:

- Cellulose in leaves (cabbage), roots (carrots, beets), bran, whole wheat, and beans

- Hemicellulose in seed coverings (bran, whole grains)

- Lignin in stems, leaves, and peel

Does a fiber-rich diet lower cholesterol? Yes. Soluble fiber, such as pectin (in apples) and beta-glucans (in oats and barley), dissolves to form a gel in your stomach that appears to carry cholesterol out of your body and lower the amount left circulating in your blood, which may be why a diet rich in soluble dietary fiber such as the fiber in oat bran appears to offer some protection against heart disease.

Does eating fiber prevent constipation? Yes. The *New England Journal of Medicine* calls dietary fiber a "colonic broom," which is a neat way of saying, "Eat fiber, stay regular!" Insoluble dietary fiber, found in whole grains, fruit and veggie skin, and the teensy little hard thingees in pears, does not dissolves in water, and it is a natural laxative that stimulates your intestinal walls to contract and relax. These natural contractions, called *peristalsis,* move solid materials through your digestive tract. In addition, insoluble fiber absorbs water and bulks up stool. So it is important to increase fluid (primarily water) intake as you increase your dietary fiber intake.

How about other intestinal nasties? Good news here, too. By moving food quickly through your intestines, insoluble dietary fiber may help prevent or relieve digestive disorders such as constipation or diverticulosis (infection caused by food getting stuck in small pouches in the wall of your colon). Insoluble fiber also bulks up stool and makes it softer, reducing your risk of developing hemorrhoids and lessening the discomfort if you already have them.

Why is dietary fiber useful on a weight loss diet? Both soluble dietary fiber and insoluble dietary fiber come in bulky, low-cal foods that can make you feel full, even satisfied, on very few calories.

multiply by 1. If your slice of bread weighs 0.5 ounces, divide the gram total by 3.5, and then multiply the result by 0.5.

Or — let's be real about this — you can look at the nutrition label on the side of the package that gives the nutrients per portion.

Raw foods almost always have more fiber than cooked foods because cooking generally adds water, which adds weight and spreads out the fiber content. For example, a 3.5-ounce portion of dried prunes has more prunes (and thus more fiber) than a 3.5-ounce portion of stewed prunes, which gives you water as well as prunes.

By the way, the amounts on this chart are averages. Individual brand-name products (bread, some cereals, cooked fruits and vegetables) may have more (or less) fiber per serving.

The high-carb diet for athletes

The relatively small amount of stored glucose in your blood and cells provides the energy you need for daily cellular transactions. The 400 grams of glycogen stored in your liver and muscles provides enough energy for ordinary bursts of activity.

But what happens if you have to work harder or longer than that? What if you are a long-distance athlete? Simple: If you stick to your normal high-carb diet, you will run out of glucose before your "work" (or competition) is done. The best example is the well-known "wall" that marathoners hit at 20 miles, 6 miles short of the finish line.

If you are stuck without food for a long period of time, say a month, your body will begin to pull energy first out of your stored fat. When that energy is used up, the body begins to digest its own muscle tissue. But converting fat to energy or digesting muscles require lots of oxygen, an element that is likely to be in short supply when you're involved in athletic competition. So athletes must find another way to leap the wall. They have. They call it *carb loading*.

Carb loading is not a diet for every day. Nor will it help people competing in events lasting less than an hour. It's strictly for events lasting longer than 90 minutes, a meal plan designed to increase temporarily the stores of glycogen in your muscles. For the best results, says the University of Maine's Alfred A. Bushway, Ph.D., you start a week in advance. Exercise to exhaustion to pull as much glycogen as possible out of your muscles. Then, for three days, you eat foods high in fat and protein and low in carbohydrates, to keep your glycogen level from rising again.

Three days before the Big Day, switch to carbs to build and conserve glycogen stores with a diet comprising about 70 percent carbohydrate with 6 to 10 grams of carbohydrate for every kilogram (2.2 pounds) of body weight. And not just any carbohydrates, mind you. You want to cram down the starchy carbs (pasta, potatoes), not the sugary ones (fruit, candy).

By the way, you'll notice that the word "sugar" — as in table sugar or candy bar — has not been mentioned here. Why? Because if you eat plain sugar during a race, it will give you a smart short burst of energy as your body quickly converts the sugar to glucose and speeds it to your muscles. But then, whoops! The hydrophilic (*hydro* = water; *philic* = loving) sugar will pull liquids from your body tissues into your stomach and intestines, triggering dehydration and (worse yet) making you feel queasy. This fact explains why sweetened athletic drinks, which provide fluids plus energy, are more reliable than candy bars.

Building Your Own Carb-Based Weight Loss Plan

Time to cut the mustard, which, I might point out, is a plant and, therefore, a high-carb food. Now that you've read about the different kinds of high-carb diets (if you read the preceding section), it's time to put together your very own high-carb weight loss plan.

You will find this a cinch because, like the lovable but pompous hero of Moliére's *Bourgeois Gentilhomme,* who discovered he had been speaking prose all his life without knowing it, you probably always used a high-carb diet without even realizing it whenever you tried to lose weight in the past.

The weekly carb-based diet chart

Your CD-ROM has three one-week diet charts based on the USDA Food Guide Pyramid. Table 6-4 is for a 1,200 calories-a-day plan. Table 6-5 is for a 1,500 calories-a-day plan. Table 6-6 is for a 1,800 calories-a-day plan. Print the one that interests you and stick it on your refrigerator.

Table 6-4	1,200 Calories/Day Plan						
Food Group (Servings)	*Mon.*	*Tues.*	*Wed.*	*Thurs.*	*Fri.*	*Sat.*	*Sun.*
Bread group (5)							
Fruit group (2)							
Vegetable group (3)							
Milk group (2)							
Meat group (5 ounces)							

Table 6-5	1,500 Calories/Day Plan						
Food Group (Servings)	*Mon.*	*Tues.*	*Wed.*	*Thurs.*	*Fri.*	*Sat.*	*Sun.*
Bread group (6)							
Fruit group (3)							
Vegetable group (3)							
Milk group (2)							
Meat group (6 ounces)							

Table 6-6	1,800 Calories/Day Plan						
Food Group (Servings)	*Mon.*	*Tues.*	*Wed.*	*Thurs.*	*Fri.*	*Sat.*	*Sun.*
Bread group (8)							

(continued)

Table 6-6 *(continued)*

Food Group (Servings)	Mon.	Tues.	Wed.	Thurs.	Fri.	Sat.	Sun.
Fruit group (4)							
Vegetable group (4)							
Milk group (2 – 3)							
Meat group (7 ounces)							

The servings chart

Print two copies of Table 6-7, which is on the CD that accompanies this book. Tape one copy to your fridge and use it when you are preparing meals at home. Fold the second copy small enough to fit it into your wallet and use it when you're eating out. No, no, no — don't pull it out at the table. You want your friends to notice that you're getting slimmer, but reading your list at the table is kind of gross, doncha think? Sneak a peek on the way to the restaurant, or check it out when you're powdering your nose, or simply memorize the whole darned thing, so you're cool when they pass the menus around.

Table 6-7	What's a Serving Size?
Food Group	*Serving Size*
Grains	
	1 slice of bread
	1-ounce ready-to-eat cereal
	½ cup cooked cereal
	½ cup cooked rice or pasta
	5 to 6 small crackers
Vegetables	
	1 cup raw leafy vegetables
	½ cup chopped raw vegetables
	½ cup cooked chopped vegetable
	¾ cup vegetable juice
Fruits	
	Medium piece of fresh fruit

Food Group	Serving Size
	½ cup cooked or canned fruit
	¾ cup fruit juice
Milk products	
	1 cup skim/lowfat milk
	1 cup skim/lowfat yogurt
	1½ ounces lowfat cheese
Meat, fish, poultry, dry beans, eggs, nuts, seeds	
	2 to 3 ounces cooked lean meat
	2 to 3 ounces cooked lean skinless poultry
	2 to 3 ounces cooked fish
	½ cup cooked dry beans
	1 egg*
	2 tablespoons peanut butter
	⅓ cup nuts or seeds
Fats, oils, sweets	
	No specific amount; very little

* No more than 4 egg yolks a week.
Source: Dietary Guidelines for Americans 2000, U.S. Departments of Agriculture and Health and Human Services, Home and Garden Bulletin 232 (Washington, D.C.: Government Printing Office, 2000).

For those who know what a serving is but don't know what it looks like, it's time to play with your food.

1. **Assemble some test food: Boil ½ cup of rice in one cup of water. Open a can of fruit cocktail or canned veggies (peas are good). Broil a boneless chicken breast.**

2. **Find a ½ cup measuring cup and a deck of regular playing cards.**

3. **When the food's ready, measure it.**

   Scoop ½ cup cooked rice into a bowl or mush it into a golf ball size globe. That's one serving of rice (or cooked cereal or mashed potatoes). Spoon ½ cup fruit or veggies into a second bowl. That's one serving, too. Trim the chicken to the size of the deck of cards. That's one serving of meat, fish, or poultry.

Memorize the sizes. It's easy to dish up reasonable portions at home. But what happens when you eat out? Disaster! Disaster! For example, one serving of pasta is ½ cup, but restaurants typically dish up 4 to 6 cups, a whopping 4 to 12 servings. To survive, use your own "attached" measuring tools, your fist (one cup) and the palm of your hand (the deck of cards). Is this system perfect? Nope. Will it do in a pinch? Absolutely. And you can always take home the remainder for the next couple of days.

Putting it together

Depending on which calorie level you have chosen, you will want to figure out how many servings of each kind of food you need (and want) each day. When you consume a serving, mark the chart with an X or a check mark or gold stars, if you prefer. When the number of Xs or check marks or stars equals the numbers of recommended daily servings, you're done for the day.

The virtue of this plan is that once you decide how many calories you want for the entire day, you're done with the math. All you have to count is servings.

Building a weight loss plan based on high-carb foods

✔ Enables you to meet your nutritional requirements

✔ Makes it possible to lose (or control) weight without counting calories

✔ Gives you plenty of tasty food choices

As a final check, review Table 6-8 and Table 6-9.

Table 6-8	Calorie Sources for Carb-Based Weight Loss Plans		
	Daily % of Calories		
Source	**Carbohydrates**	**Protein**	**Fat (Total)**
Dietary Guidelines for Americans	60%	*	<30%
The American Diabetes Association	50 – 60%	10 – 20%	<30%
The American Heart Association Step I and Step II**	50%+	*	<30%
Pritikin diet	65 – 80 %	10 – 20%	10 – 15%
Ornish diet	70 – 75%	15 – 20%	<10%

Source	Daily % of Calories		
	Carbohydrates	Protein	Fat (Total)
Popular high-carb weight loss plans	***	***	***
Your personal high-carb weight loss diet			

* Whatever is left after carbs and fat calories are counted.
** The AHA Step I diet holds cholesterol to less than 300 mg a day; the Step II diet to less than 200 mg.
*** Depends on the specific diet.
Sources: Dietary Guidelines for Americans 2000; American Diabetes Association
`www.americanheart.org;` *The American Heart Association Cookbook, 5th ed.;*
`www.pritikinfl.com;www.healthyheart.org/Educational/Conferences/`
`990609/Abdavis.htm.`

Table 6-9   Food Choices for Carb-Based Weight Loss Plans

Source	Fruit, Veggies, Legumes	Grains	Dairy	Meat, Lean	Fish	Poultry (No Skin)	Other (On Occasion)
Dietary Guidelines for Americans	Yes	Yes	*	Yes	Yes	Yes	Sweets, unsaturated fats, dressings, coffee/tea, alcohol
The American Diabetes Association	Yes	Yes	Yes	Yes	Yes	Yes	Limited sweets, coffee/tea,
The American Heart Association Step I & Step II	Yes	Yes	*	Yes	Yes	Yes	Sweets, unsaturated fats, dressings, coffee/tea, alcohol
Pritikin diet	Yes	Yes	**	***	Yes	Yes	Soy milk, alcohol
Ornish diet	****	Yes	*****	No	No	No	Full-fat tofu, flaxseed

(continued)

Table 6-9 (continued)

Source	Fruit, Veggies, Legumes	Grains	Dairy	Meat, Lean	Fish	Poultry (No Skin)	Other (On Occasion)
Popular high-carb weight loss plans	Yes	Yes	******	******	******	******	Variable
High-carb for athletes	Yes	Yes	Yes	Yes	Yes	Yes	
Your personal high-carb weight loss plan							

* Lowfat or fat-free dairy products, no more than 4 egg yolks a week
** Lowfat or fat-free only, egg whites
*** Very lean only
**** Only whole fruit/vegetables, no juice
***** Nonfat only; egg whites only
****** Depends on specific diet
Sources: Dietary Guidelines for Americans 2000; The American Diabetes Association; www.americanheart.org; The American Heart Association Cookbook, 5th ed.; www.pritikinfl.com;www.healthyheart.org/Educational/Conferences/990609/Abdavis.htm.

Flash! Hold the presses! Just as these very pages were being edited to go off to the printer to be made the book you are holding in your hands, the U.S. Department of Agriculture releases a statement naming carb-based diets as your very best bet for long-term weight control. Click onto your CD-ROM for a copy of the statement. Then click onto the Web and type in www.nutrition.gov for the new USDA-sponsored site with oodles of information and charts and "backgrounders" (special press releases for us newsies) on what's Good to Eat. When *For Dummies* say they bring you the best, fastest, boy, do they mean it!

Chapter 7

Praising Protein

· ·

In This Chapter

▶ Defining proteins

▶ Explaining how your body uses proteins

▶ Rating the different kinds of proteins

▶ Evaluating high-protein weight loss plans

· ·

*H*igh-protein weight loss plans — more accurately described as low-carbohydrate, high-protein diets — are popular because they produce quick weight loss. Unfortunately, most of the weight that melts away is *water weight,* fluid lost when your body is forced to process proteins rather than carbohydrates for energy. That means your fast slimming is, well, temporary.

In addition, nutrition experts often turn thumbs down on high-protein plans because the meals emphasize animal foods high in saturated fats and cholesterol known to clog arteries and raise your risk of heart disease. As you read this, USDA is beginning studies designed to find out whether low-carb, high-protein meal plans are safe and effective weight loss tools. The final results won't be in for a while, but a statement issued by USDA in January 2000 strongly leans toward carb-based diets as best balanced and best for your health. Click onto your CD-ROM for a copy of the executive summary of the USDA report.

After reading that report, should you still try a low-carb, high-protein plan anyway? To paraphrase the slogan of one cable TV network: "I report. You — and your doctor — decide."

Protein Power

It's baaaaaaack! Like those nasty poltergeists that chased little Carol Ann around the TV in the movie, the low-carb, high-protein weight loss plan sticks its head up every couple of years, hitting the top of the bestseller lists and picking up new friends and foes along the way.

What precisely is a low-carb, high-protein weight loss plan? Easy: The exact opposite of the carb-based meal plans that I describe in Chapter 6. For example:

- The carb-based plan emphasizes plant foods (fruits, vegetables, grains) with small amounts of foods from animals (meat, fish, poultry, eggs, and dairy). The high-protein plan emphasizes foods from animals and small amounts of foods from plants.

- The carb-based plan is lowfat. The high-protein weight loss plan is high-fat.

- The carb-based weight loss plan relies on measured servings. The high-protein weight loss plan simply says to dig in — so long as you dig into protein foods.

- The carb-based plan is endorsed by the U.S. Departments of Agriculture and Health and Human Services, the National Institute of Health, the American Dietetic Association, the American Heart Association, the American Diabetes Association, the American Society of Bariatric Physicians, and so on. The high-protein plan isn't.

Right now, the current list of popular low-carb, high-protein weight loss plans include

- Dr. Atkins' New Diet Revolution

- The Carbohydrate Addict's Diet

- Protein Power

- Sugar Busters!

The news about these weight loss plans comes in three varieties: Good, Bad, and Interesting. First, the Good News. Low-carb, high-protein weight loss plans:

- Fill your RDA for protein, an essential nutrient.

- Serve up foods with fat, which means you feel full faster and may actually consume fewer calories than usual.

- Make meal-planning a cinch: You just pile on the proteins and leave off the carbs.

- Help people who have failed at high-carb dieting to lose several pounds in just a few days, a phenomenon explained later in the section titled "How Do Low-Carb, High-Protein Weight Loss Plans Work?"

- Often fill in the blanks in your meal plan with lowfat (low starch) veggies.

The Bad News about low-carb, high-protein weight loss plans is that they

✔ Emphasize foods from animals, which means you get more total fat, more saturated fat, and more cholesterol each day, a combination that may raise your risk of cardiovascular disease (high blood pressure, heart attack, or stroke), a fact that turns many nutrition experts — and dieters — off these plans.

✔ Prohibit or severely restrict your consumption of whole categories of foods, such as grains, cereals, vegetables, and fruit. The diets may not provide sufficient amounts of dietary fiber, vitamins, minerals, and the newly identified heart-protective, anti-cancer phytochemicals (*phyto* = plant) found only in plant foods.

✔ Take off weight fast, but may not keep it off.

The Interesting News about low-carb, high-protein weight loss plans is that after several decades of claim ("You lose weight!") and counterclaim ("It's not safe!"), the nutrition gurus at the U.S. Department of Agriculture have decided to subject these weight loss plans to serious scientific evaluation. In January 2001, USDA conducted trials at several medical centers across the United States to determine whether sticking to a low-carb, high-protein weight loss plan is a safe and effective way to lose weight. The study will track volunteers for one, two, and three years to see whether they accomplish their weight loss goals. Results will start rolling in by 2002; the trials end in 2004. Even longer term studies will be needed to see the effect on heart disease and cancer, cataracts, age-related macular degeneration, and so on.

In the meantime, before you can decide whether you should put your body on a low-carb, high-protein weight loss plan, you should know what proteins are and how they work in your body. Yes, impatient readers may be excused to skip this section, but I would be shirking my responsibility if I did not point out the value of knowing how proteins work before you try a protein-based weight loss plan.

What Are Proteins, and How Do You Use Them?

Principle Numero Uno in the Protein Primer is that protein is an essential nutrient, just like fats and carbohydrates. In fact, the name protein comes from the Greek word for "of first quality," a real clue to how important protein is to your body.

The protein molecule is a long chain of units called *amino acids,* also known as "the building blocks of protein." Amino acids are made of carbon, hydrogen, oxygen, and nitrogen, which is what *amino* means, an element essential in making proteins. As a result, when people talk about how much protein you need, what they really mean is how much nitrogen you need to make proteins while doing all the other work that proteins normally do, such as

✔ Make new cells.

✔ Maintain body tissues.

✔ Synthesize *enzymes,* specialized proteins that perform specific jobs, such as digesting food and assembling or dividing molecules to make new cells and chemical substances.

✔ Synthesize *hormones,* more specialized proteins that also perform specific tasks, such as keeping your reproductive functions functioning.

✔ Synthesize *neurotransmitters,* a third group of specialized proteins — the chemicals that enable your nerve cells to transmit messages from your brain to your body and vice versa ("move that muscle," "taste that food," "hear that music," "see that movie").

✔ Creating *DNA (deoxyribonucleic acid),* the material in the nucleus of every cell in your body that carries your genes and chromosomes, the genetic structures that make you who you are.

A question of quality

All proteins are not created equal. Some are *high quality.* Some are not. Some are *complete.* Some are not. What sets one group of proteins apart from the other is whether they provide sufficient amounts of all the essential amino acids.

To manufacture specialized proteins such as enzymes, hormones, neurotransmitters, and so on, you need 22 different amino acids. Nine of these amino acids are ranked *essential* because you cannot synthesize them in your own body. You have to get them from food. The other 13 are labeled *nonessential,* not because you don't need them, but because if you don't get them from food, you can make them yourself from fats, carbs, and other amino acids.

Essential amino acids:

✔ Histadine

✔ Isoleucine

✔ Leucine

✔ Lysine

✔ Methionine

- Phenylalanine
- Threonine
- Tryptophan
- Valine

Nonessential amino acids:

- Alanine
- Arginine
- Aspartic acid
- Citrulline
- Cystine
- Glutamic acid
- Glycine
- Hydroxyglutamic acid
- Hydroxyproline
- Norleucine
- Proline
- Serine
- Tyrosine

Where to find high-quality protein

An animal's body is similar to yours, so the proteins you get from meat, fish, poultry, eggs, and dairy foods are also similar to yours and contain all the essential amino acids. This explains why proteins from animal foods are called *high-quality proteins* or *complete proteins*. You absorb them easily and use them efficiently to make new proteins every day.

On the other hand, your physiology has very little in common with a petunia's or a potato's, so the proteins in plant foods are not like yours. They often have less than optimal amounts of one amino acid or another, which is why proteins from plant foods are labeled *incomplete*. These proteins are also called *limiting*, because they can be used to build only as much tissue as the smallest amount of the "limiting" amino acid they contain. In short, proteins from plant foods may "limit" protein production in your body.

Unfortunately, although proteins from animal foods have the right combination of amino acids, they are also high in fat, with saturated fat and cholesterol that clog your arteries and raise your risk of heart disease. Plant foods are lowfat, low in saturated fat, and have no cholesterol, but their proteins are less than perfect.

What a dilemma! The foods with the best proteins may be bad for your heart. What to do? Improve the proteins in plants, of course.

Making proteins better

You can improve the quality of incomplete (limiting) proteins from plant foods by judiciously combining foods. The trick is to eat a food that is deficient in one amino acid with a food that has plenty of the missing compound. This process — putting foods together to create complete proteins — is called *complementarity.* Yes, that's spelled right. My editors always ask, "Don't you mean complementary?" No, I say, I mean *complementarity,* which is the process of matching complementary foods.

Let me show you how it works:

- Rice has a plentiful supply of the essential amino acid methionine, but limiting amounts of the essential amino acid lysine. Beans have lots of lysine, but limiting amounts of methionine. Eating rice with beans creates a dish with complete proteins. And a great flavor.

- Pasta has limiting amounts of the essential acids lysine and isoleucine; milk products such as cheese have abundant amounts of both. Shaking parmesan onto pasta creates a higher quality protein dish. And more great flavor.

 In both examples, serving foods together makes their proteins more valuable. Other examples of complementary protein dishes are peanut butter with bread, and milk with cereal. As you can determine, many complementary combinations are staples of the normal diet in places throughout the world where animal proteins are scarce or very expensive. They are also the backbone of a vegetarian diet. P.S. These foods don't have to be eaten at the same moment.

Eat these foods together to make complete protein dishes:

- Whole grains + legumes (beans and peas)
- Whole grains + dairy products
- Legumes (beans and peas) + nuts and/or seeds
- Legumes (beans and peas) + dairy products
- Nuts and seeds + dairy products

Your protein requirements

As Chapter 6 explains, your body stores carbohydrates as glucose (blood sugar) or glycogen (animal starch). As Chapter 8 explains, you store fat as, well, fat. You can go a couple of days without carbs or fat and still have a supply to draw from.

Proteins are a different story. Every day, your body uses up more protein than you get from the food you eat, so you need a continuous supply to keep going.

If your weight loss plan does not provide enough protein, you will eventually begin to break down and digest the proteins in your body cells and tissues, including those in your muscles. The sad result of this kind of desperate activity is described in Chapter 10, which explains that, while people who starve to death have serious problems with lack of water and minerals, they eventually die when protein deprivation finally stops the heart (a muscle) from beating.

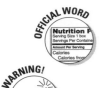

To satisfy daily protein requirements, an average healthy adult (male or female) needs about 0.8 grams of protein a day for every kilogram (kg) of body weight. One kilogram equals 2.2 pounds, so you can also express this requirement as slightly less than 0.4 grams of protein per pound of body weight ($0.8/2.2 = 0.36 = 0.4$).

Fatally incomplete

In 1976, a book called *The Last Chance Diet* turned out to be exactly that for several dozen readers. The diet was based on a 400-calorie per day protein formula called Prolinn, plus vitamin and mineral supplements. The promise was that, if you stuck to the Prolinn diet, you would lose more than 20 pounds in a month. It seemed too good to be true, but people consuming only 12,000 calories a month (400 calories × 30 days) versus the 45,000 calories (1,500 × 30 days) provided by a standard low-cal weight loss meal plan, did lose pounds as well as water weight.

Unfortunately, the protein in Prolinn was very low quality, derived from beef hides and animal hooves, horns, and underbellies, a combination you could probably match by sucking your thumb, biting your nails, and chewing your hair. Prolinn did not provide all the essential amino acids, and within two years, at least 50 people who had stayed on the weight loss plan for up to three months developed muscle weakness and eventually irregular heartbeat, leading to death.

To protect consumers, the Food and Drug Administration ruled in 1980 that all protein supplements used for weight loss must contain vitamins and minerals and carry a warning label, which appears today on all modern protein formulas. For more about modern weight loss meal replacement products, check out Chapter 13. And remember, too good to be true usually means just that.

The following examples show how to calculate your daily protein requirement:

> ✔ **Example #1:** How much protein does a 130-pound person need each day?
>
> 130 pounds (59 kg) × 0.4 grams of protein per pound body weight = 52 grams of protein
>
> A 130-pound person needs about 52 grams of protein a day.
>
> ✔ **Example #2:** How much protein does a 160-pound person need each day?
>
> 160 pounds (73 kg) × 0.4 grams of protein per pound body weight = 64 grams of protein
>
> A 160-pound person needs about 64 grams of protein a day.

Table 7-1 lists the current Recommended Dietary Allowances (RDAs) for protein for 18 different groups of people. Run your finger down the list and you will see that infants, children, and adolescents need more protein per kg/lb of body weight than adults do. That's because young people are making lots of new tissue. Adolescent boys need more protein per kg/lb than adolescent girls because boys make more muscle tissue. Women who are pregnant need more protein to build fetal tissue; women who are nursing need more protein to provide milk. By the way, anyone — young, old, male, female — who has been injured and must build new tissue also needs more protein; in cases of serious injury, this protein is often provided through IV (intravenous) fluids. But most people's diets contain more than enough protein.

Table 7-1	How Much Protein Do You Need Each Day?		
Gender	**Age (Years)**	**Protein (Grams per kg Body Weight)**	**RDA (Grams per Day)**
Boys and girls	0.0–0.5	2.2	13
	0.1–1.0	1.6	14
	1–3	1.2	16
	4–6	1.1	24
	7–10	1.0	28
Males	11–14	1.0	45
	15–18	1.0	59
	19–24	0.9	70
	25–50	0.8	63
	51+	0.8	63

Gender	Age (Years)	Protein (Grams per kg Body Weight)	RDA (Grams per Day)
Females	11–14	1.0	46
	15–18	0.8	44
	19–24	0.8	46
	25–50	0.8	50
	51+	0.8	50
Pregnant			+10
Nursing			+15

Source: *Adapted with permission from* Recommended Dietary Allowances *(Washington, D.C.: National Academy Press, 1989).*

Wait! Before you move on to the next section, did you notice a category of human beings missing from Table 7-1? If you jog, walk, or work out each day and take your exercise really seriously, you're likely to wonder where the RDA for athletes is. After all, don't really active people need extra protein to build all those muscles?

The definite answer is, sort of. Some research says, forget the extra protein. Other studies hint that athletes may benefit from an extra 0.5 grams of protein per kilogram of body weight per day — 31 grams of extra protein for a 135-pound gal and 40 grams of extra protein for a 175-pound guy. But that's no big deal. Two cups of yogurt, a slice or two of whole-wheat bread, and there you go. The thing to keep in mind is that, while protein is a major component of muscle tissue, exercise alone can increase muscle mass. An athlete's bulging biceps are a product of his workout regimen, not his diet.

Getting the protein you need

Fulfilling your protein RDA is a snap. The easy way to meet the average adult requirement of 50 to 60 grams is to wolf down two to three 3-ounce servings of lean meat, fish, or poultry (21 grams each). The more interesting way is to combine servings of different kinds of high-protein foods, many of them with less fat than meat, fish, or poultry.

For example, a vegetarian can get 50 grams of protein from any combination of:

- ✔ 2 eggs (12–16 grams protein)
- ✔ 2 slices of fat-free cheese (10 grams protein)
- ✔ 4 slices of bread (3 grams protein, each)
- ✔ 1 cup yogurt (10 grams protein)

Nonvegetarians can use this list, too, of course, combining these foods with a serving or two of meat, fish, or poultry.

How Do Low-Carb, High-Protein Weight Loss Plans Work?

People on low-carb, high-protein weight loss plans do lose weight, sometimes very fast, at least at the beginning. But they may also experience side effects related directly to the plan's lack of carbohydrates or its abundance of proteins. This section explains how these weight loss plans work and lays out some of the potential problems.

Controlling calories

First things first. People who write low-carb, high-protein diet books may say that people lose weight on *their* meal plans because of complicated carbohydrate chemistry. Yes, reducing your carb consumption has specific chemical and physical effects (which I explain later in this chapter). But nutrition experts who evaluate the low-carb, high-protein weight loss plans have a simple explanation for your weight loss. Eating foods high in fat makes you feel full longer. So you eat less. So you're getting fewer calories. So you lose weight. Ho-hum.

Losing weight versus losing water

When you talk about losing weight, what you mean is losing body fat. But the initial weight loss that you experience on low-carb, high-protein diets is a result of water loss, not fat loss.

Your body runs on the energy supplied by glucose (sugar). The easiest way to get the glucose you need is to metabolize carbohydrates (see Chapter 6). When you cut back on carbs, your body turns to fat and proteins for energy. But pulling energy out of fats and protein is hard work that requires lots of water produced when your body tried to pull energy out of fat and protein. That's why a low-carb, high-protein weight loss plan makes you urinate more often and more copiously than usual.

This produces a fast, satisfying weight loss, perhaps as much as 7 pounds in four days. But how much of the weight loss is real fat and how much is water? Obviously, the amount varies from person to person, but on average, if you do drop 7 pounds in four days on a low-carb, high-protein weight loss plan, you can reasonably assume that

✔ One or 2 pounds are fat.

✔ Five or 6 pounds are water, muscle tissue, and other nutrients, such as minerals.

The fat pounds may stay off, but the water loss is strictly temporary. After you start eating carbs again, your body will happily revert to pulling energy from the carbs and conserving water. You seem to gain back weight, but you're simply re-establishing your normal fluid balance, a definitely beneficial development. You need water to

✔ Digest food, dissolve nutrients so they can pass through the intestinal cell walls into your bloodstream, move food along through your intestinal tract, and carry off waste products. (Did your low-carb, high-protein weight loss plan make you constipated?)

✔ Provide a medium in which biochemical reactions occur.

✔ Transmit electrical messages between cells.

✔ Regulate body temperature.

✔ Lubricate your moving parts.

Water weight

On average, when you step on the scale, approximately:

✔ Sixty percent of your weight is water.

✔ Thirty percent of your weight is fat if you're a woman, slightly less if you're a man.

✔ Ten percent of your weight is a combination of protein, carbohydrates, the major minerals in your bones (calcium, phosphorus), smaller amounts of other minerals (potassium, sulfur, sodium, chloride, magnesium), and infinitesimal amounts of trace elements (iron, zinc, selenium, manganese, copper, iodine) and vitamins.

Sugar shock: A dubious proposition

When you eat carbohydrates, your pancreas secretes *insulin,* a hormone you need to digest starches and sugars. This release of insulin is sometimes called "an insulin spike" (which means the same thing as "secretes insulin" but sounds a whole lot more sinister).

Eating simple carbohydrates, such as *sucrose* (table sugar), provokes higher insulin secretion than eating complex carbohydrates, such as starch. If you have a metabolic disorder, such as diabetes, which prevents you from secreting adequate amounts of insulin, you must monitor your diet to be sure that you don't take in more carbs than you can metabolize at one time because unmetabolized sugars circulating through your blood can make you dizzy and maybe even trip you into a diabetic coma.

Some people who don't have diabetes may also have problems with sweet foods because they are *insulin resistant,* meaning that they do not handle sugars efficiently. For them, eating sugary foods may trigger a rise in *trigylcerides* (fats in the blood), thus increasing the risk of heart disease.

But most healthy people don't have any problems metabolizing even very large amounts of sugary foods. Their insulin secretion rises to meet the demand and then quickly settles back to normal.

Nonetheless, the mantra of the current low-carb, high-protein enthusiast is, "Eating carbs raises your blood-sugar level, which provokes your body to release lots of insulin, which makes you hungry, which makes you eat, which makes you fat."

This sentence has three true statements but they are connected by an untrue assumption that invalidates the cause-and-effect relationship among them:

1. Yes, eating carbs increases the amount of sugar in your blood.

2. Yes, eating carbs causes your body to secrete insulin.

3. No, there is no evidence to show that secreting insulin makes you hungrier.

4. Yes, if you eat more, you'll gain weight, but . . . see sentence 3.

Does this stop low-carb, high-protein aficionados from pushing right ahead with the sugar/insulin/fat theory? Nah.

In fact, to make it easy for folks to identify the bad carb foods, most low-carb, high-protein boosters rely on the Glycemic Index (*gly* = sweet; *emia* = in the blood), a dietary tool developed at the University of Toronto in 1981 as a nutritional aid for people with diabetes. The Index rates foods by how quickly they affect blood-sugar levels. The reference point is either glucose or white bread (depending on which lab does the testing), which are arbitrarily rated 100.

The following table gives you an idea of how several foods rate on this scale. To date, only about 300 foods have been tested, so the list is clearly incomplete. But the rule is, the higher the score, the faster you metabolize the food to glucose (blood sugar).

A Representative Sample of Food Ratings on the Glycemic Index

Glycemic Score	Food
100	Glucose
98–95	Parsnips, potatoes, white bread

Glycemic Score	Food
94–90 (white & brown)	Carrots, pasta (white & wheat), rice
89–70	Cold cereals, dried beans
69–65	Barley, cantaloupe, raisins

Source: Jane Kirby, Dieting For Dummies. *(Foster City, CA:Hungry Minds, Inc.,1997);* members.nbci.com/_XMCM/hexaquad/health3h.htm.

Does the Glycemic Index work as a weight loss system for healthy people? Probably not. Healthy people have no problem with carb-based weight loss plans; people with metabolic disorders should seek their physician's advice in setting up a weight loss plan, not rely on any pop weight loss book. Not even this book.

Messing with your muscles

A low-carb, high-protein weight loss plan may play havoc with your muscles. What? Aren't muscles mostly protein? Yes, they are. But if you don't get enough carbs for energy, your body will begin to pull energy out of fats and proteins, including — in extreme cases — the protein in your own muscle tissue.

A weight loss plan that provides sufficient amounts of carbohydrates keeps your body from digesting muscle tissue, which is why a carb-rich diet is sometimes called *protein sparing*. A medically supervised fast, done in a hospital setting under a doctor's direction, spares protein, too, because it provides sufficient amounts of essential nutrients. Check it out in Chapter 9.

How many carbohydrates do you need to protect your muscles? The USDA/HHS Dietary Guidelines for Americans 2000 recommends that you get 60 percent of your calories from carbs. Only one low-carb, high-protein regimen comes close to this: The Carbohydrate Addict's Diet suggests getting 40 percent of your calories from carbs.

✔ **Example:** How many grams of carbs do you get a day if you follow a 1,500-calorie, carb-based weight loss program as laid out by the Dietary Guidelines for Americans 2000?

1,500 calories × 60 percent = 900 calories

1 gram of carbohydrates = 4 calories

900 calories = 225 grams of carbohydrates

4 calories per gram

> ✔ **Example:** How many grams of carbs do you get a day on a 1,500-calorie, low-carb, high-protein weight loss plan with 40 percent of total calories from carbohydrates?
>
> 1,500 calories × 40 percent = 600 calories
>
> 1 gram of carbohydrates = 4 calories
>
> 600 calories = 150 grams of carbohydrates
>
> 4 calories per gram

Most best-selling high-protein weight loss plans give you even smaller amounts of carbohydrates, sometimes as little as 4 grams a day. Flex your biceps if you hear hissing from the Nutrition Corner.

Keeping an eye on ketone levels

Ketones are compounds produced when you burn fats without sufficient amounts of glucose, a likely situation when your diet is low in carbohydrates. Producing high concentrations of ketones (a condition known as *ketosis*) alters the *pH* (acid/alkaline balance) of your blood and may trip you into a potentially fatal coma.

Plain low-carb, high-protein weight loss plans are unlikely to produce such dramatic effects, but they can churn out enough ketones to:

> ✔ Make your urine smell like acetone (nail polish remover).
>
> ✔ Turn your breath and perspiration really stinky.
>
> ✔ Make you sick to your stomach.
>
> ✔ Increase your loss of sodium and potassium, which raises your risk of irregular heartbeat.
>
> ✔ Increase your production of *uric acid* (a compound produced during protein metabolism), raising your risk of kidney stones.
>
> ✔ Increase your loss of calcium, raising your risk of osteoporosis.

Will you still lose weight? Sure. But at what price?

Sugar FAQs

You may be surprised at how many things "everyone knows" about sugar are not true. For example:

✓ **Sugar is unnatural.** Sucrose, or white sugar, is a sweet compound composed of glucose and fructose (fruit sugar), both found naturally in plants. What makes white sugar unnatural is that its color has been removed to make it a prettier product. But nutritionally speaking, it is no more or less valuable than honey or the natural sugars in fruits and vegetables. In fact, you could make a small case for the idea that brown sugar is equally unnatural because it is refined sugar with molasses added for color. Cup for cup, it does have more of some nutrients, but given how little sugar we use, the amounts are negligible.

✓ **Sugar causes diabetes.** No, but eating sugary foods can increase the risk of complications in people who already have diabetes, don't secrete sufficient amounts of insulin, or can't metabolize lots of sugar at once.

✓ **Sugar is fattening.** Well, sure, if you eat so much sugar that you pile on the calories, you'll gain weight. That's what happened to lots of people who went on lowfat weight loss plans and started wolfing down lowfat but high-sugar, high-calorie cookies. Control your sugar intake, and you control your calories, which means you control your weight.

✓ **Sugar is bad for the heart.** For some carb-sensitive people, eating sugar leads to higher levels of blood fats, which means an increased risk of heart disease. People not sensitive to carbs have no problems metabolizing sugar, although keeping sugar intake to 10 percent of your daily calories is smart nutrition.

✓ **Sugar makes people (especially kids) hyper.** No. According to Vanderbilt University pediatrics professor Mark Wolraich, statistics drawn from a total of 23 studies show no stimulating effects of sugar in children. In fact, as you can see in Chapter 6, all carbs are calming chemicals.

✓ **Sugar causes cavities.** Oh, yeah. No question about it. So brush your teeth. And floss. After every meal. And maybe in between.

Choosing a Low-Carb, High-Protein Weight Loss Plan

If you've decided to try a low-carb, high-protein weight loss plan, which one works for you? Check out this section to pick one that suits your style.

Dr. Atkins' New Diet Revolution

Robert Atkins is the modern father of the high-protein, low-carb weight loss plan that says that eating carbohydrate foods stimulates your body to produce more insulin than you need, that producing this insulin makes you hungry, that being hungry makes you eat, and that (surprise!) eating makes you fat.

The Atkins diet has no set calorie count. Instead, it tells you to Eat! Eat! — as long as you eat high-protein foods. On this regimen, you are really supposed to eat as much protein food as you can actually cram into your mouth. Meat, eggs, full-fat cheese and dairy foods — all the treats forbidden on a carb-based, lowfat weight loss plan are welcome here, while the usual Good Guys — grains, fruit, veggies — are banished to the proverbial dog house.

At its most restrictive, during the first ("induction") phase, the Atkins diet allows from 4 grams of carbs (about what you get from a 3-cup salad) to 20 grams a day. At its most relaxed, Atkins permits 25 to 90 grams of carbs per day, which provides 100 to 360 calories, 7 to 24 percent of the calories in a 1,500 calorie diet. Without the carbs, you can't burn fat efficiently so you produce the ketones that I mention earlier in the section "Keeping an eye on ketone levels." The results are generally unpleasant: gastric annoyances, such as constipation and nausea; headache; and a characteristic stinky breath and perspiration.

But eating all that high-fat food can make you feel fuller than eating lots of carbohydrates. (Remember the old jokes about being hungry an hour after you eat Chinese food?) So you are likely to eat less than usual. In fact, if you add up the calories you consume each day on this meal plan, you will probably find that you are consuming fewer than you did before you started. You are also losing fluids.

So you will lose weight.

The Carbohydrate Addict's Diet

The Atkins diet advocates a low-carb, high-protein meal plan as a way to cut calories and lose weight. *The Carbohydrate Addict's Diet* by Rachel F. Heller and Richard F. Heller turns your natural enjoyment of and physiological need for carbs into — gasp! — an addiction.

This weight loss plan says, "Give up your carbs and you won't want them anymore." You get two high-protein meals and one high-carb, high-protein combination meal. If you absolutely, positively must have another serving of carbs, you have to have another serving of protein, a strategy that may increase your calorie intake and paradoxically cause you to put on weight.

Otherwise, this weight loss plan works just like the Atkins diet, taking weight off via water loss and calorie control. The question to ask here, as with all low-carb, high-protein weight loss plans, is why you should deny your body an essential nutrient in pursuit of short-term weight loss. Yes, cutting back the carbs is one way to cut back on calories, but the important element is the calories not the carbs. See Chapter 5.

Protein Power

Protein Power, created by Michael R. Eades and Mary Dan Eades, also buys into the carb/insulin/weight gain connection. But when these authors say protein power, they're not kidding. Their weight loss plan cuts carb intake to a lower level than any other popular low-carb, high-protein plan, allowing you no more than 30 grams a day, regardless of your total calorie intake. One gram of carbohydrate has 4 calories, so 30 grams gives you 120 calories. The Dietary Guidelines for Americans recommend getting 60 percent of your calories from carbs. On the Protein Power diet, 30 grams of carbohydrates provide

- Ten percent of the calories on a 1,200-calorie weight loss plan
- Eight percent of the calories on a 1,500-calorie weight loss plan
- Seven percent of the calories on a 1,800-calorie weight loss plan
- Six percent of the calories on a 2,000-calorie weight loss plan

These levels may be low enough to provoke some of the low-carb problems described in the last section.

Sugar Busters!

Like the other low-carb, high-protein weight loss plans, Sugar Busters! targets insulin and the high-carb foods it says make you secrete more hormone, which makes you fat. This weight loss plan was created by not one, not two, but four authors, plus an editor who gets his name on the cover of the book.

This weight loss plan doesn't fool around. It prohibits all insulin-stimulating foods, such as sugars, white flour, high-starch veggies (corn, potatoes), high-sugar veggies (carrots, beets), grains, and high-sugar fruits (all fruits). Sugar Busters! also says no to products made from these foods. One example is beer, which is made from grain and has 13 grams of carbs in a 12-ounce glass. On the other hand, unless I missed it, there was no ban on wine, which is made from grapes and has 2.8 grams of carbs (red wine) or 1.4 grams (white wine) per 5-ounce glass. No mention of the fact that there are no carbs, not a single one, in any size serving of spirits (gin, vodka, rum, or whiskey), which are also made from grains or other plants. Oh, well.

According to the International Food Information Council (IFIC), the average daily calorie allowance for this diet is about 1,200 calories. Thirty percent of those should come from carbohydrates, 32 percent from protein, and 28 percent from fat. If I've added that up right, there is 10 percent left over for . . . whatever. But not for something to drink with dinner. Sugar Busters! says that drinking fluids while you're eating dilutes digestive juices so that you can't digest your food. Given the fact that your gastric juices contain hydrochloric acid, this last theory is not generally accepted in the scientific community.

On a personal, admittedly picky note: While I enjoy an exclamation point now and then myself, I have to say I'm a tad put off by finding one in a medical or nutritional recommendation where it seems to shout, "Hey! You there! Do this! Do it now! Or else!" See what I mean?

The Zone

Da-de-da-da. Da-de-da-da. This Zone has no connection to the one inhabited by Rod Serling. It was created by Barry Sears who visualizes it as a metabolic state where your body and mind are relaxed and strong.

To project the dieter into his or her very own zone of contentment, this moderately low-carb, high-protein plan prescribes a neat set of numbers clear enough to calm the heart of anyone who loves Real Rules:

- ✔ Your calories should be a 40-30-30 ratio of carbs to protein to fat.
- ✔ Your meals should have no more than 500 calories.
- ✔ Your snacks should have less than 100 calories.
- ✔ You should get about 1,300 calories a day.
- ✔ Your protein portions should be the size of your hand.

What with all the figuring and paperwork, it may take you a minute or two to see that on this weight loss plan you will almost certainly be eating less than you normally do. Much less, says Salge Blake, nutrition columnist at the Web site www.thriveonline.com, who says: "If you followed The Zone to the letter, you would eat less than 1,000 calories a day."

And lose weight.

Table 7-2 summarizes the amounts of carbohydrates and calories recommended on each of these five low-carb, high-protein diets, comparing these numbers with the recommendations of the USDA/HHS Dietary Guidelines for Americans 2000.

Table 7-2	Carbohydrates for Low-Carb, High-Protein Weight Loss Plans	
Plan	*Carbohydrate Grams*	*% of Daily Calories (1,700-Calorie Diet)*
Dr. Atkins' New Diet Revolution	4–90	1–24%
The Carbohydrate Addict's Diet	*	*
Protein Power	30+	7%
Sugar Busters!	**	30%
The Zone	**	40%
Dietary Guidelines for Americans 2000	**	60%

*Not specified
**Varies with calorie intake
Sources: Dietary Guidelines for Americans 2000; Jane Kirby, Dieting For Dummies. *(Foster City, CA: Hungry Minds, Inc., 1998);* www.thriveonline.com/eats/experts/joan/ joan.12-13-96; *and* www.ivillage.com/diet/features/dietsaz/.

For more info on low-carb, high-protein diets, check out the official Web sites listed in Table 7-3, which offer explanations and encouragement, plus menus, meal plans, special foods, and items such as meal replacement bars — and maybe T-shirts and bumper stickers, too.

Table 7-3	Web Sites for Low-Carb, High-Protein Weight Loss Plans
Weight Loss Plan	*Web Site*
Dr. Atkins' New Diet Revolution	www.atkinscenter.com
The Carbohydrate Addict's Diet	www.carbohydrateaddicts.com
Protein Power	www.eatprotein.com
Sugar Busters!	www.sugarbusters.com
The Zone	www.zoneperfect.com

So What Happens on a Low-Carb, High-Protein Weight Loss Plan?

The easiest way to explain what happens when you try a low-carb, high-protein diet is this: "Hold the carbs. Pile on the proteins." My, that sounds easy. But wait: When you hold the carbs, that means cutting back on fruits and veggies, not to mention grains. Doing that cuts back on basic nutrients: vitamins, minerals, and fiber found naturally in fruits, veggies, and grains. For this reason, most low-carb, high-protein plans include an admonition to take a multivitamin every day. Your doctor may already advise you to do that, but with a low-carb, high-protein regimen, it's practically required.

Table 7-4 lays out the food choices allowed on five popular low-carb, high-protein weight loss plans as compared with the Dietary Guidelines for Americans meal suggestions. What an interesting comparison!

Table 7-4	Food Choices for Low-Carb, High-Protein Weight Loss Plans			
Plan	*Fruits*	*Vegetables*	*Grains*	*Dairy*
Dr. Atkins' New Diet Revolution	Limit	Limit	Avoid or limit bread & pasta	Limit milk & yogurt; Unlimited eggs & butter
The Carbohydrate Addict's Diet	Limit	Limit	Avoid or limit bread & pasta	
Protein Power	Limit	Limit	Avoid or limit bread & pasta	
Sugar Busters!	Unlimited high-fiber, low-sugar fruits; Limit high-glycemic index fruits	Unlimited high-fiber, low-starch vegetables; Limit high-glycemic index vegetables	Avoid or limit bread & pasta	Unlimited egg whites

Plan	Fruits	Vegetables	Grains	Dairy
The Zone	Limit high-glycemic fruits (bananas); Unlimited high-fiber, low sugar fruits	Limit high-glycemic vegetables (carrots); Unlimited olives, nuts, peanuts, & high-fiber, low-starch vegetables	Avoid or limit bread & pasta	Unlimited egg whites
Dietary Guidelines for Americans	2 servings per day	3 servings per day	5–11 servings per day	2 servings (lowfat) per day

Plan	Meat, Fish, Poultry	Special Gimmick
Dr. Atkins' New Diet Revolution	Unlimited	Extremely low-carb initial phase
The Carbohydrate Addict's Diet		One reward meal a day
Protein Power		No more than 30 g of carbohydrates a day
Sugar Busters!	Unlimited lean meat	No liquids with meals
The Zone		40-30-30 ratio of carbs to protein to fats
Dietary Guidelines for Americans	2–3 3-ounce servings per day	None

Chapter 8

Fiddling with Fats

. . . .

In This Chapter

▶ Identifying the fats in your food

▶ Naming fat's functions in your body

▶ Losing weight by manipulating fats

▶ Figuring out how much fat you need

. . . .

*T*his chapter explains why you need fat in your diet, how your body uses fats, and how to manage the amount of fat you get each day from food. Does that make your eyes glaze over because it sounds so boring? Think again. Without fats, you can't absorb and use fat-soluble nutrients, such as the vitamin A that protects your eyes and your vision. In other words, if you don't get the fats you need, eventually your eyes really will glaze over — reason enough to read this chapter.

The Facts about Fat

Fats are in the fire. In the last few years, *dietary fat* (the fats in food) has been blamed for numerous health problems ranging from obesity to heart disease to certain kinds of cancer. But warnings aren't the whole story. Fats are also good for you. In fact, no healthy body can function without them.

You need food components such as carbohydrates, proteins, and fats to build tissues and maintain your body. Fat from food is used to build adipose (fatty) tissue that:

✔ Contains "fat cells" that hold stored energy.

✔ Insulates your body and prevents heat loss in cold climates.

✔ Cushions your internal organs if you trip and fall.

✔ Provides a natural cushion for your skin and bones.

✔ Gives you a shape (think breasts, hips, and buttocks).

The name game

The chemical family name for fats and related compounds such as cholesterol is *lipids* from *lipos,* the Greek word for fat. Liquid fats are called oils; solid fats are called, well, fat.

And that's just half the list. You also need dietary fats (including the dreaded cholesterol) to:

- Enable you to use fat-soluble vitamins such as A (which protects eyes, skin, and mucous membranes) and E (super for your heart and arteries) and to manufacture vitamin D when sunlight hits the fat stored just under your skin.

- Help your gallbladder produce *bile acids,* digestive chemicals that allow you to absorb fats and fat-soluble nutrients such as vitamin A, vitamin D, vitamin E, and vitamin K.

- Maintain *cell membranes* (the outer "skin" that holds your body cells together).

- Build *myelin,* the fatty material around each nerve cell that makes it possible to zap electrical messages back and forth so that you can think, see, speak, move, and do all the miraculous tasks a living body performs.

- Sustain your brain (which is loaded with fats such as cholesterol).

- Assemble molecules called *phospholipids,* which carry other molecules into your cells.

- Create fat and protein molecules called *lipoproteins,* the particles that haul fats, including cholesterol, around through your bloodstream.

- Produce steroid hormones such as testosterone.

Nutrition note: These activities are so important to your health that if you don't take in enough cholesterol, your body will just go right ahead and produce cholesterol on its own. In fact, most of the cholesterol in your tissues is built right in your own liver, which churns out about 1 gram (1,000 mg) a day from the raw materials in the proteins, fats, and carbohydrates you consume. If you eat less cholesterol in food, your liver will just make more, which is why it can be such a chore to lower your cholesterol levels through diet alone. Some people must also use drugs called *statins,* which work by lowering your liver's production.

How Much Fat Do You Need?

You probably need less fat than you're getting now. In the United States, a "normal" diet often provides more — much more — than enough fat to fulfill all your bodily needs. The real question isn't how much is enough, but how much is too much.

The "correct" answer to that one seems to depend on who you ask. For example:

- ✔ The U.S. Department of Agriculture/Health and Human Services Guidelines for Americans 2000, recommends that no more than 30 percent of your total daily calories come from fat.

- ✔ On the other hand, a strict lowfat regimen, such as the Pritikin Diet described in Chapter 6, pushes fat consumption down to a measly 10 percent of your total daily calories.

- ✔ On the third hand (what? no third hand?), an eat-all-you-can-wolf-down high-protein meal plan such as the Atkins diet (it's in Chapter 7) has no — that's *no* — limit on how much fat you can eat.

Who's right?

Who knows?

Until recently, the answer was The Government — for example, the U.S. Departments of Agriculture and Health and Human Services, which firmly endorses the 30-percent solution. Their rationale and professional consensus is that a diet with lots of fat increases your risk of obesity, diabetes, heart disease, and some forms of cancer. (The risk of colon cancer seems to be tied more clearly to a diet high in fat from meat than fat from dairy products.) Ditto for those pushing very lowfat diets.

But people promoting a protein-based diet with unrestricted amounts of fat say, piffle! They insist that eating lots of fat makes you full so that you eat less, which means you lose weight which lowers your risk of . . . well, the same list of medical nasties you just read in the preceding paragraph.

Today, after years of fighting back and forth between the pro- and anti-fat folks, the USDA has now decided to decide. In 2001, the agency will begin a three-year study to determine whether a diet with unlimited amounts of fat is an effective, safe way to lose weight (more about that in Chapter 7).

What's that fat in my soup?

Ninety-five percent of the fats in your food are triglycerides. The rest are phospholipids and sterols, plus some diglycerides and monoglycerides and free fatty acids.

Triglycerides are compound molecules that contain one unit of glycerol and three (tri=three) fatty acids. *Glycerol* is a small, water-soluble carbohydrate that carries fats through blood; *fatty acids* are chains of carbon atoms with hydrogens attached. (Relax. That's all the chemistry you have to absorb here.) You digest triglycerides into glycerol and fatty acids, which are burned for energy to build adipose tissue.

Phospholipids have one unit of glycerol, two fatty acids, and a phosphate unit (made from the

mineral phosphorus) that enables phospholipids to dissolve in water. This is important because it enables phospholipids, such as lecithin, to serve as microscopic rafts that carry hormones and fat-soluble vitamins (A, D, E, K) through your bloodstream and across cell membranes.

Sterols, such as the newly identified healthful fats in soybeans, are circular fat and alcohol molecules that do useful biochemical jobs but provide no calories. Vitamin D is a sterol. So is the sex hormone testosterone. And so is cholesterol, which — contrary to common wisdom — is not a useless substance. In fact, your body uses cholesterol to build hormones and vitamins.

Naming the Fats in Food

This section defines the different kinds of fats in foods. Yes, it can be heavy slogging at times, but what you read here will make it easier for you to manage fats in any weight loss plan you choose. If you want to skip ahead to the practical stuff — setting up a fat-alert meal plan — okay, be my guest. But do come back and read this section later.

All dietary fats contain chain-like molecules (some short, mostly long, and a few in between) called *fatty acids.* When you are considering how much fat you should include in your diet, understanding how nutritionists characterize different kinds of fatty acids can help you make the "right" food choices. Here are three basic questions nutrition experts ask when classifying fatty acids:

✔ Is this fatty acid essential or non-essential?

✔ Is this fatty acid saturated or unsaturated?

✔ Is this unsaturated fatty acid an omega-3 or an omega-6?

What an essential fatty acid is

Like essential amino acids (check it out in Chapter 7), *essential fatty acids* are compounds your body cannot manufacture on its own. You have to get essential fatty acids (and essential amino acids) from food.

The two clearly essential fatty acids are *linoleic acid* and *linolenic acid.* If you get enough linoleic acid from food, then your body can make all kinds of good things, including another fatty acid, arachonidonic acid. If you get sufficient amounts of linolenic acid, you can make *eicosapentaenoic acid (EPA)* and *docosahexaenoic acid (DHA),* two additional important fatty acids.

Because you can manufacture them in your own body, arachonidonic acid, EPA and DHA are not labeled "essential." But it takes a lot of energy to produce these fatty acids. As a result, most nutritionists recommend that you get them from food. Table 8-1 shows you the food sources of the essential fatty acids.

Table 8-1	Where to Find Essential (And Almost Essential) Fatty Acids
Fatty Acid	*Food Source*
Linoleic acid*	Corn oil, safflower oil, sesame oil, soybean oil, sunflower oil
Arachidonic acid**	Beef, pork, lamb
Linolenic*	Canola oil, soybean oil, walnut oil, and margarine and shortening made from these oils
Eicosapentaenoic acid (EPA)	Fatty fish (Anchovies, haddock, herring, mackerel, salmon, sardines, scallops, tuna)
Docosahexaenoic acid (DHA)	Human milk

*Essential
**Almost essential
Source: Eleanor Noss Whitney, Corinne Balog Cataldo, Sharon Rady Rolfes, Understanding Normal and Clinical Nutrition *(Minneapolis/St. Paul: West Publishing Company, 1994).*

What quantities of essential fatty acids do you need to include in your diet? Surprise! You probably don't have to worry about that at all. In the United States, essential fatty acid deficiencies are virtually unknown except among infants or institutionalized patients fed formula foods lacking all polyunsaturated fatty acids for long periods of time. This situation occurred years and years ago and, once identified, has never been seen again.

But some people really need a number to hang their nutrition hats on. Okay, how about this? The National Academy of Sciences recommends that 1 to 2 percent of your total calories come from linoleic acid. But knowing this percentage is not useful information, unless you have a reference book identifying the exact amount of linoleic acid in the various foods you eat and a calculator to total up your daily total.

The better way is to follow the advice of the American Heart Association and the Dietary Guidelines for America, both of which suggest having at least a tablespoon of veggie oil or margarine a day. That's easy. And it's enough.

Sat fats versus unsaturated fatty acids

Chemically speaking, a fatty acid is a chain of carbon atoms (each with hydrogen atoms attached) plus a carbon-oxygen-hydrogen group (the unit that makes the molecule an acid) at one end of the chain.

Now here's one short (very short) chemistry lesson. When nutritionists describe fatty acid molecules as being saturated, monounsaturated, or polyunsaturated, they are telling you what kinds of bonds (links) the carbon atoms in the fatty acid molecule have to their fellow atoms. Carbon atoms have four bonds available. In fatty acids:

- Carbon atoms with four single bonds to other atoms are *saturated*. (Depending on where the carbon sits in the fatty acid chain, the four single bonds may be either to three hydrogen atoms and one carbon atom or to two hydrogen atoms and two carbon atoms.)
- Carbon atoms with two single bonds (one to a hydrogen atom and one to a carbon atom) plus a double bond to the next carbon atom in the chain are *unsaturated*.

Fatty acids with one unsaturated carbon atom are *monounsaturated* (mono = one). Fatty acids with two or more unsaturated carbon atoms are *polyunsaturated* (poly = many). Whether a fatty acid is saturated, monounsaturated, or polyunsaturated tells you much about its effect on your body, described later in this chapter in the section on creating a fat-conscious diet.

Figure 8-1 shows the difference between a saturated and an unsaturated carbon in a fatty acid chain. Notice that the unsaturated carbon has a double bond to the next carbon atom in the chain.

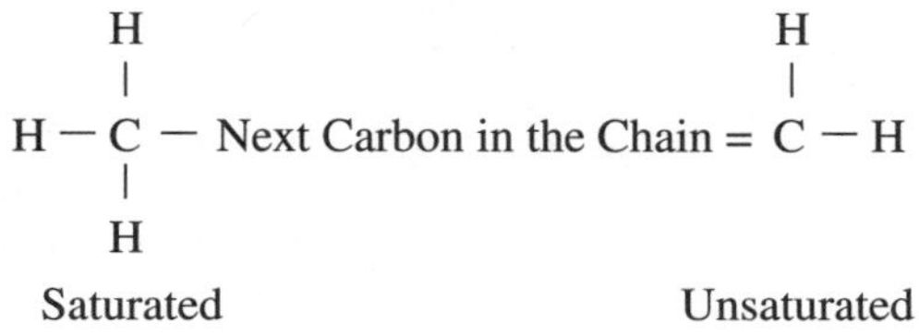

Figure 8-1:
Saturated
versus
unsaturated
carbon
atoms.

```
       H                              H
       |                              |
  H — C — Next Carbon in the Chain = C — H
       |
       H
  Saturated                    Unsaturated
```

Saturated and unsaturated fatty acids differ not only in how many carbons have how many atoms attached, but also in their physical characteristics that predict how they will behave in your body (actually in your arteries). The most important is whether they are liquid or hard at a certain temperature:

- Saturated fats such as lard are solid at room temperature and harden when chilled.
- Monounsaturated fats such as olive oil are liquid at room temperature and thicken (but do not solidify) when chilled.
- Polyunsaturated fats such as canola oil are liquid at room temperature and stay liquid even when chilled.

How to tell the good guys from the baddies? All fats and oils contain both saturated and unsaturated fatty acids, but nutritionists classify them as saturated, monounsaturated, or polyunsaturated based on which fatty acids are most plentiful. The system works like this:

- A saturated fat, such as butter, has mostly saturated fatty acids.
- A monounsaturated fat, such as olive oil, has mostly monounsaturated fatty acids.
- A polyunsaturated fat, such as corn oil, has mostly polyunsaturated fatty acids.

But wait! Margarine — which is made from unsaturated fats such as corn and soybean oil — is solid. How can that be? Ah, as the DuPont commercial used to say, "Better living through chemistry." The naturally polyunsaturated fats in margarines have been artificially saturated by food chemists who tack extra hydrogen atoms on to their carbons. This process, called *hydrogenation,* turns an oil, such as pourable oil, into a spreadable fat: margarine. A fatty acid with extra hydrogens is called a *hydrogenated fatty acid.*

Table 8-2 is a list of saturated and unsaturated fats and oils. Canola oil, with more than half its fatty acid content monounsaturated, is a *monounsaturated oil.* On the other hand, although nearly 25 percent of the fatty acids in corn oil are monounsaturated, the percentage of polyunsaturated fatty acids is higher, so corn oil is considered *polyunsaturated*.

Wait! One thing more. Yes, I know that some of the totals below do not add up to 100 percent. Why? Because all fats and oils contain small amounts of other fatty acids that have no effect on whether the fat/oil is classified as saturated.

Table 8-2	Comparing the Fatty Acids in Fats and Oils		
This Contains	*This Percentage of:*		*So It Is Labeled:*
	Saturated *Monosaturated*	*Polyunsaturated*	
Canola oil	7	53	22	Monounsaturated
Corn oil	13	24	59	Polyunsaturated
Olive oil	14	74	9	Monounsaturated
Palm oil	52	38	10	Saturated
Peanut oil	17	46	32	Monounsaturated
Safflower	9	12	74	Polyunsaturated
Soybean	15	23	51	Polyunsaturated
Soybean-cottonseed oil	18	29	48	Polyunsaturated
Butter	62	30	5	Saturated
Lard	39	45	11	Saturated*

*There is always an exception: Because more than ⅓ of its fats are saturated, lard is called saturated.
Source: Nutritive Value of Foods (Washington, D.C.: U.S. Department of Agriculture, 1991); "Food and Life" (New York: American Council on Science and Health, 1990).

Omegas and You

Linoleic acid and arachidonic acid have a structure chemists name an omega-6 fatty acid. Linolenic acid and the hormone-like substances called eicosapentaenoic acid (EPA) and docosahexaenoic acid (DHA), which are made from linolenic acid, are omega-3 fatty acids.

The number tacked on to an omega fatty acid's name — 3 or 6 — indicates the position of the first double bond between carbon atoms in the fatty acid chain. The omega-3 has its first double bond 3-carbons in from the end; the omega-6 has its first double bond six carbons in from the end. Figure 8-2 shows a diagram of these patterns.

```
        H   H   H
        |   |   |
 H — C — C — C = C — ETC.
        |   |   |
        H   H   H
```

Omega-3 Fatty Acid

```
        H   H   H   H   H   H
        |   |   |   |   |   |
 H — C — C — C — C — C — C =
        |   |   |   |   |
        H   H   H   H   H
```

Omega-6 Fatty Acid

Omega-3 and omega-6 fatty acids are found primarily in fish and shellfish. They appear to reduce inflammation, perhaps by turning off an enzyme called COX-2, which has been associated with inflammatory diseases such as rheumatoid arthritis and skin cancer.

According to the Arthritis Foundation, omega-3s relieve joint inflammation in people with rheumatoid arthritis. Studies at Purdue University show that omega-3s may also prevent the natural breakdown of bone tissue and increase production of a bone-protecting growth factor that steps up new bone formation — at least in laboratory rats whose ovaries have been removed, cutting off their natural supply of bone-protecting estrogen (a condition analogous to menopause in women).

Although they are chemical cousins, the omega-6 fatty acids have not yet been shown to carry the benefits associated with omega-3s.

How much omega-3 do you need? There are no rules yet, but some experts (including the American Heart Association) now suggest three or more servings of fatty fish a week, a common diet pattern in Mediterranean countries such as Greece. Table 8-1, earlier in this chapter, shows you which foods have what fat.

Choosing a Fat-Conscious Diet

If I suggest setting up a "carbohydrate-based" diet or a "low-carbohydrate, high-protein diet," you get a quick, clear picture of what I'm talking about.

The first gives you lots of grains, fruit, and veggies with smaller amounts of red meat and dairy products. The second promotes a meal plan with everything reversed. Now you get plenty of meat, fish, and poultry, with smaller (sometimes much smaller) portions of grains and starchy veggies.

But if I say "fat-based" diet, what in the world do I mean? Bowls of whipped cream? Tablespoons of butter? Mayonnaise sandwiches? Fat may be tasty, but it's not a useful base on which to build a nutritious diet. So forget "fat based." Think "fat conscious" instead.

What's your preference?

Fat-conscious meal plans come in small, medium, and really, really large. In plain English, these categories translate to:

- A very lowfat diet
- A moderate lowfat diet
- An unlimited fat diet

Lowfat diets and moderately lowfat diets are discussed in Chapter 6; you can find everything you need to know about an unlimited fat diet in Chapter 7. But I've included short catch-up explanations here so that you create a workable fat-conscious diet without having to flip back and forth between pages. First up: very lowfat meal plans.

Very lowfat diets

With the exception of cholesterol (which has no calories and provides no energy), fats are high energy nutrients with more than twice as much energy (calories) per gram as carbohydrates or proteins. One gram carbs or protein has 4 calories; one gram fat, 9 calories. A bit of simple math — dividing 9 by 4 — shows you can eat slightly more than two servings of carb or protein food and get the same number of calories as one equivalent serving of fats (say two ounces versus one ounce).

If the easiest way to lose weight is to cut back on calories, the easiest way to cut back on calories is to cut way back on fats. Very lowfat diets such as the Pritikin Diet or the Ornish Diet (check out Chapter 7) or a vegan diet (lots of plant foods, no foods from animals at all) may cut your fat intake down to 10 percent or less of your total daily calories.

Moderate lowfat diets

Many experts, including the fat-aware American Heart Association, think you will also be bored out of your gourd by a very lowfat diet because the diet is just too restrictive for you to stay with it for any length of time. So they opt for a moderate lowfat eating plan, such as that proposed by the Dietary Guidelines for Americans and virtually every other Good Nutrition organization.

A moderate lowfat diet limits your calories from fat to no more than 30 percent of all the calories you eat each day. And it emphasizes the good fat/bad fat notion — for example, unsaturated fats (good) versus saturated fats (bad). According to the Guidelines, no more than 10 percent of your total daily calories should come from artery-clogging saturated fats (the 10 percent is part of the 30 percent, not an extra amount).

If you usually take in about 2,000 calories a day, this advice means that you should get

- ✔ 600 calories or fewer from fat (30% × 2,000 calories = 600 calories).
- ✔ 200 calories or fewer from saturated fat (10% × 2,000 calories = 200 calories).

And did I forget to say that moderate lowfat diets also suggest limiting your cholesterol intake to no more than 300 mg a day from food, regardless of your calories? Now I've said it. Whew!

Unlimited fat diets

This kind of diet, usually called "low-carb, high-protein," says, "Who cares about fat. Eat all you want!" For the lowdown on this meal plan, skip to Chapter 7. All you need to know here is that people who are enthusiastic about an unlimited fat diet say that it helps you lose weight because eating fats makes you feel full, a physical sensation called *satiety*. Then, because fat is digested more slowly than proteins or carbohydrates, you feel fuller longer. Which means you eat less, eat less often, and . . . well you get the picture. I won't bore you by repeating the details here (as I said, they're all spelled out in Chapter 7).

Setting Up a Daily Fat Record

This is the Real Deal, the part of the chapter that justifies calling this book *The Weight Loss Kit For Dummies* instead of, say, the *Weight Loss Encyclopedia* or *The Weight Loss Guide* or *The Weight Loss Book*.

First, choose the diet you plan to follow: Very lowfat, moderate lowfat, or unlimited fat. Of course, if you pick the eat-all-the-fat-you-want diet, you can just forget the chart and zip right ahead to the next chapter.

Still here? Then your next step is to print the chart you will use to track the fats. Then you will want a list that gives you a general idea of which foods have more (or less) fat. And finally, because virtually all nutrition tables and labels list fat content in grams, you need to know how to translate grams of fat into fat calories.

1. **Choose a diet.**

    Refer to the previous section and choose the diet you want. Remember, picking the unlimited fat diet means skipping the rest of this chapter.

2. **Print the chart.**

    Click onto your CD-ROM to locate Table 8-3. Print a copy of the chart and set it aside for a minute, and I will give you the info you need to fill in the chart. By the way, I have abbreviated grams to g and calories to cal.

Table 8-3		Tracking the Fat			
My diet is					
I can have this many fat calories a day:					
I can have this many sat fat calories a day:					
	Food	**Total fat (g/cal)**	**Sat fat (g/cal)**	**Total fat (cal/% day's cal)**	**Total sat fat (cal/% day's cal)**
Sunday					
Monday					
Tuesday					
Wednesday					
Thursday					
Friday					
Saturday					

3. **Choose the foods you plan to eat.**

    Keep the following pointers about fat in mind when you're choosing the foods you'll eat:

- Fruits and vegetables have only traces of fat, primarily unsaturated.

- Grains have small amounts of fat, up to 3 percent of their total weight.

- Dairy products vary. Cream is a high fat food. "Regular" milks and cheeses are moderately high in fat. Skim milk and skim milk products are lowfat foods. Most of the fat in any dairy product is saturated fat.

- Meat is moderately high in fat, and most of its fats are made up of saturated fat acids.

- Poultry (chicken and turkey) is relatively low in fat — so long as you serve it without the skin.

- Fish is relatively low in fat, and its fats are composed primarily of unsaturated fats such as omega-3s.

- Vegetable oils, butter, and lard are high-fat foods. Most of the fats in vegetable oils are unsaturated; most of the fats in lard and butter are saturated.

- Processed foods, such as cakes, breads, and canned or frozen meat and vegetables dishes, are generally higher in fat than plain grains, meats, fruits, and vegetables.

Table 8-4 is a short but representative sampler of how much fat you find in different foods. For more detailed info, check out Appendix A, which lists the specific nutrient content (including fats) of ordinary servings of more than 200 common foods.

Table 8-4	Fat Content of Common Foods
Food	*% Fat*
Bread, cereals, grains	
Breads	2–4
Cereals	trace–2
Pasta (plain)	1–2
Fruit	*trace*
Exception: Avocado	17
Vegetables	*trace*
Exception: Olives	20

(continued)

Table 8-4 *(continued)*

Food	% Fat
Meat, Poultry, Fish	
Beef	
Stewed	
Lean only	15
Lean & fat	29
Ground	19
Roast (rib)	
Lean only	15
Lean & fat	31
Chicken breast, roasted, without skin	3
Turkey, light and dark, no skin	5–20
Shellfish	1–2
Fatty fish	6–10
Dairy products	
Butter	81
Egg yolk	33
Cheese	
American	32
Cottage (creamed)	4
Cottage (lowfat)	2
Swiss	28
Milk	
Whole	3.2
Lowfat	2
Nonfat (skim)	0
Vegetable oils	100
Margarines	80
Nuts	50–70

Source: Nutritive value of foods, Washington: U.S. Department of Agriculture, 1991.

4. Translate the grams of fat to fat calories.

Pick a food, any food. Flip to the Nutrient Data chart in Appendix A. Locate the food in the list. Run your finger across the page to find the column with the grams of total fat in the food and the grams of sat fat. To turn these numbers into calories, simply multiply by 9 (the number of calories in a gram of fat). By the way, feel free to round off to the nearest whole number.

Here are some examples for you:

Example #1: One medium fresh pear has 0.66 grams total fat and 0.04 grams sat fat.

$0.66 \times 9 = 5.94 = 6$ calories total fat

$0.04 \times 9 = 0.36 = 0.4$ calories sat fat

Example #2: One (average) slice of white bread has 1.62 grams total fat and 0.32 gram sat fat.

$1.62 \times 9 = 14.58 = 15$ calories total fat

$0.32 \times 9 = 2.88 = 3$ calories sat fat

Example #3: A 3-ounce broiled extra lean beef burger has 13.88 grams total fat and 5.46 grams sat fat.

$13.88 \times 9 = 124.92 = 125$ calories total fat

$5.46 \times 9 = 49.14 = 49$ calories sat fat

To figure the percentage of calories you get from fat, divide your total fat intake (in calories) by the number of calories your diet provides each day.

Example: Your moderate fat diet allows you 2,000 total calories a day. Today, your meals had 600 calories from all fats with 120 calories from sat fat.

$\dfrac{600 \text{ calories total fat}}{2,000 \text{ calories}} = 30$ percent calories from fat

$\dfrac{120 \text{ calories sat fat}}{2,000 \text{ calories}} = 6$ percent calories from sat fat

And that's it, everything you need to track the fats in your daily diet. To give you an idea of how simple the process is, I have filled in a sample column in Table 8-5 to show you how to calculate the fat content of one meal, a bland but common breakfast of orange juice, white toast, and a pat of margarine. Obviously, you will get a larger total when you count up all the grams and calories in a full day's menu. By the way, they are abbreviated to g for grams and cal for calories.

Table 8-5				Tracking the Fat	
My diet is					
I can have this many fat calories a day:					
I can have this many sat fat calories a day:					
	Food	*Total fat (g/cal)*	*Sat fat (g/cal)*	*Total fat (cal/% day's cal)*	*Total sat fat (cal/% day's cal)*
Sunday	Slice white bread	1.5/13.5	0.2/1.8		
	Tsp soft margarine	3.78/34	0.66/5.9		
	Cup, orange juice	0.5/4.5	0.06/0.5		
				21.8/1%	8.2/0.4%

Chapter 9

A Diet Grab Bag

*B*oy, oh boy, did I ever pick the best title for this chapter. It really is a grab bag of weight loss programs that don't fit into well-known categories such as "low-calorie, carbohydrate-based" or "low-carb, high-protein" or "low-fat" or "high-fat" or "fat-free" or "controlled-fat."

In other words, the weight loss plans that I describe here are, well, unusual. For example, they may require you to limit your food choices so strictly that the list often seems neither reasonable nor palatable. Or they may direct you to eat certain foods at certain times during the day or with certain other foods (or without certain other foods) — and predict dire consequences if you stray from the path. Or they may suggest (actually insist) you check out your body type before ordering lunch. Or they may promise to free your body of toxins. Or they may tell you to stop eating. Period.

As a result, the nutrition community, including the U.S. Departments of Agriculture and Health and Human Services and important professional organizations such as the American Dietetic Association and the American Heart Association, tend to regard these plans as

✔ Nutritionally inadequate.

✔ Misleading in their promise of weight loss.

✔ Potentially harmful to your body.

Of course, it's a free country, and no one can force you to choose one diet over another or even to pass up a diet that does not appear to provide the nutrients you need to stay healthy while losing weight. But it's always smart to protect yourself by checking with your doctor before starting a new diet, particular as it seems different for the Good Weight Loss Diet, that boring old regimen that:

✔ Provides a full complement of nutrients: vitamins, minerals, protein, fat, carbohydrates — and more.

✔ Includes lots of different foods.

✔ Advises you to exercise while dieting.

✔ Promises to help you lose weight at a slow, but steady pace.

✔ Comes with your doctor's Seal of Approval.

One-Food Weight Loss Plans

Do you like grapefruit? Are you bananas for cabbage soup? Are you nuts about bananas? Do you like these foods so much that you are willing to base your whole weight loss plan on one of them?

Aw, c'mon.

The grapefruit meal plan was hot stuff when your mother (maybe your grandmother) was a teenager. The cabbage soup regimen is this generation's update. Bananas seem to come and go. But no matter what food you pick, a weight loss plan that emphasizes one food everyday or at every meal is like the "one-horse sleigh" in *Jingle Bells* (okay for a quick trip to Granny's but not meant for the longer haul).

Relying on a single food is a bad weight loss choice because it's:

✔ Boring

✔ Nutritionally inadequate

✔ Poor training for a lifelong weight control program

I can just hear your answer: "Aw, c'mon yourself. Look how much weight I'm losing with this diet." Well, no surprise there: You're cutting back on calories, and as you can plainly see in Chapter 5, that's one sure way to drop the extra pounds. But getting to your new slim, trim self by cutting out a whole list of foods may cost more, nutrition-wise, than you want to spend.

The American Heart Association (AHA), among others, has warned that even a short-term reliance on a one-food plan can lead to vitamin and mineral deficiencies. Worse yet, most one-food plans ignore long-term dietary changes and regular exercise. Check out Chapter 1 and Chapter 17 for the real skinny on changing your attitude toward food and incorporating exercise into your daily schedule.

Finally, when you're trying to lose weight, variety really is the spice of life. It's tough enough to cut back on calories and favorite foods without eliminating everything that makes mealtime fun, which enables you to stick with your diet.

An effective weight control program is one that enables you to stay at a healthful weight for longer than a week or even a few months. Done right, it should be good forever.

Plain grapefruit? Cabbage? Bananas?

Baloney.

Food-Combining Weight Loss Plans

Think of the food-combining weight loss plan as a variation on the one-food weight loss plan. The meal plans in this diet are about 70 percent fruits and veggies, plus one or two servings of starchy carbohydrates and some animal protein foods.

So far so good. But the food-combining plan allows you to eat more than one food (or one kind of food), but not necessarily at the same time.

According to the authors of combination weight loss books such as *The New Beverly Hills Diet*, Marilu Henner's *Total Health Makeover,* and Suzanne Somers' *Get Skinny on Fabulous Food,* when you try to digest different foods at the same time, your body produces toxic substances that make you gain weight. So to stay in step with a combination weight loss plan, these books may tell you to:

- ✔ Eat only fruit for breakfast.

- ✔ Have no more than six different fruits and veggies at any one meal.

- ✔ Never eat carbohydrates and proteins at the same time. (I guess that rules out tuna sandwiches!)

- ✔ Wait four hours after eating protein before eating carbohydrates. (I guess you eat the meatballs at lunch and the spaghetti at dinner?)

There's more, but you get the idea. What you may not get is the fact that this is interesting but nutritionally ridiculous. Oh, heck, of course you got that.

If you follow a food-combining meal plan to the letter, you are likely to drop some pounds. However, according to a study in the April 2000 issue of the *International Journal of Obesity and Related Metabolic Disorders,* you won't lose any more weight with a combination weight loss plan than with a controlled-calorie balanced diet consisting of "normal" foods (their words), where you get more than 40 percent of your calories from carbs, 31 percent from fats, and 25 percent from protein.

A (very) short course in human digestion

Carnivores (meat-eating animals such as lions) thrive on meat, but their intestines are not long enough to pull nutrients out of many plants. *Herbivores* (plant-eating animals such as cows) are just the opposite. They have long intestinal tracts, sometimes with more than one stomach, and are perfectly adapted to drawing nutrients out of plants, even some as tough as alfalfa and hay. *Omnivores* (plant- and meat-eaters, such as you and me) have middle-size digestive tracts — long enough to get nutrients out of many plants.

You can find a complete discussion of the digestive process in my book, *Nutrition For Dummies* (published by Hungry Minds, Inc.). But for now, all you need to know is that your body pulls vitamins, minerals, and other important substances out of food via a two-part digestive process that includes

- Mechanical digestion — that is, mashing the food physically (chewing it in your mouth; churning it in your stomach)

- Chemical digestion — that is, attacking it with enzymes and gastric juices at every point in your digestive tract

You need a good set of choppers for starters. More important, you need to be able to secrete the different enzymes required to digest different kinds of food:

- Proteases digest proteins.

- Lipases digest fats.

- Amylases digest starches.

- Specific enzymes digest specific carbs: For example, gastric alcohol dehydrogenses begins digesting alcohol in your stomach.

These enzymes are released at specific sites along the digestive tract, from your mouth — where saliva contains amylases that begin the digestion of carbs — to your stomach and your intestines.

Some people are unable to produce some of the enzymes they need to digest certain foods. One common example is the inability of many adults to make sufficient amounts of *lactase,* the enzyme required to digest lactose, a sugar in milk. This condition is treated by eliminating or modifying consumption of some foods. However, other people have more serious metabolic disorders that prevent them from digesting fats or carbohydrates; these relatively uncommon conditions may be life-threatening and require medical attention.

But healthy adults have no trouble coming up with all the enzymes needed to digest proteins, fats, and carbohydrates. And your gastric juices — liquids secreted in your stomach, pancreas, and small intestine — are equal opportunity destroyers that can chew their way through virtually anything you toss down, short of iron nails.

Why do you lose weight on a food-combining plan? For one thing, the rules are so complicated that you could spend hours trying to set up your three square meals a day. That activity alone reduces your calorie intake.

Food-combining plans often emphasize fresh fruits and veggies. Not only is this sound nutritional advice, but it also cuts back on calories.

And because these plans suggest that you don't eat protein with carbs, you're likely to be getting just one or two servings of meat, fish, or poultry a day, a practice in line with the Dietary Guidelines for Americans (published in 2000) and the American Heart Association recommendations. That's the good news.

The not-so-good news is that some food-combining plans recommend that you give up meat and/or dairy products entirely. Doing so makes your food-combining plan a vegan plan. (*Vegetarians* eat dairy foods that come from animals, such as eggs, milk, and cheese; however, *vegans* don't eat any dairy foods from animals.) Eating less meat and full-fat dairy products is okay. But if you don't eat meat *and* give up even lowfat dairy products, your may miss out on some of these essential nutrients:

- Calcium, iron, and zinc (easier to absorb from animal foods than from plants)
- Vitamin B12 (only in animal foods)
- Vitamin D (only in eggs, milk, and fish)

Another potential problem with food-combining plans is the occasional recommendation to eat nothing but fruit for days at a time. Yes, eating lots of fresh fruit is good. But eating lots and lots of fresh fruit can set off gastric rumbles. What kinds of rumbles? Trust me, you'll know when it happens.

But the worst news about food-combination plans is that the people presenting these plans sometimes misinterpret basic nutrition facts. Trying to lose weight is hard enough, but trying to lose weight without factual information about how your body works is no fun.

Eating-to-Type Weight Loss Plans

Eating to type, also known as niche dieting, a relatively new entry in the weight loss sweepstakes, is the guiding principle behind such books as *Eat Right 4 Your Type* and *Your Body Knows Best.*

The people who came up with these weight loss plans have assimilated snippets of information from the following disciplines and have come up with an eating plan made Just For You:

- ✔ Anthropology (Where did your ancestors live?)
- ✔ Chemistry (What's your blood type?)
- ✔ Physiology (What's your body shape? How fast is your metabolism?)

It's nice that someone cares that much. But is this sort of plan healthful or nutritionally valid?

To paraphrase Hamlet, "That's the question, alright." But not the only one. Eating-to-type weight loss plans try to answer some of the following questions:

- ✔ Do you come from a cold or warm climate?
- ✔ What's your blood type?
- ✔ How fast is your metabolism?

"Do you come from a cold or warm climate?"

If your ancestors came from a really cold climate, the niche-diet folks say your body will work best on lots of meat and calorie-dense foods high in protein and fat (which your ancestors needed to protect themselves from the cold). Your reasonable answer to this statement might be: "Even if I now live in Florida?"

"What's your blood type?"

According to the type-diet gurus:

- ✔ Type O means you come from hunters and have lots of stomach acid needed to digest meat.
- ✔ Type A (or Type AB) means you come from an agricultural background and are designed to eat carbs.
- ✔ Type B means you are somewhere in the middle, less meat-friendly than a Type O, less carb accommodating than a Type A.

To which you might well answer: "I'm Type A, my sister's Type B, my mother's family came from Sweden, and my father's folks are from Southern Spain." Help!

"How fast is your metabolism?"

Do you know how fast you burn food? What?, You don't know your metabolic rate, which is another way of saying *burn food?*

If you can eat anything that doesn't bite back and still stay slim, you burn food fast and efficiently. On the other hand, if you gain weight just reading about food, your metabolic rate is definitely slower. Eating-for-type plans say

✔ Fast burners need meat to feed their furnaces, while slow burners should stick to lower fat poultry and fish — which sounds good until your read through some calorie charts and find that some meat is lower in fat than some poultry and fish. Ooops.

✔ Carb loading is only for fast burners because it will make slow burners fat by stimulating insulin secretion, a theory that underlies some low-carb, high-protein diets as I explain in Chapter 7.

That's interesting, but if you lose weight on a made-for-your-type plan, check out the calorie count. I bet it's lower than your usual diet, a prescription that works for any type.

Toxic-Waste Weight Loss Plans

Your body is efficiently designed to eliminate waste through

✔ Respiration (breathing out)

✔ Perspiration

✔ Urination

✔ Defecation

The main action occurs in your stomach and your small and large intestines where, with the assistance of your liver, pancreas, and gallbladder, usable (digestible) material from food is digested (broken apart) into simple compounds your body can easily absorb. Excess water produced by digestion is funneled to the kidneys to be eliminated as urine. Indigestible solid material is carted off to the colon where excess water is squeezed out and the material descends to the rectum and is eliminated as feces.

Mentioning the unmentionable

Fecal matter is solid waste composed of indigestible material from food, cells from the lining of the intestine, and friendly bacteria from your intestines. The friendly bacteria that live happily in your intestinal tract churn out Vitamin B12 and Vitamin K, digest carbs, break down proteins, and excrete the smelly gas that sometimes embarrasses you. The brown color of feces is due to pigments from bile, one of the gastric juices used to digest food.

Weight loss plans that claim to help you lose weight by "cleansing" your system usually rely on either diuretics (also known as water pills) to make you urinate more often, or laxatives (you know what they do) as well as diuretic or laxative herbs and foods. You can find a list of diuretic herbs in Chapter 14; laxative herbs and foods include senna, prunes, and anything high in fiber.

Needless to say, the weight you lose is mostly water — so when you stop the diet, you gain weight. In addition, abusing diuretics or laxatives may cause problems such as dehydration, diarrhea, or a severely irritated colon. In severe cases, losing lots of fluids may unbalance your supply of electrolytes (minerals that help transmit impulses from cell to cell), and interfere with electrical signals that keep your heart beating; this is definitely not a good thing!

Fasting: The Last-Resort Diet

When you choose to go without food, you call your behavior *fasting*. When a catastrophe such as war or famine keeps you from getting food, that's called *starvation*. Politically and socially, fasting and starvation are totally different phenomena, one voluntary, one not. But to your body, no food means no food. Period. Sensing danger, you involuntary set off all kinds of internal alarms as basic metabolic defenses spring into action. The resulting physiological brouhaha may have distinctly unpleasant consequences. Read on.

As you can plainly see in Chapter 5, your body uses 79 percent of the energy (calories) you consume each day to run its organs and systems: your heart, your lungs, your digestive tract, and last, but definitely not least, your brain.

Your body runs on glucose, the end product of metabolism. The foods most easily metabolized to glucose are carbohydrate foods, the plant foods such as fruits, veggies, and grains. Fat foods are second choice, a less efficient but still useful source of glucose. Under normal circumstances, there is no third choice. Except in emergencies, you use protein foods only to build and repair body tissues, not as a source of energy.

You can store carbs as glycogen, which is easy to change to glucose. You can store fat as, well, fat. When it's crunch time — you're stuck on an ice floe in the Arctic with no supply ship in site — the fat breaks down into fatty acids from which your body extracts small amounts of *glycerol* (a fatty substance), which yields little bits of glucose. So if you miss a couple of meals, you can get by for a day or so on your carb and fat reserves.

But yoo-hoo! Look here! This is the important part. Without adequate supply of carbs, your body looks for a new glucose mine, and what it finds is the protein in your muscles and organs. To compensate for the lack of protein, your body will literally begin to digest itself, breaking the proteins in muscle and organ tissue into amino acids, which yield *pyruvate,* a compound that can be used to manufacture glucose. Well, that sounds good. But it's not.

How your body responds to fasting

You can store carbs, and you can store fat, but you can't store protein. You need a new supply every day. Without it, you cannot make the red blood cells you need to carry oxygen to every tissue. You cannot make enough new cells to compensate for your natural daily loss of muscle tissue or the natural daily loss of cells lining your digestive tract. And without sufficient protein, you won't have enough *albumin,* a protein in blood that helps maintain fluid balance (the amount of liquid inside and outside each cell).

As a result,

- ✔ You feel weak (not enough oxygen).
- ✔ Your muscles thin down (not enough new cells).
- ✔ Your digestion is bollixed up (ditto).
- ✔ Your belly swells (too much fluid retained).
- ✔ You are light-headed (not enough liquid to keep blood flowing to the brain).

Literary fasting factoid

Upton Sinclair, the author of *The Jungle* — a novel whose revolting depictions of meat-packing plants in Chicago led to the creation of the first meat inspection laws — wrote another, deservedly less famous book called *The Fasting* *Cure* in which he claimed that long-term fasting could cure asthma, cancer, colds, kidney and liver disease, syphilis, and TB, thus proving that great novelists don't necessarily know beans about nutrition.

Another problem with using protein for energy is that to process the protein your body needs lots of water. As a result, while you lose weight, most of the weight you lose is liquids your body needs for essential functions, like breathing, and digesting, and . . . well, all that good stuff.

Like protein depletion, water depletion, a.k.a. dehydration, has serious consequences. Feeling thirsty is a signal that you've lost an amount of liquid equal to about 1 percent of your body weight. When that doubles to 2 percent, your circulation slows for lack of water in blood cells and blood plasma (the liquid around the cells inside the blood vessels).

If your water loss doubles again, to 4 percent of your body weight (5 pounds for a 130-pound woman; 7 pounds for a 170-pound man), you have less water in your body tissues so

- ✔ You feel sick to your stomach.
- ✔ Your temperature rises.
- ✔ You are very tired.
- ✔ You breathe faster.
- ✔ Your heart beats faster.

When your water loss equals 10 percent of your body weight, you're dizzy, with muscle spasms, on the verge of kidney failure. At 20 percent, it's goodbye, Charlie.

If this list of problems isn't enough to make you swear off fasting until your start to nibble at your own muscles, consider this: When your body turns to your muscles and organs for energy, it eventually runs into a wall. You've only got so much protein tissue available. In the end, it will be used up, your heart will stop, your brain will shut down, and you will die of starvation. If dehydration doesn't get you first.

Sorry about that.

Medically sanctioned fasting

Given the bleak picture I've painted of fasting, you may be surprised, no, astonished to hear that there are situations in which going without food can be good medicine. The key is the phrase "medically supervised." Patients fasting in a hospital under a doctor's care don't just stop eating. They get specially prepared products sold only to doctors and hospitals that contain sufficient amounts of glucose and protein to protect vital muscles and organs. These products also contain nutrients such as vitamins and minerals to prevent deficiency disease.

Political-fasting factoid

Mohandas Karamchand Gandhi (1869–1948) was an Indian political and spiritual leader who created and led the passive resistance movement which brought about India's independence from Great Britain in 1947. Often jailed by the Brits, Gandhi was a pacifist whose threats to fast until death forced the British to release him back to his work, which was to peacefully toss them out of his country.

Like the Very Low Calorie diet program described in Chapter 5, medically supervised fasting is meant only as a short-term program for people who meet very specific criteria:

- ✔ They are more than 100 pounds overweight.
- ✔ They have a BMI higher than 30.
- ✔ They have a BMI 27 to 30, but also have weight-related health problems such as diabetes or high blood pressure.

Neither fasting nor Very Low Calorie diets are recommended for

- ✔ Women who are pregnant or breast-feeding.
- ✔ Children or adolescents.
- ✔ People who have medical conditions or are using medication that makes it difficult to tolerate the side effects of severe calorie cutting.

Supervised fasting is a short-term option that must be carefully monitored to prevent serious health risks such as heart failure. Although fasting can jump-start a weight loss program, experts value it for its long-term weight control. In other words, as they say on those daredevil TV car commercials, don't attempt this one at home.

By now, it should be clear that this fasting is a last resort weight loss stratagem that should be used only with a doctor's advice and consent. Message delivered.

Religious-fasting factoids

Observant Jews fast from sundown to sundown at Yom Kippur, the Day of Atonement, when all repent of their past year's sins.

Muslims fast from dawn to dusk during the 29 or 30 days of Ramadan, the ninth month of the lunar Muslim calendar, a time of forgiveness and the settlement of debts. The daily fast is followed by feasting during the night hours.

Christians are more likely to abstain from specific foods at certain times of year rather than to fast. For example, during Lent, the 40-day period between Ash Wednesday and Easter Eve that commemorates Jesus' fasting in the wilderness, a Christian may fast or more likely abstain from eating one or more of his or her favorite foods.

In all these cases, the young, the old, the sick (including pregnant women), and travelers (including soldiers) are excused from fasting. Other religious and/or spiritual groups occasionally promote fasting as a way to "cleanse the body" or reach a higher state of consciousness. The first effect is easy to explain: When you don't put anything in, nothing comes out. The second, a lightheadedness, is a physiological phenomenon due to a slowing supply of oxygen to the brain — which who's to say you can't interpret it as a metaphysical moment. Peace.

Part III
Strategic Food Choices

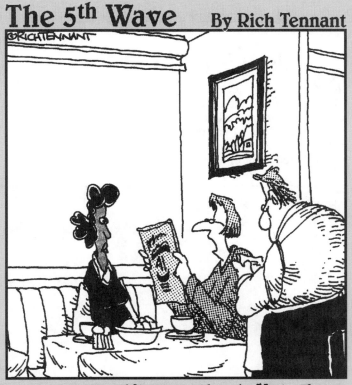

The 5th Wave   By Rich Tennant

"I'll have the 'Healthy-Heart-High-Fiber-Lowfat-I'll-Just-Have-A-Bite-Of-My-Neighbor's-Eggs-Benedict Breakfast.'"

In this part . . .

Okay, you've decided to lose, and you've chosen a weight loss plan. Now you need to implement your choice by understanding your nutritional needs, making the best choices when you eat out, buying the right food for meals made at home, or discovering when it makes sense to use (gasp!) food substitutes in place of real food.

Chapter 10

Nutrition for Dieters

• •

In This Chapter

▶ Discovering the nutrients your body needs

▶ Finding out what the Recommended Dietary Allowances (RDA) are

▶ Knowing what happens if you don't get the nutrients you need

▶ Choosing a supplement product

• •

*W*hen you go on a weight loss program, you may cut back on calories, but your body still says, "Hey, send down the nutrients I need." No sweat. (That comes later, in Chapter 18.) This chapter spells out exactly what those nutrients are. It shows how to balance your calories from protein, fats, and carbs and lists the precise amounts of vitamins, minerals, and other chemical goodies you need to stay healthy while losing weight.

I have to tell you in advance that this chapter runs longer than I expected. The problem is that I am a nutrition junkie. Nutrient numbers turn me on, and, like some who craves potato chips, I can't eat — I mean write about — just one. If you don't share my obsession, please feel free to skim a bit here, turn to another chapter for a while, and come back when you're ready for more. All these nutrient nuggets will be here waiting when you're ready for more.

How Much Nutrition Do You Need?

A healthful diet provides sufficient amounts of calories, protein, fat, carbohydrates, dietary fiber, and all the vitamins and minerals your body needs. Don't worry about how to cram this into a meal plan right now; I get to creating menus and shopping for nutritious diet meals in Chapters 11 and 12. Right now, your assignment, if you choose to accept it, is just to sop up some basic data on good policy for getting the calories, protein, fat, carbs, vitamins, and minerals your body needs.

Changing your diet in order to lose weight should never mean cutting back on essential nutrients. To find out how to apply the information you've just read about nutrients to your everyday life, see Chapter 11, which talks about planning weight loss meals.

Calories, protein, fat, and carbohydrates

Dealing with these four — calories, protein, fat, and carbohydrates — is a cinch. Chapter 5 is a detailed, and I mean mi-nute-ly detailed, explanation of exactly how many calories your require each day to keep on truckin'. Chapters 6 through 8 lay out the rules for diets that manipulate protein, fats, and carbs, including dietary fiber, to come up with New! Special! Guaranteed! weight loss plans.

I'll start here with recommendations from the U.S. Department of Agriculture/Health and Human Services Dietary Guidelines for Americans 2000 for reasonable daily consumption of fat, saturated fat, total carbohydrates, and dietary fiber.

The Guidelines say that:

- **The total amount of fat in your diet should not be more than 30 percent of all the calories you get each day.**

  Example: If your weight loss diet gives you 1,500 calories, no more than 450 calories should come from fat.

  1,500 x 0.30 (30 percent) = 450

- **No more than 10 percent of the calories you consume should come from saturated fat.**

  Example: If your weight loss diet provides 1,200 calories a day, no more than 120 calories should come from saturated fats.

  1,200 x 0.10 (10 percent) = 120

- **Carbohydrates (primarily the complex ones from fruits, vegetables, and whole grains) should account for 60 percent of your daily calories.**

  Example: If your weight loss diet provides 2,000 calories a day (yes, that sounds high, but it is just about right for a 220-pound man trying to get down to 200 pounds), 1,200 calories should come from carbs.

  2,000 x 0.60 (60 percent) = 1,200

- **You should get 11.5 grams of dietary fiber for every 1,000 calories you consume.**

  Example: On a 1,500 calorie diet, that means 17.25 grams of dietary fiber.

1,000 calories = 11.5 grams dietary fiber 500 calories = 1/2 11.5 = 5.25 grams dietary fiber

11.5 + 5.25 = 17.25 grams dietary fiber

Table 10-1 shows the number of calories from fats and carbs the Guidelines recommend for three common controlled-calorie weight loss regimens. Because the nutrition facts label at the supermarket lists nutrients in grams, the chart also lists the approximately equivalent number of grams. For your own reference,

✔ One gram of protein has four calories.

✔ One gram of fat has nine calories.

✔ One gram of carbohydrates has four calories.

✔ One gram of dietary fiber has 0 calories. (Your body does not absorb fiber.)

Table 10-1	Your Fat and Carb Allotments			
Total Calories Per Day	**Calories from Fat (total)**	**Saturated Fat**	**Carbohydrates**	**Dietary Fiber**
1,200	360 (40g)	120 (13g)	720 (180g)	0 (13.8g)
1,500	450 (50g)	150(17g)	900 (225g)	0 (17.3g)
2,000	600 (67g)	200 (22g)	1,200 (300g)	0 (23g)

Source: Adapted from Dietary Guidelines for Americans 2000.

Wait! What about protein? I'm glad you asked. Your protein requirements are set in terms of grams of protein per kilogram (2.2 pounds) of body weight. Because the average man weighs more than the average woman, his RDA for protein is higher than hers. The protein RDA for an average adult male, age 25 to 50, is 79 grams; for an average adult woman, age 25 to 50, it is 63 grams.

Vitamins and minerals

When you first think of nutrients, you probably think of vitamins and minerals. The most familiar set of recommendations for vitamins and minerals are the Recommended Dietary Allowances (RDA) created 60 years ago by the Food and Nutrition Board, a branch of the National Research Council, which is part of the National Academy of Sciences in Washington, D.C. RDAs exist for 18 vitamins and minerals:

✔ Vitamin A

✔ Vitamin D

✔ Vitamin E

- ✔ Vitamin K
- ✔ Vitamin C
- ✔ Thiamin (vitamin B1)
- ✔ Riboflavin (vitamin B2)
- ✔ Niacin
- ✔ Vitamin B6
- ✔ Folate
- ✔ Vitamin B12
- ✔ Calcium
- ✔ Phosphorus
- ✔ Magnesium
- ✔ Iron
- ✔ Zinc
- ✔ Iodine
- ✔ Selenium

In each case, the RDA has two special characteristics:

- ✔ **The RDA is an amount that can prevent but does not cure a specific nutrient deficiency.** For example, the correct RDA for vitamin C is 60 mg for women and men. Getting this amount of vitamin C will give you a sufficient reserve. If you already had scurvy, you would need much higher amounts of the vitamin to cure it.

- ✔ **RDAs are averages, not daily requirements.** For example, the RDA for vitamin C is 60 mg, about half the vitamin C in one 8-ounce glass of fresh orange juice. To meet this RDA, you can drink one 8-ounce glass of juice on Monday, skip Tuesday, drink another glass on Wednesday, and be just fine. Maybe even a bit better than fine. Two 8-ounces glasses of fresh OJ have 240 mg vitamin C. Divide that by 60 (the RDA), and you get 4, which means a 4 $\frac{2}{10}$th day's allotment. Whew! But wait! The time slot has to be reasonable. You can average three days, but you can't take 600 mg one day and then forget about Vitamin C for 10 days. A good rule: Be reasonable.

RDAs are not the only important numbers for vitamins and minerals. A second set of Food and Nutrition Board nutrient recommendations is the list of Adequate Intakes (AIs), originally known as Estimated Safe and Adequate Daily Dietary Intakes (ESADDI). You might say that AIs are high level guesswork, safe amounts of seven nutrients considered absolutely vital for your health, even though nobody knows exactly how much of each one you need. The nutrients in this category are

- ✔ Biotin

- ✔ Chromium

- ✔ Copper

- ✔ Fluoride

- ✔ Manganese

- ✔ Molybdenum

- ✔ Pantothenic acid

The Food and Nutrition Board's third nutrient brainchild is the Dietary Reference Intake (DRI). This set of numbers was created in 1993 by Food and Nutrition Board Dietary Reference Intake panels charged with re-examining the RDAs with an eye to the latest research and nutrition information. I bet you're not surprised to hear that the panel's first order of business was to establish a new standard for nutrient recommendations called — hold onto your hat here! — the Dietary Reference Intake.

Actually, the DRI is a catchall category that includes all the other categories of nutrient info such as:

- ✔ **Estimated Average Requirement (EAR):** The amount that meets the nutritional needs of half the people in any one group (such as teenage girls or people older than 70). Nutritionists use the EAR to figure out whether an entire population's normal diet provides adequate amounts of nutrients.

- ✔ **Recommended Dietary Allowance (RDA):** The average for individuals that ensures adequate supply but doesn't cure nutrient deficiency.

- ✔ **Adequate Intake (AI):** The recommended amount of a nutrient for which no RDA has yet been set.

- ✔ **Tolerable Upper Intake Level (UL):** The highest amount of a nutrient that you can consume each day without risking an adverse effect.

The Dietary Reference Intakes panels' first report, listing new recommendations for calcium, phosphorus, magnesium, and fluoride, appeared in 1997. Its most notable change was to increase the calcium RDA from 800 mg to 1,000 mg for adults age 31 to 50 and postmenopausal women taking estrogen and to 1,500 mg for postmenopausal women not using hormone replacement therapy.

The second DRI panel report, in 1998, had new recommendations for thiamin, riboflavin, niacin, vitamin B6, folate, vitamin B12, pantothenic acid, biotin, and choline. The most important revision was increasing the folate recommendation to 400 mcg a day based on evidence showing that folate reduces a woman's risk of giving birth to a baby with spinal cord defects and lowers the risk of heart disease for both men and women.

A third DRI report, in 2000, deals with the antioxidant nutrients vitamin C, vitamin E, selenium, and beta carotene. Citing inadequate information, the report cautioned against excessive use of beta carotene supplements. The report also recommends

- ✔ An increase in the RDA for vitamin C from 60 mg for all adults to 75 mg for women and 90 mg for men.

- ✔ An increase in the RDA for vitamin E from 8 mg for women and 10 mg for men to 15 mg (22 International Units [IU]) for adults.

- ✔ A daily intake of 55 mcg selenium for adults, with an upper limit (UL) of 400 mcg.

You can expect to see more DRI reports published through 2003 with recommendations for vitamin A, vitamin K, several trace elements (minerals) such as zinc, and other food components such as phytochemicals (phyto = plant; chemicals = chemicals, so for example, chemicals from plant). The complete new set of numbers is also expected by 2003.

Tables 10-2, 10-3, 10-4, and 10-5 show the current RDAs for adults, including those on weight loss diets. Table 10-6 shows the current ESADDIs for adults, including those on weight loss diets. The numbers in parentheses are the recommendations from Dietary Reference Intakes panels reports, which will almost certainly be incorporated into the next set of RDAs.

The tables use the following abbreviations:

- ✔ **g:** gram
- ✔ **RE:** retinol equivalent
- ✔ **mg:** milligram
- ✔ **a-TE:** alpha-tocopherol equivalent
- ✔ **mcg:** microgram
- ✔ **NE:** niacin equivalent
- ✔ **kg:** kilogram

Table 10-2			The RDAs		
Age (Years)	Vitamin A (mcg/RE)	Vitamin D (mcg)	Vitamin E (mg/IU)	Vitamin K (mcg)	Vitamin C (mg)
Males					
19–24	1,000	10	10	70	60 (90)
25–50	1,000	5	10	80	60 (90)
51+	1,000	5	10	80	60 (90)

Age (Years)	Vitamin A (mcg/RE)	Vitamin D (mcg)	Vitamin E (mg/IU)	Vitamin K (mcg)	Vitamin C (mg)
Females					
19–24	800	10	8	60	60 (75)
25–50	800	5	8	65	60 (75)
51+	800	5	8	65	60 (75)

Source: Adapted with permission from Recommended Dietary Allowances (Washington D.C.: National Academy Press, 1989), and interim DRI panel reports.

Table 10-3			The RDAs		
Age (Years)	Thiamin (Vitamin B1) (mg)	Riboflavin (Vitamin B2) (mg)	Niacin	Vitamin B6 (mcg/NE)	Folate (mcg)
Males					
19–24	1.5	1.7	19	2.0	200
25–50	1.5 (1.2)	1.7 (1.3)	19 (16)	2.0 (1.3)	200 (400)
51+	1.2	1.4	15	2.0	200
Females					
19–24	1.1	1.3	15	1.6	180
25–50	1.1	1.3 (1.1)	15 (14)	1.6 (1.3)	180 (400)
51+	1.0	1.2	13	1.6	180

Source: Adapted with permission from Recommended Dietary Allowances (Washington D.C.: National Academy Press, 1989), and interim DRI panel reports.

Table 10-4			The RDAs		
Age (Years)	Calcium (mg)	Phosphorus (mg)	Magnesium (mg)	Iron (mg)	Zinc (mg)
Males					
19–24	1,200	1,200	350	10	15
25–50	800 (1,000)	800 (700)	350 (420)	10	15
51+	800	800	350	10	15

(continued)

Table 10-4 *(continued)*

Age (Years)	Calcium (mg)	Phosphorus (mg)	Magnesium (mg)	Iron (mg)	Zinc (mg)
Females					
19–24	1,200	1,200	280	15	12
25–50	800	(1,000)	800 (700)	280 (420)	12
51+	800	800	280	10	12

Source: Adapted with permission from Recommended Dietary Allowances (Washington D.C.: National Academy Press, 1989), and interim DRI panel reports.

Table 10-5   The RDAs

Age (Years)	Iodine (mcg)	Selenium (mcg)
Males		
19–24	150	70
25–50	150	70
51+	150	70
Females		
19–24	150	55
25–50	150	55
51+	150	55

Source: Adapted with permission from Recommended Dietary Allowances (Washington D.C.: National Academy Press, 1989), and interim DRI panel reports.

Table 10-6	Estimated Safe & Adequate Daily Dietary Intakes				
Age (Years)	Biotin (mcg)	Pantothenic Acid (mg)	Copper (mg)	Manganese (mg)	Fluoride (mg)
Males					
19–24	30–100	4–7	1.5–3.0	2.0–5.0	1.5–4.0
25–50	30–100 (30)	4–7 (5)	1.5–3.0	2.0–5.0	1.5–4.0
51+	30–100	4–7	1.5–3.0	2.0–5.0	1.5–4.0
Females					
19–24	30–100	4–7	1.5–3.0	2.0–5.0	1.5–4.0
25–50	30–100 (30)	4–7 (5)	1.5–3.0	2.0–5.0	1.5–4.0
51+	30–100	4–7	1.5–3.0	2.0–5.0	1.5–4.0

Age (years)	Chromium (mcg)	Molybdenum (mcg)	Choline (mcg)
Males			
19–24	50–200	75–250	Not determined
25–50	50–200	75–250	Not determined
51+	50–200	75–250	Not determined
Females			
19–24	50–200	75–250	Not determined
25–50	50–200	75–250	Not determined
51+	50–200	75–250	Not determined

Source: Adapted with permission from Recommended Dietary Allowances (Washington D.C.: National Academy Press, 1989), and interim DRI panel reports.

What Happens If You Don't Get the Necessary Nutrients?

Nutrient deficiencies are serious stuff. For example, you need vitamin D in order to absorb calcium for strong bones. If you don't get enough vitamin D, your bones may suffer no matter how much calcium you swallow.

Luckily, many balanced weight loss diets, such as a controlled calorie regimen that encourages you to eat lots of fruits and vegetables, may actually provide more vitamins and phytochemicals (the newly identified goodies in plants) than your regular eating plan. Getting minerals such as calcium and iron from plant foods is a tad more difficult. On the other hand, many lower fat, lower calorie dairy products such as skim milk or fat-free yogurt actually have slightly more calcium than the full-fat version, and virtually all grain products sold in the United States are fortified with B vitamins and iron.

On the other hand, diets that emphasize one food or one nutrient while excluding others may be deficient in one or more nutrients. Some animals, such as cows and goats, are *herbivores* (from the Latin words for plant and eat). They have multiple stomachs and a long digestive tract that enables them to pull nutrients out of really complex plants like alfalfa. Others, such as lions and tigers, are *carnivores* (from the Latin words for meat and eat). They have one stomach and a short gut that requires meat, which gives up its nutrients in a flash. Human beings are *omnivores* (from the Latin word for all and . . . well, you know what). They have one stomach and a medium length gut that enables them to extract nutrients from animal foods (meat and dairy), as well as many plants. A diet that ignores one group of foods or another may make it hard to get the nutrient you need from food alone.

Table 10-7 lists the unpleasant effects that may occur when people don't get sufficient amounts of vitamins. Table 10-8 is an equally unpleasant list of problems associated with getting insufficient amounts of minerals.

Meeting RDA requirements protects you against nutrient deficiency. If your odd symptoms linger even when you follow a balanced diet with plenty of nutrients, something other than a vitamin or mineral deficiency may be to blame. When in doubt, don't guess. Don't self-medicate. Check with your doctor to be sure.

Table 10-7	Symptoms of Vitamin Deficiency	
If You Don't Get Enough Vitamin . . .	*Found In*	*Your Body May Show These Signs of This Deficiency*
Vitamin A	Yellow and green fruits and vegetables	Difficulty seeing in dim light; dry, rough or cracked skin; dry mucous membranes and eyes; slow wound healing; nerve damage; lessened sense of taste, hearing, and smell; reduced perspiration; and increased risk of respiratory infections.

If You Don't Get Enough Vitamin . . .	Found In	Your Body May Show These Signs of This Deficiency
Vitamin D	Fish, enriched milk	*Adults:* Osteomalacia (soft, porous bones that fracture easily). *Children:* Rickets (weak muscles, delayed tooth development, and soft bones).
Vitamin E	Nuts, seeds, oils	Reduced absorption of fat.
Vitamin C	Citrus, fruits, vegetables	Scurvy (bleeding gums; tooth loss; nosebleeds; bruising; painful or swollen joints; shortness of breath; increased susceptibility to infection; slow wound healing; muscle pains; and skin rashes.
Thiamin (vitamin B1)	Grain foods, meat, seeds	Poor appetite; unintended weight loss; upset stomach nausea, vomiting; depression; and loss of concentration.
Riboflavin (vitamin B2)	Grain foods, liver, milk	Inflamed mucous membranes, cracked lips, sore tongue and mouth, "burning" eyes; skin rashes; and anemia.
Niacin	Grain, meat, fish, poultry	Pellagra (diarrhea); inflamed skin and mucous membranes; mental confusion and/or dementia.
Vitamin B6	Grains, meat, fish, poultry	*Adults:* Anemia; convulsions; skin rashes; and upset stomach and increased risk of heart disease. *Infants:* Nerve damage.
Folate	Grains, vegetables, fruit	Anemia and increased risk of heart disease and fetal birth defects.
Vitamin B12	Meat, fish, poultry, milk	Pernicious anemia (damaged red blood cells; neurological/psychiatric symptoms due to nerve cell damage; increased risk of stomach cancer due to damaged stomach lining).

Sources: Recommended Dietary Allowances (Washington D.C.: National Academy Press, 1989).

Table 10-8	Symptoms of Mineral Deficiency	
If You Don't Get Enough of This Mineral . . .	*Found in*	*Your Body May Show These Signs of This Deficiency*
Calcium	Dairy products	Increased risk of osteoporosis; high blood pressure; and impaired blood clotting.
Phosphorus	Dairy products	Fragile bones and weak muscles.*
Magnesium	Grain foods, beans, nut, seeds	Weak muscles; cramps, tremor; irregular heartbeat; loss of memory; and confusion.*
Iron	Grains, meat, fish, poultry	Anemia (fatigue, greater sensitivity to cold temperatures)
Zinc	Grains, meat, poultry, oysters	Loss of appetite, decreased sense of taste; increased risk of infection; impaired wound healing; and impaired sexual function (male).
Iodine	Iodized salt, seafood	Goiter (swollen thyroid gland).
Selenium	Seafood, meat, organ meats, eggs	Muscle pain and weakness.

* Rare in the United States
Sources: Recommended Dietary Allowances (Washington D.C.: National Academy Press, 1989).

Vitamin and Mineral Supplements

Every year, Americans buy nearly $3 billion worth of *dietary supplements*, products the Food and Drug Administration defines as any pill, tablet, capsule, powder, or liquid you take by mouth that contains a dietary ingredient.

Clearly, vitamin and mineral products fill the bill. But is the bill worth paying? Some people say, yes. They like using supplements for "nutritional insurance" because they think the RDAs are just too low. Others regard them as a quick and easy way to get vitamins and minerals without the pesky fat and sugars in ordinary food. As you might expect, most nutrition professionals, including such prestigious practitioners as the American Dietetic Association, the National Academy of Sciences, and the National Research Council, generally prefer that healthy people invest their time and money whipping up meals and snacks that supply necessary nutrients via a balanced, tasty diet.

This stance is not mere academic pomposity: Learning how to use food intelligently — which means getting the nutrients you need — pays enormous dividends in the long run. It's like riding a bicycle. Once you've mastered the principles of preparing meals that give you the correct amount of vital nutrients, you never forget the basics.

But older people and people at any age who are on a weight loss diet, cutting back on food, and juggling meal plans, using a multivitamin and mineral product may be the simplest way to make sure that you meet your RDAs. To make it easy to pick an effective product, the Food and Drug Administration has come up with a consumer-friendly label for vitamin and mineral products similar to the Nutrition Facts label you find on food (which I talk about in Chapter 11).

FDA's supplement labels

The new supplement labels for vitamins and minerals must

- ✔ List every ingredient in the product, including "fillers" such as starch and sugar.
- ✔ Show the amount of the vitamin or mineral in each dose.
- ✔ Show the %DV for each vitamin and or per dose (translation: the *percentage daily value* — for example, the percentage of the RDA).

The label for any product that includes other dietary ingredients such as *botanicals* (herbs) or *amino acids* (the building blocks of protein) must

- ✔ Show the quantity per serving.
- ✔ Tell you there are currently no RDAs for these ingredients.
- ✔ Tell what part of the plant a botanical comes from (for example, leaves, flowers, roots — you name it).

This informative label is a good guide to what's in the package. Next question: Which package should you pick?

Choosing a vitamin and mineral supplement

Buying a vitamin, mineral, or combination supplement is just a matter of using your bean. For example, your common sense tells you to:

- ✔ **Choose a well-known brand.** Generally speaking, a respected name on the label gives you some assurance of quality product.
- ✔ **Read the ingredient list.** That way, you can to be certain that the product has the specific nutrients you want.

✔ **Choose a product with sensible doses.** Unless your doctor prescribes a dietary supplement as medicine, you probably don't need products marked "therapeutic," "extra-strength," or any variation thereof. Your best choice is one that follows the RDAs.

To find them, check out the column on the label that shows the DV%, the percentage of the Daily Value (RDA) the supplement provide. Yes, it's true, the old RDAs are lower than some newer recommendations. For example, the DV (RDA) for vitamin C is currently 60 mg for an adult, but the new RDI (thumb back a couple of pages to find a definition) is 75 mg for a woman and 90 mg for a man. A product that contains 60 mg vitamin C is described as having 100%DV, but you and I know that won't be true in a few years when the new RDAs are released. On the other hand, it's close enough for comfort.

✔ **Look for the initials USP.** They stand for U.S. Pharmacopoeia, a thoroughly reputable testing organization.

✔ **Check out effectiveness statements.** Under current law, the Feds can't require the safety and effectiveness tests on dietary supplements that they run on prescription or over-the-counter drug products. Phrases such as "release assured" or "proven release" may be your only guide.

✔ **Look for an expiration date.** Well-known brands, including store brands, usually move quickly off the shelves so that you get a fresh product, but here's another way to ensure freshness: Pick the package with the expiration date furthest from today. Naturally, you will pass up products ones that expire before you can use up all the pills, such as the 100-pill bottle whose expiration date is 30 days from now.

✔ **Check the storage requirements.** Even if you buy a product with the correct expiration date, it may be less effective if you don't keep it in the right place. Some supplements must be refrigerated; the rest should be stored, like any food product, in a cool, dry place. Never put dietary supplements in a cabinet over the stove or the refrigerator — true, the fridge is cold inside, but the motor pulsing away inside emits heat.

Finally, exercise good judgment. If a supplement label makes promises that sound good to be true — "Buy me! You'll live forever" — the reality is, it's too good to be true. FDA won't let supplement marketers say their products cure or prevent disease (that would make them medicines which is a whole other ball of wax and testing rules). But the agency does permit claims about how a product works, such as "maintains your cholesterol" rather than the medical claim that the product "lowers your cholesterol."

Chapter 11

Shopping for Weight Loss Meals

• •

In This Chapter

▶ Scheduling food purchases

▶ Balancing calories

▶ Filling your plate

▶ Adapting meals for different diets

• •

*T*his chapter is one long list of shopping tips, so if you already make a list before you trundle off to the supermarket or if you can read a Nutrition Facts Label at 50 feet, or if you already know how to choose your fruits and veggies, move on! On the other hand, if you're the kind of shopper who's often seduced by specials or those nifty fattening impulse items at the check-out counter, considers apples the only acceptable fruit, and often returns from shopping minus the carrots but with duplicates of items already in your kitchen cabinet, Stop! Read! Discover!

Oh, boy, that sounds like a march. Which, I might add, also helps take off pounds, as explained in Chapter 18.

What to Do Before You Shop

Supermarkets are designed to trap you into buying things you never thought you'd need (and probably don't). The aisles are cleverly arranged to highlight unusual items like, oh, canned chocolate-coated octopus. (Hey, if you were stuck with ten cases of that dubious special, you'd try to snare unwary shoppers, too!)

To avoid the traps, you need to plan ahead. That means

✔ Choosing a daily calorie allowance

✔ Making a shopping list

✔ Setting a realistic shopping schedule

Calorie-conscious food shopping

Most weight loss programs begin with a daily calorie allowance. Once you've settled on the number of calories you can consume each day, figuring out your shopping list is as easy as one-two-three:

- ✔ To determine your calorie allowance, check out Chapter 5. Hint: The most common calorie allowances for people who are trying to lose weight are 1,200 calories, 1,500 calories, and 1,800 calories. Caution: Less than 1,200 is considered unhealthy and possibly unsafe for adults.

- ✔ To find out how many servings of which kinds of food you get with your calorie allowance, run your finger over to Table 11-1, which is based on the Departments of Agriculture/Health and Human Services Food Guide Pyramid. (Chapter 6 has a picture of the Pyramid.)

Table 11-1	Recommended Daily Servings		
Food Group	*Number of Servings*		
	1,200 cal/day	*1,500 cal/day*	*1,800 cal/day*
Bread group	5	6	8
Fruit group	2	3	4
Vegetable group	3	3	4
Milk group	2	2	2 to 3
Meat group	5 oz.	6 oz.	7 oz.

Source: International Food Information Council Foundation; US Department of Agriculture, Food Guide Pyramid (1995).

Making a list

Okay. After you know what you need, you should be making a list, checking it twice, gonna find out what's naughty and . . . ooops! Right sentiment, wrong song.

But making lists is definitely *de rigueur* (that's French for "the right thing to do") when you need to control your supermarket purchases. The idea is to create a shopping list that ensures getting enough food from each group to meet your daily requirements. You probably eat lunch out or at your desk, so that means

✔ 7 breakfasts

✔ 2 lunches

✔ 6 dinners (Yes, you should treat yourself to a night on the town once a week. Maybe twice.)

Here are three ways to make lists:

✔ **Just make a list.** Buy one of those magnetic note pads; stick it on your refrigerator door; and write down things you need to buy when you go food shopping. Be sure to include the basics every week: bread, fruit, veggies, milk, and so on.

✔ **Click onto your CD-ROM and print Table 6-5 (daily food servings for a person on a 1,200 calorie diet) or Table 6-6 (ditto, 1,500 calories) or Table 6-7 (ditto, 1,800 calories).** Fill in what you need to buy to provide the right number of servings. Use that as a shopping list.

✔ **Click onto your CD-ROM for the Food Guide Pyramid shopping list.** Print one copy (see Figure 11-1). No, make that two, one for the door of your fridge and one for your purse. Oh, heck, print three. That way you'll have an extra, and you won't have to print it out again.

Once you've printed the Pyramid, write the number of your daily servings in each space. During the week, fill in the blanks. For example, if you run out of pasta, write that in the box for grains at the bottom of the Pyramid. Parmesan cheese goes into the dairy box. Olive oil into the space for fats and sweets. And so on. When you're ready to shop, check the Pyramid. Add or subtract items as required to bring your purchases into line with the Pyramid's recommended number of servings. When the whole thing looks about right, that's your shopping list, with — please note — room for a small number of goodies at the tippy-top. Oh, goodie!

Shopping on a schedule

As I said, groceries and supermarkets are out to get you to buy what they want to sell, which is not necessarily what you need to take home. (Yes, canned chocolate-covered octopus — or some variation on the theme — is waiting for you!) So your Mission Possible, should you choose to accept it, is to maneuver through the maze and arrive at the checkout counter with your shopping list intact.

One way to accomplish this task is to schedule shopping trips twice a week and stick to the schedule like glue. No random food runs. No, I-just-have-to-get-there-because-I'm-out-of-milk-for-my-cereal expeditions that end with your being loaded down like the yaks that ferry climbers' gear up Mt. Everest. You know as well as I do that going out for a quart of milk means coming back with cookies and ice cream. Shopping twice a week avoids that while giving you two passes at the perishables such as fresh fruits and veggies. Two trips. No kidding. No cheating.

A second sound stratagem is to eat before you shop. Yes, that's right — nibble on something healthy, take a nosh, have a piece of fruit or a slice of toast with lowfat cheese or a cup of yogurt. Taking the edge off your appetite makes you less susceptible to the blandishments of the marketplace, including the free tidbit samples at the deli counter.

Now all you have to do is get through the aisles.

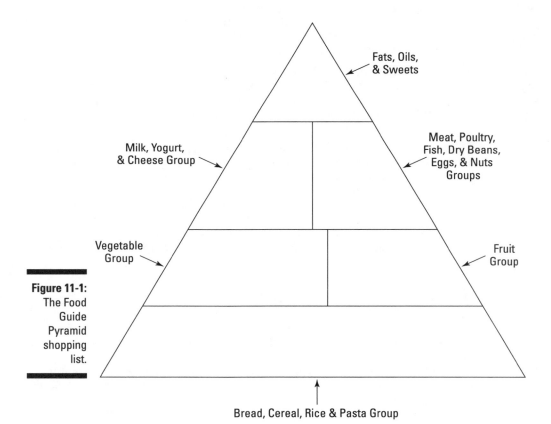

Figure 11-1:
The Food
Guide
Pyramid
shopping
list.

Surviving the Supermarket

Otherwise serious weight losers have been known to lose it totally when faced with a freezer case. Men and women who spend their working hours calculating orbits for space shuttles crumble when faced with the weekly Specials! circular. All those colors, all those lights, all that music, all that food!

Making it through the market with your shopping list (not to mention your self-esteem) intact means learning to use the tools of the trade, nutrition facts, health claims, and your own common sense ability to recognize a healthful food.

The nutrition facts food label

Peter Pan had Tinker Bell. You've got nutrition facts right there on the package. For example, there you are at the freezer case, irresistibly drawn to double dark chocolate ice cream (lots of fat, saturated fat, cholesterol, and a whopping 230 calories per ½ cup serving). But then, just as your hand is moving straight through the case, ready to reach for the ice cream, suddenly, out of the corner of your eye, you see the Nutrition Facts chart on the label of the lowfat but equally irresistible chocolate sorbet. It says, "No fat, no saturated fat, no cholesterol, and only 90 to 130 calories per serving." When you put the label side by side, is there any question which one comes out the winner?

I am not going to go into boring detail about exactly what's on the Nutrition Facts Label because all the info is in my book *Nutrition For Dummies.* But I can't pass up the chance to explain why the quantities on the Nutrition Facts label are listed in metric terms such as the gram rather than the more familiar (to American eyes) ounce and pound.

The gram and its smaller sisters, the milligram (¹⁄₁₀₀₀ gram) and the microgram (¹⁄₁₀₀₀th milligram), are practical terms with which to describe very, very small quantities such as the amount of vitamins, minerals, and other nutrients. For example, an ounce of dry matter, such as a soyburger or a breast of chicken, equals 28 grams. If the burger and the breast have 5 grams of protein per serving, it's easier on the brain to translate the protein content as "5 grams" rather than "⁵⁄₂₈ ounce."

Grams, milligrams, and micrograms also play a role in determining the % daily value (%DV), the amount of your daily requirement of a nutrient supplied by one serving of a particular food based on your total calorie consumption. If you read the nutrition facts label carefully, perhaps while standing in endless

Friday night or Saturday morning checkout lines, you will see that %DVs are based on diet providing 2,000 calories a day.

Why 2,000, you may ask. It's a fat story, I answer. The U.S. Departments of Agriculture/Health and Human Services' Dietary Guidelines For Americans recommend limiting your daily consumption of saturated fat to no more than 10 percent of your total calories. A diet with 2,000 calories a day permits 20 grams of saturated fat (10 percent×2,000). This amount appears to be low enough to protect older folk, particularly female Senior Citizens, the ones most vulnerable to heart disease. Because younger men and women often require more calories each day, food packages may also carry %DV for a 2,500 calorie diet if there's room on the label.

Of course, grams aren't the only quantities you will encounter in your search for a healthy diet. Table 11-2 is a handy guide to abbreviations and equivalents used on food labels (and in this book).

Table 11-2	Abbreviations and Equivalents
Abbreviation	*Equivalent*
oz	ounce
g	gram
mg	milligram
mcg	microgram
1 oz	28 grams (dry weight) or 30 grams (liquid weight)
1 g	1,000 milligrams or 1,000,000 micrograms
1 mg	1,000 micrograms

Health claims

Now what about those wonderful health claims you see on food packages? You know, the statement that one food or another can lower cholesterol, slim you down, turn your hair blonde — whatever. Well, those claims are regulated by law. Table 11-3 shows you what they mean.

Table 11-3	Health Claims	
This Term	*Applied to These Nutrients*	*Means the Food Has*
Free	Fat	Less than 0.5 g per serving
	Saturated fat	Less than 0.5 g per serving
	Cholesterol	Less than 0.5 g per serving
	Sugar	Less than 0.5 g per serving
	Calories	Fewer than 5 per serving
Low	Fat	3 g or less per serving
	Saturated fat	1 g or less per serving
	Sodium	140 mg or less per serving
	Cholesterol	20 mg or less per serving
	Calories	40 or less per serving
Reduced	Calories, all nutrients	Contains at least 25 percent fewer calories or less of a nutrient than the standard product
Light	Calories	⅓ fewer than the standard product
	Fat	50 percent less than the standard product
	Sodium	50 percent less than the standard product
Less*	Calories, all nutrients	25 percent less than the standard products
Lean	Meat, fish, poultry	Less than 10 g fat and 0.5 g or less saturated fat and less than 95 mg cholesterol per 100 g serving
Extra lean	Meat, fish, poultry	Less than 5 g fat and less than 2 g saturated fat and less than 95 mg cholesterol per 100 g serving
High	All nutrients	20 percent of more of the % Daily Value per serving

(continued)

Table 11-3 *(continued)*

This Term	Applied to These Nutrients	Means the Food Has
More	All nutrients	At least 10 percent more of a particular % Daily Value than the standard product
Good source	All nutrients	10 to 19 percent of the % Daily Value for a specific nutrient

"Fewer" is a synonym for "less."
Source: "The new food label," FDA Backgrounder, April 1994.

USDA and FDA have also approved specific statements about how a food or nutrient influences your risk of certain medical conditions. Table 11-4 lists approved claims.

Table 11-4 **Approved Food Label Health Claims**

Food/Nutrient	Health Claim
Calcium	That a food/diet high in calcium protects and reduces the risk of osteoporosis.
Fat	That a food/diet low in fat, saturated fat, and cholesterol reduces the risk of heart disease and some forms of cancer.
Dietary fiber	That a food/diet high in dietary fiber may reduce the risk of heart disease and some forms of cancer.
Sodium	That a food/diet low in sodium may reduce the risk of high blood pressure.
Fruits/vegetables	That a diet high in fruits and vegetables may reduce the risk of some forms of cancer.

The common-sense guide to unlabeled food

Some foods such as fresh meat, poultry, fish, fruits, and vegetables come without labels. It's up to you to recognize what's good to eat on your own. No problem:

✔ One 3-pound chicken yields four individual servings (two breast quarters and two leg/thigh quarters). As a result. a chicken is a wonderful diet food. You can chop it up, pull off the skin (all that fat and cholesterol), and freeze it in quarters for cooking later in the week. Can't stand dismembering the bird? Oh, go ahead: Buy cut-up quarters (legs and breasts).

✔ Fish has heart-healthy fatty acids (check out sat fat and unsaturated fat in Chapter 7), and is tasty, too. Some people keep fish overnight. I like to cook it the day I buy it.

✔ Americans love red meat. But does it have to be beef? Try lowfat frozen soy burgers or ground turkey (cook it way past medium, please!) as substitutes. Must have beef? Pick very, very lean ground round. For steak, choose sirloin; it's got less fat per ounce than other steak cuts. If you've got really strong teeth, pick *bracciola,* an Italian version of thinly sliced round, not as tender as sirloin, but steak nonetheless. For people with strong teeth. Or did I mention that already?

✔ Frozen entries do have labels, but I include them here because they come to mind when you're looking at main dishes. The frozen plates offer a quick respite from cooking on days when you just can't drag yourself to the stove. Give in once in a while. Just pick the lowfat entry. With veggies. Add a salad. Eat.

✔ Fruits and vegetables should register by color. Your best bet, nutrition-wise, are the greens and deep yellows. Plus the crucifers (onions, garlic, cauliflower, and other relatives of broccoli, Brussels sprouts, and cabbage).

Dishing Up Dinner

Arranging your own plate is a cinch. You check how many servings of which foods you should consume each day and stack up the food accordingly. But what happens when you're cooking for more than one, and the other individual does not want to be on your diet? How to dish up meals for him/her/them without breaking the rules for you?

The trick is to choose adaptable dishes.

✔ With roast chicken, you get the lowfat, skinless breast quarter with baked potato plus a salad with fat-free dressing. Your Significant Other(s) get the legs and thighs, plus a pat of butter or margarine on mashed potatoes, and regular dressing on the salad.

✔ With spaghetti, you get tomato sauce and a tossed salad; they get tomato sauce with a meatball and dressed salad. Your bread is warm but naked; theirs has garlic oil.

✔ You all get turkey burgers, but theirs come with a small side of fries. You get a baked potato.

Table 11-5 lists several such pairings that make it possible to serve the same meal two ways.

The pleasure principle

Repeat ten times after me: "Variety is the spice of (weight loss) life. Besides, I deserve a reward!"

Cutting calories is trying enough. Boring meals would be intolerable. And, yes, you do deserve a reward for working so hard to plan healthful menus. So isn't it nice to know that fat-free frozen yogurt actually counts as a source of calcium? Add fat-free chocolate syrup in small amounts, plus a sliced banana or some berries, and you've got one daily fruit serving, too. Oh, wow.

Table 11-5	Alternative Food Pairs	
Food	*For You*	*For Them*
Pasta	Basic tomato sauce	Basic tomato sauce plus a meatball and Parmesan cheese
Vegetables	Plain veggies	Veggies with butter
Salad	No-fat dressing	Regular dressing
Fruit	Fresh	Fresh with cream
	Poached (canned) no sugar	Poached (canned) with sugar syrup
Poultry	Skin-free	With skin
	White meat	White and dark meat
Dessert	Fat-free frozen yogurt	Ice cream
	Fat-free chocolate sauce	Hot fudge sauce
Coffee	Espresso	Cappuccino

Chapter 12

Eating Thin When Eating Out

· ·

· ·

*W*hen you're trying to lose weight, eating out can be a trying experience. All those choices! All those confusing menu terms! All those *big* portions! As you have guessed from the title, this chapter lays out stratagems to help you avoid diet disasters and control fat and calories as you make you way through the Menu Maze.

Adapting the Menu to Your Diet

In restaurants, people on a low-carb, high-protein weight loss plan have an easy time deciding what to eat. All they have to do is say yes to meat, fish, and poultry, and no to bread and starchy veggies.

People counting calories on a standard carb-based, lowfat weight loss diet face more complicated choices because they must keep on eye on portion sizes while hunting for hidden hazards such as cream in the sauce or butter in the veggies. The following guidelines should help.

Start smart

A carb-based, lowfat diner can enjoy the full Monty — no, not nude dining, but a full three- or four-course dinner — by starting with the right appetizer. What's right? Aw, c'mon, you know I mean a tasty but low-calorie, lowfat dish such as clear soup, a salad with lemon juice dressing, or shellfish such as shrimp cocktail (10 to 30 calories per shrimp) with catsup or horseradish sauce. Making this choice lets you continue ordering down the menu.

Pick an appetizer as your main course

Choosing an appetizer as a main course is another way to reduce fat and calories. With the increased popularity of lowfat, low-cal seafood, many restaurants serve an appetizer of a really big (and I mean *huge*) bowl of steamed mussels in their shells in a tomato-based sauce with one crusty piece of French bread underneath to sop it up with. Salads are also good choices. (Just hold the dressing or ask for a lowfat version.) Add a glass of cold, dry white wine, and one more piece of bread, and this "appetizer" can be a meal in itself. — with a lot fewer calories and less fat than many entries on the menu, including fish. It's cheaper, too.

Don't butter the bread

Don't oil it, either. Now that everybody knows vegetable oils are lower in sat fats than butter, many restaurants from pizza parlors to the fanciest white tablecloth establishment cater to their patrons sense of sophistication by substituting a small bowl of olive oil for the standard plate of butter pats. Before you reach for the oil, though, consider this: Vegetable oils, including the ubiquitous olive oil, are not an unmitigated blessing. Yes, the oils have less saturated fat than butter. True, they are cholesterol-free. True, they are rich in heart-healthy monounsaturated fatty acids. But the bad news is that all dietary fats — butter, margarine, oils — have about the same number of calories per serving, 100 to 125 calories per tablespoon. Sorry about that.

By the way, don't assume that your bread is lowfat just because you didn't butter it. Some breads come pre-buttered or oiled. One example is the Italian thick bread, focaccia. Another is the all-American popover. And don't forget muffins.

To test the fat content of your bread, pick up a piece and put it on your napkin. Hand sticky? Oil spots on the napkin? You know what that means.

Serve the veggies naked

Victorians boiled vegetables into a yucky muck — no color, no texture, no taste. Then came butter, cheese, and cream sauces, often broiled to a tasty brown crust. Sorry, but these are not for you if you're lowfat, carb-based. Instead, you want a dish for which the cook relies on herbs and spices or *reduced* (boiled down and thickened) fat-free bouillons or imaginative treatments such as purees and kabobs or lowfat stir-fry to make vegetables tasty but trim, a culinary technique leading to dining heaven and nutrition joy. The vegetable flavors come through loud and clear, while the calories stay very, very, very low.

Minimize the main dish

Lowfat, carb-based diners know fried or sauced foods are verboten. Best bet? Something broiled, baked, or roasted — without added fat and with the drippings siphoned off. You can further reduce the fat content of any meat or poultry main dish by wielding a mean knife and fork to cut away any visible fat. Yes, that means the crisp skin, too.

Another possibility is to order the main course without the main part. In other words, have your protein food (meat, fish, poultry) in your small-serving appetizer (remember those meaty mussels) and then assemble a main course of veggies or, again, a salad. It may cost a bit more to have a special dish assembled, and you may have to beg a bit, but most reputable restaurants will work with you. Especially if you point out that your strategy is allowing you to order three dishes — appetizer, main dish, and dessert (well, at least something sweet. More about that later) — instead of one.

What you want are all the nifty little extras that come with the real main dishes. No boring steamed stuff. No veggies so raw they have no flavor. (The difference between raw cauliflower and cauliflower that's been steamed for 30 minutes, then dusted with dill, is so fabulous that anyone who insists on passing the cold version should be charged with vegetable abuse). Instead, demand tiny boiled onions. Call for baby peas with mint. Pickled beets or red cabbage. Sugared unbuttered carrots. Darling little boiled or baked potatoes with a crust of paprika or cumin, the more, the merrier. The result? Fewer calories, more fiber, less fat, and a wider variety of vitamins, minerals, and phytochemicals. Oh, wow.

Control the portions

When it comes to serving sizes, restaurants can be hazardous to your diet. For example, according to the U.S. Departments of Agriculture/Health and Human Services Food Guide Pyramid, one serving of pasta is ½ cup. But not at your favorite Italian restaurant, where the standard serving of pasta, with or without sauce and parmesan, is typically four to six cups, a whopping 8 to 12 USDA/HHS servings.

You can check out Chapter 6 for a clear picture of how to measure standard serving sizes at home. But unless you are a true fanatic, you're probably not going to haul your measuring spoons along to your favorite restaurant. You need reasonable alternatives. Naturally, I have them. The Food Guide Pyramid serving size for most fruits and veggies is ½ cup — a portion about the size of your fist (okay, half the size of a really large fist). The serving size for a protein food such as meat, fish, or poultry is a deck of cards, about the size of the palm of your hand. (Yes, yes, a little smaller than a really big hand.)

Neat-o.

Sideline the sauce

Exercise some restraint. Ask your waiter to bring the sauce on the side. Take a teaspoonful. Hand back the rest. Out of sight, out of mind. Down 100 calories or more.

Share dessert — or substitute espresso

After a heavy meal, your body naturally craves something sweet. (You need the carbs to burn the food you've eaten; see Chapter 6.) One way to have your cake and eat it, too, without the fat and calories is to split a dessert. Another is to choose a sweet but fat-free treat such as berries. Or you can ask for fat-free sweetened espresso, Greek, or Turkish coffee. Hate coffee? Have a special tea or a soda.

When the Menu Says, "Eat Me, I'm Healthy," Ask for Proof

The people who make and market the foods you buy at the supermarket are required by law to detail ingredient labels on their packages (more about that in Chapter 11). Restaurants are ordinarily exempt. They don't have to tell you exactly what's in the "beef Stroganoff" or "vegetable stir-fry."

However, the exception is a dish for which the restaurant makes a health claim. If the menu copy says "lowfat" or "heart healthy" or has a cute little red heart next to the item, the Nutrition Education and Labeling Act requires backup. The backup can be an ingredient list on the menu, or the restaurant can simply keep on hand a notebook that:

- ✔ Lists the nutrient content of each labeled dish, or
- ✔ Shows that the dish was made according to a recipe from an authoritative professional association or dietary group such as the American Heart Association, or
- ✔ Demonstrates that the nutritional values for the dish are based on a reliable nutrition guide, such as the U.S. Department of Agriculture's voluminous Handbook #8, several volumes with perhaps a thousand pages of nutritional analysis for all kinds of food. (The abbreviated version of Handbook #8 appears in Appendix A, and it's online, as you can see in Chapter 20.)

As with the labels on food packages, this policy is designed to make sure that any food that claims to be "healthy" really is.

Exploring the Food Map

Every country in the world and some regions, too, has its own food fashions. Despite their differences, virtually all these places have meal plans that share some common features:

- ✔ A basic grain staple (bread, rice, pasta)

- ✔ A basic protein staple (meat, fish, poultry, and milk products)

- ✔ A basic seasoning pattern regarded as "ours" — basil and oregano in Italy, soy sauce plus wine and vinegar in China, tomatoes and chili peppers in Mexico, peanuts in some parts of Africa, or sour cream and dill and paprika in Eastern Europe

Best of all, every single one of these cuisines has something tempting to offer an adventurous gourmand. Alas, what's tempting may not fit into every diet. Table 12-1 is a simple guide to what works on a lowfat, carb-based meal plan.

Table 12-1	Choosing Lowfat/Carb-Based Ethnic Dishes
Chinese Food	**French Food**
Bean curd (not fried)	Au vapeur (steamed)
Moshu chicken/pork	En brochette (broiled)
Fresh noodles	Grille (grilled)
Seafood	
Shrimp & lobster sauce (minus egg yolks)	
Steamed dumplings	
Vegetarian dishes	
Velvet sauce (egg-whites)	
Indian Food	**Italian Food**
Chutney	Pasta
Dal (lentils)	Picata (lemon/wine sauce)*
Masala (curry)	Tomato sauces
Matta (peas)	Vegetable or seafood salad
Pilau (rice)	Wine sauces
Raita (yogurt & cucumbers)	

(continued)

Table 12-1 *(continued)*

Japanese Food	Mexican Food
Clear broth	Black beans and black bean soup
Miso soup or dressing	Ceviche (marinated seafood)
Mushimono (steamed)	Enchiladas, burritos, fajitas (minus cheese and/or sour cream)
Nimono (simmered)	Gazpacho
Sashimi	Rice & beans
Sushi (raw fish)	
Udon (fresh noodles)	
Yaki (broiled)	
Yakimono (grilled)	

*Ask them to make the meat/chicken without breading.

Did I mention that you can also edit many individual dishes? Consider the pizza. For a family whose dinner is divided by diet, pizza can be a noncombat zone where lowfat carb-based dieters:

- Switch to lowfat or fat-free cheese.
- Skip the cheese entirely.
- Add lowfat protein foods such as grilled chicken.
- Pile on the lowfat low-cal veggies such as broccoli or onions or mushrooms or — your choice.

Surviving on Fast Food

As you can see in Chapter 22, which lists diet-friendly fast-food choices, being on a weight loss diet doesn't mean you have to pass up fast food.

If that surprises you, the reason may be that you haven't actually stood there in a burger heaven trying to read the teensy little type on the nutrition chart pasted on the wall just about two inches higher than your eyes can see.

Well, I say, try harder. Drag a chair over to the wall, climb up, and read the thing. True, some of these places only have chairs welded to the tables. Yes, if you try to move one over to the wall, the manager will start sidling up to see what the heck you're doing. But be polite. Explain to him that you just want to choose the most diet-friendly item on his yummy menu. Smile. If he's a Good Guy, he'll pull out a printed brochure with the info in it, and you can read it as you eat your meal.

You'll be happy you took the time to do it. A fast-food burger (with roll for lowfat carb-based dieters, without roll for low-carb, high-protein aficionados), plus a salad, and a small lowfat milk or a cup (8 ounce) milk or a small diet cola may not sound like great nutrition, but the version served up in most fast-food restaurants is actually a pretty good meal. Table 12-2 compares the nutrient values of three basic McDonald's burger meals. Although all three have more carbs and less protein than most low-carb high protein diets recommend, they meet current USDA recommendations for lowfat high-carb diets: No more than 30 percent of your total calories should come from fat, although Meal No. 1 is slightly high in saturated fat, which should provide only 10 percent of total calories. The meals all meet USDA/HHS cholesterol guidelines and give you lots of vitamin A and vitamin C. Meal No. 1 and Meal No. 2 are also good sources of calcium. To define terms:

- The *burger* is the basic, small no-frills hamburger.

- The *garden salad* includes one packet of fat-free herb vinaigrette dressing.

- The *shake* is a small 414 ml (about 14 ounces) vanilla shake.

- The *milk* is an 8-ounce container of lowfat (1 percent) milk.

- The *cola* is a 16-ounce cup (small).

By the way, the initials *DV* stand for *daily value,* a nutritional guideline suggesting how much of each nutrient you should get each day from a 2,000 calorie diet. For the complete skinny on the DV and how it is used on food labels, check out Chapter 11.

Stop! Before you bite into that burger, remember that Table 12-2 is only a guide. Menus and ingredients often change, so check the nutrition charts at your local fast-food heaven.

Table 12-2	Nutritious Fast-Food Meals		
Nutrient Values	*Burger, Garden Salad, Small Lowfat Vanilla Shake*	*Burger, Garden Salad, Milk*	*Burger, Garden Salad, Small Cola*
Calories	710	450	490
% calories from fat	24%	24%	16%
% DV saturated fat	47%	26%	17%

(continued)

Table 12-2 *(continued)*

Nutrient Values	Burger, Garden Salad, Small Lowfat Vanilla Shake	Burger, Garden Salad, Milk	Burger, Garden Salad, Small Cola
% DV cholesterol	23%	13%	10%
% DV dietary fiber	22%	21%	21%
% DV vitamin A	130%	130%	120%
% DV vitamin C	50%	50%	45%
% DV calcium	50%	45%	15%

Source: The McDonald's Corporation.

If no brochures are at your local store, you may want to turn to Appendix A and click your way into the USDA Nutrition Database to call up nutrition info for brand name products, including fast-food items. Or you can click the companies directly. Table 12-3 lists Web site addresses for selected fast-food chains.

Table 12-3   Fast-Food Web Sites

Restaurant	Web Site
Au Bon Pain	www.aubonpain.com
Arby's	www.arbys.com
Burger King Corporation	www.burgerking.com
Dunkin' Donuts	www.dunkindonuts.com
Kentucky Fried Chicken	www.kentuckyfriedchicken.com
McDonald's Nutrition Information Center	www.mcdonalds.com
Pizza Hut	www.pizzahut.com
Subway	www.subway.com
Wendy's International Inc.	www.wendys.com

Flying High

What can you say about airplane food? Or should I ask, what can you say *good* about airplane food?

True, Air France has pretty good wine and a yummy Asian veggie meal. Yup, the lowfat tea sandwiches on British Air are to die for. But more often than not, especially on domestic flights, meal time is not a happy foodie moment, and it's not much better for diet-conscious flyers.

Yes, the portions are so small their effect may be negligible, but if your diet is lowfat, low-cholesterol, low-salt, or low-calorie, you can call ahead and reserve a special meal that, by law, must conform to the standards set by the Food and Drug Administration as listed in Table 12-4.

Did you know that when writing about quantities of nutrients (or anything else), the scientific shorthand for *more than* and *less than* is an open arrow? The arrow points to the right (>) for *more* and to the left (<) for *less*. In print, the symbol looks like this:

>1 = more than 1

<1 = less than 1

Now you know.

Table 12-4	Measuring Low-Cholesterol, Lowfat, and Low-Sodium
Term	*Meaning*
Low-calorie	<120 calories per serving*
Lowfat	<3 grams fat per serving*
Low-cholesterol	<20 mg cholesterol per serving*
Low-sodium	No more than 140 mg sodium per serving

* One serving = 100 grams/3.5 ounces
Source: Food and Drug Administration.

But not even the government can guarantee taste and flavor, so when we fly, my husband and I tote along out own provisions for our preferred carb-based, lowfat diet.

The night before a flight, we toss a couple of individual gelatin or pudding desserts into the freezer, along with lowfat cheese or sliced chicken sandwiches (on toast, with no condiments to sog the bread). Just before leaving the house, the frozen desserts and sandwiches go together into one plastic baggie. We fill a second plastic bag with fresh or dried fruit, plus napkins, plastic spoons, and small packets of mustard, ketchup, or mayonnaise. Then we drop everything into a small shopping bag. As the plane leaves the ground, we feast on nicely defrosted food. Great dining? No. But it keeps us nutritiously provisioned from here to wherever.

To assemble a lunch box at the airport, lowfat, carb-based dieters can pick a turkey sandwich with mustard or catsup. Add some fruit. A lowfat or fat-free muffin's okay. So is one of those big pretzels so long as you knock off some of the humongous salt crystals.

Or what the heck. As I said, the portions on airplane meals are so small, you can surrender this once and forget it. Just don't eat the cheesecake.

Bon voyage.

Chapter 13

Measured Meals and Formula Foods

This chapter is about practical help for the previously hopeless, people who want to lose weight but can never quite get the hang of measuring portions or figure out exactly how to cut calories and still get all the nutrients they need. Does that sound like you? Then this is your lucky day because I am about to introduce you to products that will make it easier for you to meet weight goals without your having to do anything but buy, mix, pop, or crunch. In other words, weight loss Heaven!

Measured Portions

Remember when Mom used to cut up your meat into teeny, tiny pieces you could handle without dropping stuff all over the floor?

Remember how she would put small portions of food into special places in your dinner plate so you got just enough of everything you were supposed to eat?

Well, Mom's not going to do that any more, but several people are more than willing to step in for her. At the top of the list are a gaggle of weight loss programs, which sell prepacked meals. On the other hand, the U.S. Departments of Agriculture/Health and Human Services prefers to teach you how to slice up calories yourself. After all, when it comes to serving food, size counts.

Here's proof. In France, everyone eats everything Americans have been taught to fear: high-fat foods such as pâté de fois gras, whole milk cheese, butter-basted chicken, and on and on and on. Yet they still stay slim, and a French man's risk of heart disease, though higher in recent years, is still lower than an American's. Scientists call this the *French Paradox.* I call it plain old portion control, a variant of "everything in moderation."

So does Bonnie Taub-Dix, media representative for the New York State Dietetic Association. "When you order salmon with cheese sauce in France, you get three small pieces of salmon with a little piece of cheese in the middle," she says. "In the United States, the serving would be a piece of salmon the size of a brontosaurus bone with cheese melted all over it."

In other words, a portion in France is not the same as a portion in the United States. Actually, an American portion may not be what it once was, either. The present-day New York bagel is now a whopping four servings from the bread group represented on the Food Pyramid, and the standard cola, once six ounces, has now morphed into a 20-ounce giant. Of course, as the portions inflated, so did Americans.

How to beat the Bigs? Easy. Either learn to control your own portions, or have someone else (no, not Mom!) do it for you.

Using the Food Guide Pyramid to measure portions

Every once in a while, you may wonder exactly what you get for the tax dollars you send down to Washington. One very good example is the USDA/HHS Food Guide Pyramid, an eating plan based on "measured portions" that enables you to put together a controlled-calorie diet with lots of tasty variety and plenty of essential nutrients.

To see how easy it is to keep your diet in line, serving-size-wise, just refer to the Food Guide Pyramid in Chapter 6 where you can find a short guide to serving sizes (Table 6-8). It tells you how to mush up food into sample serving sizes (a golf-ball-size portion of rice, for example), so that you can see what a portion really looks like.

Or check out Table 13-1, which shows you the Food Guide Pyramid's recommendations for daily servings of specific portions of several basic foods. The number of servings per day is based on a diet ranging from 1,600 calories a day at the lower end to 2,800 calories a day at the top. Neat.

Table 13-1	What's One Portion?	
Food	*One Portion*	*Recommended Servings Per Day**
Fruit and vegetables	One medium whole fruit or veggie, or ½ cup chopped, sliced, or cooked	5 to 9
Grains	½ cup cereal, pasta, rice, etc., 1 slice bread	6 to 11
Meat, fish, poultry (leaned, cooked)	2 to 3 ounces	5 to 7
Dairy foods	1 cup milk/yogurt, ½ to 1 ounce cheese	2 to 3

* The lower number is for a 1,600 calorie diet; the higher number applies to a 2,800 calorie diet. Source: USDA.

The Pyramid is a blueprint for a lowfat, carbohydrate-based diet. To see how it works, you can flip back several chapters to Chapter 6 or click on to the Chapter 6 tables on your CD-ROM. These charts lay out the portion allowances for people on 1,500, 2,000, and 2,500 calorie diets. Pick the one that fits your needs and fill in the blanks. There's your measured portion diet. Wouldn't it be great if every problem were so easily solved?

Picking prepacks

Anyone who's ordered takeout or zapped a frozen dinner in the microwave knows the joy of having someone else do all the work.

Prepacked measured meals come from weight loss marketers, such as Weight Watchers, Jenny Craig, The Zone, and others, whose programs are described in Chapter 17. The primary aim is to make sure that you get just enough — and no more.

You can take it for granted that prepacked meals from reputable companies:

- ✔ Are low-cal and meet nutrition guidelines.
- ✔ Save time and energy you'd otherwise spend shopping for food and cooking it.
- ✔ Taste okay, some better than others. (What did you expect? I told you Mom's not the one in the kitchen.)

Scaling down the Pyramid for kids

USDA has created a version of the Food Guide Pyramid just for kids. As you can see, this daily guide for children 2- to 6-years-old is based on the same servings that work for you.

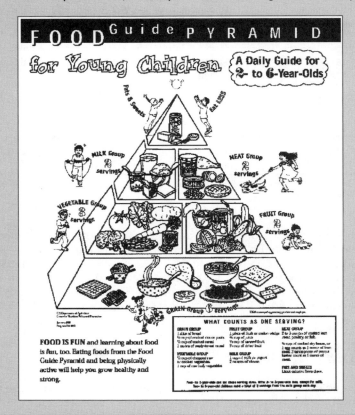

Given the diversity of plans — home delivery versus pick-it-up-in-the-supermarket-freezer — prices differ wildly. Before you take the plunge into prepacked meals, you may want to take a calculator to the supermarket (or the telephone or online Web site) and do some careful addition. Depending on your time, your tastes, and your dedication to home cooking (or your utter loathing for the kitchen), you may choose to:

✔ Go for broke and get everything ready-made.

✔ Choose a couple of prepacked meals a week and stick them in the freezer for times when you're so ragged out that you don't even have the energy to boil (calorie-free) water.

✔ Forgo the prepacks and devote one afternoon a weekend whipping up individual portions you can thaw and serve the following week (more about that in Chapter 11).

Or you may simply opt to substitute something else for one food meal a day.

Substitutes for Real Meals

Cutting back on food isn't the only way to cut back on calories.

You can also cut out food entirely, at least one meal at a time.

No, I don't mean fasting, (which I discuss in Chapter 9). I mean using food substitutes.

The old fogies in the nutrition establishment call meal substitutes *formula foods*. A generation tuned into computer lingo might call them *virtual foods,* even though you can see, taste, and feel them. Either way, what I am talking about are the powders, liquids, and bars touted as miracle "meals" in ads populated by skinny models who look like they wouldn't recognize an extra pound if it came up and bit them on the. . . . Whooooops! Almost slipped there.

But will they work for real people? The short answer is, yes. The longer answer is, if used with care.

Formula foods then and now

Early formula food products were tasteless, sometimes downright unpalatable, hard-to-dissolve high-protein powders meant to be blended into whatever liquid met your fancy. Their only benefit was protein; sometimes, not very high-quality protein (a topic discussed in Chapter 7).

The first popular liquid meal substitute was Metrecal, a 1960s product that was available in soup flavors as well as the standard vanilla and chocolate. In the pre-sat fat era, this diet product was smoothed out with palm kern/coconut oil, a highly saturated fat that clogs your arteries.

The first "candy bar" type formula food snack was actually a candy bar, the calorie-dense, nutrient-enriched block of chocolate produced by Hershey Chocolate for soldiers on the battlefield in World War II. Would you be surprised to discover that the bar was much more popular than dried out C-rations?

Today's formula food products taste better than the originals, but the format's pretty much the same:

- The quick-dissolving powders are made to be mixed with milk for a complete, lowfat, low-calorie meal. Hate milk? Choose an unflavored powder and mix it with juice.

- The liquids are complete, lowfat low-calorie meals you can shake and drink from the can as soon as you pop the lid.

- The bars come in two versions. The first is a complete, lowfat, low-calorie meal (is there an echo in here? I seem to be repeating myself). The second is a "high energy" snack, not enough nutrition for a meal, just enough to give you a boost late in the afternoon — or late in the race.

Formula powders and liquids are available under a fairly limited list of brand names, but bars seem to number in the zillions. Okay, maybe that's an exaggeration, but I did count 60 different ones in the list compiled by The Center for Science in the Public Interest (CSPI), a consumer-advocacy group, which rated meal/snack bars in the December 2000 edition of its popular publication, the *Nutrition Action Health Letter*.

To quality as a meal substitute, a bar should give you:

- A reasonable limit on calories, say around 200 calories per serving

- A respectable amount of protein (experts recommend 15 grams per serving)

- A healthy dose of dietary fiber (some bars have a healthy 5 grams per serving)

- A manageable amount of total fat (3 grams or less per serving qualifies as "low fat) and saturated fat (2 grams is okay; 1 gram — or less — is better)

For a complete rundown on formula bars, click onto CSPI's ratings, cleverly titled "Bar Exam" (cute!), at www.cspinet.org/nah/12_00/barexam.html.

Excellent ingredient lists

Package labels for Real Foods list all ingredients plus calories and nutrition data for protein, fat, sat fat, carbs, fiber, plus a couple of vitamins and minerals. Labels for formula food products are more complete: every ingredient *plus* all important nutrients.

Table 13-2 lists the ingredients in a representative formula powder, formula liquid, or formula bar meal substitute. For convenience sake, I've chosen three products from the same manufacturer. For simplicity's sake, I've grouped ingredients into just four categories in Table 13-2:

- *Protein* means the source of the protein in the product.

- *Texturizer* is a catchall label for all the ingredients from gums to oils that smooth out the texture or keep other ingredients from separating and generally make the formula food feel good in your mouth.

- *Flavoring agents* means things that make the product taste good.

- *Other* includes nutrients such as vitamins and minerals, and dietary fiber, plus non-nutrients such as coloring agents.

Table 13-3 shows you the nutrient content of the same products. Look carefully Do you see something interesting? That's right. Almost all vitamins and minerals are present in an amount listed as "35%," which stands for "35% DV," which translates to "35% Daily Value," which in this case means slightly more than one-third the RDA for a person whose diet supplies 2,000 a day.

Table 13-2	Decoding the Formula		
Products	**Powder***	**Liquid+**	**Bar#**
Protein sources	Whey protein concentrate, soy protein isolate, nonfat dry milk, sweet dairy whey	Fat-free milk	Nonfat milk, nonfat yogurt powder, soy protein isolate, milk protein isolate
Texturizers	Gum arabic, powdered cellulose,guar gum,carrageenan, soybean lecithin, cellulose gum, xanthan gum, cornstarch	Calcium caseinate, gum arabic, cellulose gel, cellulose gum, mono- and diglycerides, soybean lecithin carrageenan, canola oil	Palm kern oil, soy lecithin, calcium caseinate, partially hydrogenated soybean and/ or cottonseed oil, cellulose gel, guar gum
Flavoring agents	Sucrose, fructose, maltodextrin aspartame, artificial flavor	Sugar, cocoa, artificial flavor	Maltodextrin, dextrose, natural flavors, corn syrup, salt, brown sugar, high maltose corn syrup, honey
Other	25 vitamins and minerals, soy fiber	22 vitamins and minerals, water, caramel color,	22 vitamins and minerals, raisins, toasted

(continued)

Table 13-2 *(continued)*

Products	Powder*	Liquid+	Bar#
		FD & C Red 3, FD & C Yellow 6	rolled oats, graham cracker cookie pieces, sodium bicarbonate lemon juice, natural and artificial flavors

* Ultra Slim-Fast Strawberry Supreme
+ Ultra Slim-Fast Creamy Milk Chocolate
# Slim-Fast Meal on-the-go Oatmeal Raisin
Source: Product labels on shelves in New York City, December 2000.

Table 13-3	Comparing Representative Formula Food Meal Substitutes		
Nutrient (Per Serving)	Powder* (3 T. Plus 8-Oz. Nonfat Milk)	Liquid+ (1 11-oz can)	Bar# (1 bar)
Calories	200	220	220
Protein (g)	5	10	8
Total fat (g)	0.5	3	5
Saturated fat (g)	0	1	3.5
Cholesterol (mg)	5	5	>5
Total carbohydrates (g)	25	40	36
Dietary fiber (g)	4	5	2
Sugars (g)	20	35	19
Vitamin A	50%	35%	35%
Vitamin D	59%	35%	35%
Vitamin E	100%	--	35%
Vitamin K	25%	25%	25%
Vitamin C	50%	100%	35%
Thiamin	35%	35%	35%
Riboflavin	30%	35%	35%

Nutrient (Per Serving)	Powder* (3 T. Plus 8-Oz. Nonfat Milk)	Liquid+ (1 11-oz can)	Bar# (1 bar)
Niacin	50%	35%	35%
Vitamin B6	35%	35%	35%
Folate	30%	30%	30%
Vitamin B12	50%	35%	35%
Biotin	50%	35%	35%
Pantothenic acid	50%	35%	35%
Calcium	50%	40%	30%
Iron	35%	15%	15%
Zinc	35%	15%	15%
Phosphorus	35%	40%	25%
Iodine	35%	35%	35%
Magnesium	30%	35%	35%
Copper	10%	--	--
Selenium	25%	25%	25%
Manganese	35%	35%	--
Chromium	35%	35%	35%
Molybdenum	35%	35%	35%
Chloride	10%	--	--

-- No amount listed on label
* Ultra Slim-Fast Strawberry Supreme
+ Ultra Slim-Fast Creamy Milk Chocolate
# Slim-Fast Meal on-the-go Oatmeal Raisin
Source: Product labels on shelves in New York City, December 2000.

Will Formula Food Products Help You Lose Weight?

Absolutely. Just look at the calorie count. Your "normal" lunch probably serves up about 500 calories or more. If you switch to a formula food meal that clocks in at about 200 calories, you've just cut 300 calories off your daily

Five facts for formula food dieters

Wait! Before you rush out to buy a powder, liquid, or bar, read these rules:

Fact #1. Your doctor is the best judge of whether a formula food diet product is right for you.

Fact #2. Formula food is meant to be used in place of one meal a day, no more.

Fact #3. Formula foods don't work as "add-ons." At 200+ calories a pop, "extra" bars and drinks pile on pounds.

Fact #4. Products that look alike can have very different amounts of some nutrients such as fats. Read the label before you bite!

Fact #5. Your body needs at least 1,200 calories a day, even when you're dieting. If you're very large, you may need even more to avoid nutrition trouble, which is why Fact #1 is first on this list.

intake. To lose one pound, you have to cut back 3,500 calories. Stick to the formula lunch without increasing the amount of calories you get during the rest of the day, and you'll drop 3,500 calories and one pound in 11.6 — heck, call it 12 — days. Guaranteed.

On the other hand, formula foods probably won't help keep pounds off long term. Neither mixing a powder nor pouring a liquid nor ripping open the wrapping on a formula food bar will teach you how to whip up nutritious weight loss meals or snacks on your own. As a result, once you lose weight, breathe a sigh of relief, and toss out the substitute meal products, guess what? You're likely to gain back the weight you lost. Maybe more.

But that's a problem for another day. Or another chapter. Like Chapter 5, which tells you how to count and control calories, or Chapter 11, which shows you how to plan weight loss meals, or Chapter 17, which discusses how to change your attitudes and stay trim, or Chapter 18, which shows you how to use exercise for the same purpose.

Formulas for weight gain

I want to take a minute to talk about liquid nutritional supplements such as ENSURE, NUTRAMENT, SUSTACAL, and the less expensive but equally nutritious private label (store) brands. These products may look like petite versions of the formula weight loss products, but they're not.

One frivolous but significant difference is immediately apparent in the advertising. Ads for weight loss liquids feature foxy babes. Ads for nutritional supplements features foxy grannies. This is not surprising when you consider the second, more important difference: the calorie count. An 11-ounce can of a formula weight loss liquid gives you a measly 220 calories. An 8-ounce can of a nutritional supplement has 230. Do the math, and you'll see that the supplement has about 50 percent more calories per ounce than the weight loss product:

Example #1: Weight loss liquid

$$\frac{220 \text{ calories}}{11 \text{ ounces}} = 20 \text{ calories per ounce}$$

Example #2: Nutritional supplement

$$\frac{230 \text{ calories}}{8 \text{ ounces}} = 28.75 = 29 \text{ calories per ounce}$$

An anyone can plainly see, the target audience for the nutritional supplement isn't dieters. It's people who want to gain or maintain weight while bringing their vitamin and mineral intake up to par, such as:

- Naturally thin folks who would give a skinny arm and a leg for some round padding at hips, buttocks, and breast.

- Senior Citizens like Foxy Granny whose appetite ain't what it used to be. (Their eyes aren't, either, so they may have trouble reading that teensy little type on the label. Shame on the marketing managers!)

- People with a chronic illness that torpedoes appetite or makes it difficult to swallow solid food.

Table 13-4 lists the percentage of the RDAs in one representative product, based (as usual) on a 2,000 calorie a day diet. Look quickly, and it seems that the supplement has smaller amounts of vitamins and minerals than you get from a formula food liquid meal. But wait! Once again, do the math. Comparing the representative liquid in Tables 13-3 and 13-4 shows you that the two are pretty much equal in most vitamins and minerals.

Example #1: The 11-ounce formula weight loss drink provides 35% DV for vitamin A.

$$\frac{35 \text{ percent}}{11 \text{ ounces}} = 3.125\% \text{ DV per ounce}$$

Example #2: The 8-ounce liquid supplement provides 25% DV for vitamin A.

$$\frac{25 \text{ percent}}{8 \text{ ounces}} = 3.125\% \text{ DV per ounce}$$

Table 13-4	What's In A Formula Supplement?
Nutrient Per Serving	*8-Ounce Private Label Nutrition Supplement*
Calories	250
Protein (g)	5
Total fat (g)	6
Saturated fat (g)	0.5
Cholesterol (mg)	<5
Total carbohydrates (g)	40
Dietary fiber (g)	0
Sugars (g)	14
Vitamin A	25%
Vitamin D	25%
Vitamin E	25%
Vitamin K	25%
Vitamin C	50%
Thiamin	25%
Riboflavin	25%
Niacin	25%
Vitamin B6	25%
Folate	25%
Vitamin B12	25%
Biotin	25%
Pantothenic acid	25%
Calcium	30%
Iron	25%
Zinc	25%
Phosphorus	30%
Iodine	25%
Magnesium	25%

Nutrient Per Serving	8-Ounce Private Label Nutrition Supplement
Copper	25%
Selenium	25%
Manganese	60%
Chromium	25%
Molybdenum	50%
Chloride	10%

Source: Duane Reade Liquid Nutrition Package label on sale in New York City, December 2000.

Other food substitutes

Formula foods and supplements give you enough nutrients and calories to enable you to whack off excess calories from a whole meal or snack at one clip. Other substitute foods simply nibble at the edges of your calorie consumption. But take care of the nibbles and surprise! The pounds may take care of themselves.

For example, Table 13-5 tells you exactly how many calories you can lop off each cup of coffee or tea by using an artificial sweetener instead of sugar. Does this seem insignificant? Wait: There are 4 grams of sugar in one teaspoon. At 4 calories a gram, that equals 16 calories. Three cups of coffee a day, one teaspoon sugar per cup, equals 48 calories. Pass up those 3 teaspoons, and in just about 73 days, you will have cut back 3,500 calories, enough to skim one whole pound off your hips. Painlessly.

Table 13-5		Sweet, Sweeter, Sweetest
Sweetener	**Calories Per Gram**	**Sweetness Relative to Sugar***
Sugar (sucrose)	4	-------
Acesulfame-K	0	150 to 200 sweeter than sugar
Aspartame	4	160 to 200 times sweeter than sugar
Cyclamates	0	30 to 60 times sweeter than sugar
Saccharin	0	200 to 700 times sweeter than sugar
Sucralose	0	600 times sweeter than sugar

* The range of sweetness represents estimates from several sources.
**Yes, aspartame has 4 calories per gram, but you need so little to get a sweet flavor that you can count it as 0 calories per serving.

Do I hear some questions? Oh, you want to know if eating sugar substitutes makes you crave sweets? No, it doesn't. But eating foods sweetened with sugar substitutes can make you gain weight. Yes, you read that right. Here's why: Even though the substitutes subtract calories, the rest of the ingredients in your sugarfree treats — flours, eggs, milk, and so on — do have calories. If you eat one sugarfree cookie instead of one cookie with sugar, you subtract calories. But gobble up five sugarfree cookies instead of that one cookie with sugar, and your calorie total soars. Me, oh, my, there's just no free lunch. . . . I mean cookie.

Another substitute that will reduce your calorie intake is fake fat. These products come in four basic varieties:

✔ Carb-based products such as vegetable gums and dietary fiber that make food feel smooth and thick. (See Table 13-2 for some of the texturizers in formula foods.)

✔ Fat-based products such as olestra (trade name: Olean) whose chemical structure has been altered so that your body cannot absorb it. No absorption, no calories.

✔ Protein-based products such as Simplesse whose lush creaminess comes from egg whites or milk protein.

✔ Combination products such as the new cholesterol-lowering spreads Benecol and Take Charge, which are less than 50 percent fat. (The rest is water plus colors, flavors, and veggie solids.)

Most fat replacers are used only in processed foods such as baked goods, frozen desserts, or snacks (chips) or to fill in the space when fat is removed from processed meats or cheeses. Only the combination products are meant for your dining table, at home, on your very own breakfast toast. They won't work for baking or frying because they're less than half fat. When they melt, you get a small puddle of fatty water that would turn out soggy French Fries, not crisp ones. Sorry about that.

FDA has given olestra a clean bill of health, but fairness requires me to report that some people develop gastric upset, including potentially serious diarrhea, when they eat products made with this fat substitute. In addition, there is some concern that eating olestra may prevent your body from absorbing nutrients such as vitamin A and vitamin D, which dissolve only in fat. And finally (there is always a finally), using fat substitutes is one way to cut calories, but repeated studies show that the only way to take off weight and keep it off is to change your lifestyle (translation: exercise!) and learn to handle food intelligently.

Part IV
Other Ways to Lose Weight

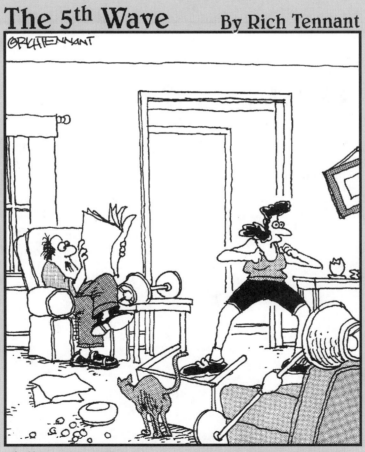

The 5th Wave   By Rich Tennant

"I'm glad kickboxing relaxes YOU!"

In this part . . .

Diet counts, but when rearranging your food choices doesn't do the job, medicine can offer two serious alternatives for people who are dangerously obese. This part explains how diet drugs work, listing their benefits and side effects. You also find info about weight loss surgery, a growing specialty for those whose weight is high enough to threaten their lives. A weighty part indeed.

Chapter 14

Weight Loss Pills and Potions

. . . .

In This Chapter

▶ Understanding the medicines that help you lose weight

▶ Finding out who should use weight loss medication

▶ Discovering the risks and benefits of weight loss drugs

▶ Becoming familiar with herbal weight loss products

. . . .

*T*his chapter is not for casual dieters. The information is pretty technical: drug names, side effects, that sort of thing. If your goal is just to peel off ten pounds so that you can slip into a slinky gown two weeks from Tuesday, your best bet is to flip back to Part II or fast forward to Part V. On the other hand, what you see here just might come in handy the next time a friend needs some advice on how to lose weight without popping fat pills. Reading it couldn't hurt.

Knowing Who Should Use Weight Loss Medication

As a general rule, obesity experts say that weight loss drugs, also known as *fat pills* or *diet drugs,* should be reserved for those men and women with serious weight-related issues such as:

✔ A need to lose 100 pounds or more.

✔ A body mass index (BMI) of 30 or higher.

✔ A BMI of 27 or higher plus such weight-related health risk factors such as diabetes, high blood pressure, or high cholesterol. (Psst! For the lowdown on BMI, check out Chapter 2.)

Is this cautious approach justified? Yes. Taking weight loss medications may take pounds off fast, but it doesn't mean you'll keep them off. According to the National Task Force on Prevention and Treatment of Obesity, weight loss medication is a long-term commitment: If you need pills to lose weight, you'll need to take pills long term to keep it off.

 Even more important, most weight loss drugs have potentially serious side effects. Most medicine is a balancing act in which the benefits sit on one side of the see-saw, and the risks sit on the other. If all you have to lose are those darned last ten pounds, this particular medical see-saw may not be weighted in your favor.

Understanding What Weight Loss Medicines Are

Broadly speaking (which may not be the right phrase to use about weight loss products), all currently approved diet drugs fall into one of two basic categories: products that reduce your craving for food or products that reduce your body's absorption of the food you eat.

Appetite busters

These medications lower your food intake either by altering brain chemistry so that you get fewer hunger signals or by making the taste of food less appealing. This group of drugs include

- Amphetamines
- Appetite suppressants
- Antidepressants
- Local anesthetics

Fat blockers

 This second group of weight loss products, called *fat blockers,* prevent your body from absorbing dietary fat (the fat in food). Caution! *Laxatives* (drugs that increase bowel movements) and *diuretics,* which are also called *water pills* (drugs that make you pee more frequently), can make you feel thinner because they eliminate water from your body. But the loss is strictly temporary; these products are not considered safe and effective weight loss drugs.

Profiling Specific Weight Loss Medications

Okay, this is the part you may find boring. It describes the different kinds of weight loss medications and how they affect your body.

Amphetamines

Amphetamines are strong stimulants. The category includes dextroamphetamine (Dexedrine) and methamphetamine (Desoxyn), which were originally introduced in the 1930s to treat a condition called *narcolepsy,* which makes you fall asleep without warning. Pretty much by accident, someone discovered that taking amphetamines made people less hungry.

Unfortunately, amphetamines are addictive substances. Your body soon adapts to the drugs, a phenomenon called *tolerance.* As a result, you need bigger doses to produce the same anti-appetite effect. Worse yet, amphetamines can make you so jittery that the slang name for this class of drugs is *speed* or uppers. Amphetamines:

- ✔ Upset your stomach.
- ✔ Keep you from sleeping.
- ✔ Elevate your blood pressure.
- ✔ Make your heart beat faster or irregularly.

Some doctors still prescribe amphetamines for short-term weight loss, but the drugs are definitely not state-of-the-art.

Appetite suppressants

Modern appetite suppressants are tailor-made to keep your body from destroying naturally occurring chemicals called *neurotransmitters,* which enable your brain cells to fire messages back and forth, including the appetite bulletin: "No more food. I'm full."

Two important neurotransmitters are *serotonin,* a calming chemical, and *norepinephrine,* a stimulant that makes you feel full. *Phentermine* (Ionamin, Fastin, Banobese, Obenix, Zantryl) and *mazindol* (Mazanor, Sanorex) increase the amount of norepinephrine available to your brain cells. A third appetite suppressant, *sibutramine* (Meridia), introduced in 1997, is a double-acting pill

that increases the amount of both serotonin and norepinephrine, calming you
down and making you feel full at the same time. In one study, volunteers
taking sibutramine lost about ten pounds more those given a placebo pill.

The side effects of appetite suppressants include

- Dry mouth
- Constipation
- Insomnia
- Dizziness
- Elevated blood pressure
- Rapid heartbeat

Fat blockers

Actually, the proper name for fat blockers is *lipase inhibitors,* which translates to "a drug that reduces the effectiveness of the enzymes [lipases] your
body uses to break down the fats in food so that they pass undigested out of
your body." Whew.

The first prescription fat blocker approved by the Food and Drug
Administration (FDA) was orlistat (Xenical), which reduces your absorption
of dietary fat by about 30 percent. Orlistat was introduced in 1999 after two
clinical trials with 1,700 volunteers in which those who got the drug along
with a low-calorie, lowfat diet and regular exercise lost nearly twice as much
weight (22 pounds versus 13 pounds) as those who dieted and exercise but
got a placebo (a look-alike dummy pill). The big message is that those who
took orlistat lost more weight than those who took a placebo. The more
subtle message is that the guys who didn't get the drug still lost weight. And
they didn't have to cope with orlistat's annoying side effects: smelly intestinal gas, frequent or oily bowel movements, and leakage from the rectum.

Chitosan (pronounced *ky-to-san*) is a nonprescription ingredient made from
chitin, a carbohydrate extracted from the hard outer skeleton of shellfish. You
can't digest chitosan, so it sips right through your body, carrying some
dietary fat along, although probably not enough to make a real difference in
your calories intake. Like other indigestible dietary fiber, chitosan absorbs
water and bulks up stool, so if you eat lots of chitosan without drinking
enough water, you may be constipated or — in rare cases — develop a bowel
obstruction.

Both orlistat and chitosan reduce your body's absorption of fat-soluble medications, as well as nutrients such as vitamin A, vitamin D, vitamin E, vitamin K,
and *beta carotene,* the deep yellow pigment in fruits and veggies credited with
reducing the risk of some kinds of cancer.

The fen-phen fiasco and the propanolamine flip

Fenfluramine (Pondimin) and phentermine (Adipix) are amphetamine-like appetite suppressants that alter the levels of neurotransmitters circulating in your brain. Beginning late in the 1980s, obesity experts decided to prescribe the drugs as a package. The combination, popularly known as *fen-phen,* was an extremely effective weight loss product.

Soon fen-phen use soared. In 1996, doctors wrote more than 18 million prescriptions for phentermine and fenfluramine as special clinics began to pop up like mushrooms just to sell these drugs, often to people who were less than 30 pounds overweight.

But in July 1997, the fen-phen bubble burst when the Mayo Clinic in Rochester, Minnesota, released a report documenting heart valve damage in 24 fen-phen users. Some needed surgery to replace the valves; some developed pulmonary hypertension, a potentially fatal accumulation of fluid in the lungs.

The Food and Drug Administration (FDA) halted sales of the fen-phen combo and in September 1997 took fenfluramine and a related drug, dexfenfluramine (Redux), off the market.

Phentermine is still an approved medication for short-term weight loss treatment.

Three years later, another blip occurred on the diet drug scene. In October 2000, an FDA advisory panel voted to recommend that FDA ban the use of the nonprescription appetite suppressant phenylpropanolamine in products such as AcuTrim and Dexatrim, as well as a variety of cold remedies and antihistamines/decongestant combinations. The following month, FDA asked manufacturers of all PPA products to voluntarily pull their products from drugstore shelves while the agency wrote new rules that would effectively ban the use of PPA.

Phenylpropanolamine is a *vaso-constrictor,* a substance that causes blood vessels to narrow, raising blood pressure, a risk factor for stroke. Since 1969, the year it began keeping stats, FDA had collected at least 44 reports of stroke linked to the use of products containing phenylpropanolamine. The FDA panel estimated that the risk of stroke for age 18 to 49 who use phenylpropanolamine products may be up to 15 times that of women who do not use the drug.

Antidepressants

When the going gets tough, some people head for the dinner table. Others stop eating. Antidepressants are not marketed as weight loss products, but some evidence indicates that these drugs, bolstered by behavior modification and nutritional counseling, can alleviate weight problems by cooling emotional turmoil. But you have to choose the right drug. Tricyclic antidepressants, a class that includes amitryptiline (Elavil), increase appetite and may cause weight gain. Fluoxetine (Prozac) and paroxetine (Paxil) may not.

Local anesthetics

Taste buds are not tiny flowers. They are sensory organs that enable you to detect the different flavors in food. Flavor signals from the food travel

Fat cells, fat signals

When you take in more calories from food than you spend as energy, the excess calories are stored as body fat. (See Chapter 5 for a detailed explanation.) The fat is stored in specialized cells called *fat cells,* which expand to accommodate extra fat and contract when you lose weight. And vice versa: When you use up the energy stored as fat, your fat cells shrink so that you look thinner.

In 1995, researchers at Rockefeller University discovered a gene in fat cells that directs the production of a hormone called *leptin* (from the Greek word for *thin*). Leptin appears to tell your body how much fat you have stored, thus regulating your need for more food to provide more energy. Leptin also regulates your hypothalamus gland's secretion of *NPY,* a hormone that signals hunger.

When the Rockefeller scientists injected leptin into specially bred fat mice, the mice ate less, burned food faster, and lost significant amounts of weight. Will this work for human beings? Only time — and some well-regulated clinical trials — will tell.

through the taste buds and then along nerve fibers to your brain, which evaluates the signals as "Yummy!" or "Yuck!"

Benzocaine is a local anesthetic that stuns your taste buds into insensibility. Since the late 1950s, it has been available as an ingredient in nonprescription weight loss products such as chewing gums and candies. Does it work? Good question. Forty years ago, a study showed that people who used benzocaine gum and candy while following a low-calorie diet lost weight. The problem is, no one is certain whether the effective agent was the benzocaine or the diet.

Herbal Remedies for Folks Who Want to Be Thin

Some herbs stimulate your desire to eat more; others claim to help you eat less. If I were talking about prescription drugs, you could bet that any product sold for one of these purposes would actually perform as promised. But that's not necessarily true with herbs and other dietary supplements.

In 1994, Congress passed and the President signed into law the Dietary Supplement Health and Education Act limiting FDA's control over dietary supplements. Under this law:

  ✔ FDA cannot require premarket tests to prove supplements are safe and effective.

  ✔ FDA cannot limit the dosage in any dietary supplement.

> ✔ FDA cannot halt or restrict sales of a dietary supplement unless there is evidence that the product has caused illness or injury when *used according to the directions on the package.*

In other words, if you experience a problem after taking slightly more or less of a supplement than directed on the label, FDA cannot help you. As a result, the agency has found it virtually impossible to take products off drugstore shelves even after reports of illness and injury. (See the next section.)

Herbal fen-phen

Herbal fen-phen is a name for a product containing ephedra and St. John's wort. The name is also used to describe other herbal products, which may or may not contain these two herbs.

Ephedra is a stimulant whose active ingredients are the central nervous system stimulants ephedrine and pseudoephedrine, the latter widely used as a *decongestant* (a drug that shrinks swollen tissues) in over-the-counter cold and allergy medication.

St. John's wort (Hypericum perforatum) is widely used in Europe to treat mild depression. The National Institutes of Health has launched a study of the value of St. John's wort for depression but not for obesity. Until now, no well-controlled clinical trials have evaluated the herb's actions and adverse effects, either alone or in combination with ephedra.

In 1991, the German Commission E approved the use of ephedra preparations to relieve mild bronchial spasms, but cautioned that ephedra should not be taken by people with:

> ✔ Anxiety disorders
> ✔ High blood pressure
> ✔ Thyroid disorders

It is definitely worth noting that ephedra, like the amphetamines, is an addictive substance whose adverse effects include

> ✔ Insomnia, restlessness, and irritability
> ✔ Nausea and vomiting
> ✔ Difficulty urinating
> ✔ Seizures
> ✔ Psychological problems
> ✔ Abnormal heartbeat and fatal heart attack

To date, more than 800 illnesses and at least 17 deaths have been reported among people taking ephedra supplements (including ephedra teas). As a result, several states have restricted their use. In 1997, the Food and Drug Administration proposed mandatory warning labels for supplements containing ephedrine and moved to lower the amount of ephedrine permitted per dose/supplement to 8 mg. However, data from a number of studies released in 1999 showed that ephedrine did not begin to produce adverse effects in doses lower than 20 mg. As a result, the General Accounting Office (GAO) concluded that while FDA was correct in trying to regulate the use of ephedra, the permissible dose should be set higher than 8 mg. As late as summer 2000, the FDA was still working on new proposals for ephedra labeling. Although ephedra is available without prescription, it makes sense to check with your doctor before using this herb.

Herbs that stimulate your appetite

If you are trying to lose weight, your response to this headline is likely to be, "Who needs 'em?" The answer is, lots of people.

Sometimes taste buds go on strike. For example, when you have a cold, food often tastes like so much damp cotton because you can't perceive the different flavors. Getting older may also impair your ability to taste your food; what seemed spicy when you are in your 20s may seem tame when you cross the 50-year line.

Herbs and spices help. First, they add more intense flavors and aromas that are easier to perceive. Second, they may irritate the lining of your mouth, make you salivate, and start a chain of physiological events that ends with your stomach sending hunger signals to your brain, a process described in full in *Nutrition For Dummies*.

Following is a list of some herbs and spiced approved as appetite stimulants by Commission E, the internationally respected agency of the German government, which evaluates the safety and effectiveness of herbal products.

- Angelica root
- Caraway seed
- Chicory
- Cinnamon
- Coriander
- Dandelion leaves
- Fenugreek

- ✔ Gentian
- ✔ Mustard
- ✔ Orange peel

Ingredients that don't work

Both the Food and Drug Administration and the Federal Trade Commission have a hand in making sure that the weight loss medications you take actually do what they promise to accomplish. FDA handles the ingredients; FTC watches over the promises.

FDA and weight loss drugs

For nearly ten years in the 1980s and 1990s, FDA painstakingly combed through the list of thousands of ingredients in nonprescription drug products, including products meant to help you lose weight. Some ingredients in weight loss products such as benzocaine and phenylpropanolamine were certified safe and effective. Others were safe but not effective. A third group was found to be neither safe nor effective. The list of those not generally recognized as safe and effective for losing weight is too long to be reprinted here. Click on the table on your CD-ROM to see the list as it appeared in the Federal Register, a record of the proceedings in the U.S. Congress. You may be surprised to see how many familiar ingredients, such as ascorbic acid (vitamin C) and vitamin A, don't make the cut.

FTC and drug advertising

While FDA is checking out the products, the Federal Trade Commission combats consumer fraud by exercising its authority to fine the manufacturers using false advertising claims to sell their products. According to FTC, one good example of this kind of flimflam occurs with fat burners, nutritional supplements that promise to rev up your metabolism to the point where you burn calories super-fast. Even while you're sleeping.

From 1994 to 1999, FTC issued at least 15 complaints, violations, or consent orders (the targeted company agreed to stop doing whatever it was doing) to companies selling fat burners. There were some very Big Names involved, but I've decided not to embarrass the offenders on the theory that by complying with FTC decisions, they have all essentially agreed to go and sin no more.

But tomorrow is another day, and who knows who is out there plotting to separate your from your hard-won cash with promises of miracle weight loss products? Not me. So fight back. If you come across a product that uses the words fat burners, take notes: Write down the company's name and address, the name of the product, the ingredients, the price, and any advertising copy that says, "Buy me! Right now! I burn away your fat!" Then click onto the

Federal Trade Commission site at www.ftc.gov. Scroll to the bottom of the page and click Complaint Form. When the form pops up on your screen, fill it out, send it off, and pat yourself on the back for being a Good Citizen.

Herbs that increase your loss of liquids

Some herbs are *diuretics* (substances that make you urinate more frequently); others are *laxatives* (you know what that means). True, people who use these herbs, either as teas or in special weight loss supplements, may lose some water weight temporarily. But diuretics may cause dehydration, and laxatives may be thoroughly debilitating, so neither is considered a safe, effective agent for weight control. Table 14-1 lists some herbs with diuretic or laxative properties.

Table 14-1	Diuretic and Laxative Herbal Products	
Herb	*Diuretic*	*Laxative*
Aloe		x
Asparagus root	x	
Birch leaf	x	
Dandelion root, leaf	x	
Flaxseed		x
Goldenrod	x	
Horsetail	x	
Juniper berry	x	
Mate	x	
Senna		x

Source: Mark Blumenthal, ed., The Complete German Commission E Monographs. Austin, TX: American Botanical Council, 1998.

The Heart of the Matter

Taking weight loss medication takes off pounds, but drugs alone are no substitute for a long-term lifestyle change that alters your approach to food and adds exercise to your daily regimen. And the adverse effects of the medications may not be worth the benefits for the moderately overweight. Hey, nobody ever said it would be easy. Sorry about that.

Chapter 15

Is This Stitch Necessary?

I was going to title this chapter "Blood and Guts," but my husband, who has a fine sense for such things, called that totally gross. Hence, the tamer title "Is This Stitch Necessary?" Of course, no matter what you call it, this chapter is serious stuff. For those who fit the criteria listed here, the procedures described are considered worth the effort. But it is well to remember that no surgery, no matter how minor it may seem, is totally risk-free. None should be undertaken lightly.

What Weight-Related Surgery Is

Two basic kinds of surgical treatment exist for weight-related problems: cosmetic surgery and gastrointestinal surgery.

> ✔ **Cosmetic surgery,** such as liposuction and abdominoplasty, improves the way your body looks but does not affect the function of your digestive organs.

> ✔ **Gastrointestinal surgery** for obesity is called *bariatric surgery,* from *baros,* the Greek word for weight. Bariatric surgery such as gastric bypass alters the size and layout of your digestive tract in an effort to help you lose weight by restricting the amount of food you can eat and the amount of nutrients, including calories, you can absorb.

All doctors who perform these surgeries are surgeons, but their specialties differ. Cosmetic surgery is generally done by plastic surgeons. Bariatric surgery is usually performed by a general surgeon who specializes in gastroenterological procedures. Starting from the top:

A surgeon is a doctor who has

- ✔ Graduated from an accredited four-year medical school.
- ✔ Completed at least three years as a resident (graduate student) in general surgery in an accredited hospital.
- ✔ Been certified by an American medical specialty board or is a Fellow of the American College of Surgery (FACS).

A plastic surgeon is a doctor certified by the American Board of Plastic Surgery (ABPS) who has

- ✔ Completed a residency in plastic surgery.
- ✔ Practiced for two years.
- ✔ Passed written and oral specialty exams.

A bariatric surgeon is a doctor certified by the American Society of Bariatric Physicians who has

- ✔ Completed a residency in gastrointestinal surgery.
- ✔ Specialized in obesity-related procedures.

 Although some cosmetic procedures are done in a doctor's office, your doctor should have practice privileges at an accredited hospital. Hey, you never know — and it pays to be prepared.

Liposuction

Liposuction, from the Greek word for fat *(lipo)* and the English word for, well, suction, is exactly what its name implies, a surgical procedure during which your doctor removes fatty tissue from under your skin at sites such as:

- ✔ Abdomen
- ✔ Hips
- ✔ Buttocks
- ✔ Thighs
- ✔ Knees

- Upper arms
- Neck
- Chin
- Cheeks

Who is qualified for liposuction?

According to the American Society of Plastic Surgeons, you qualify for liposuction if you are a healthy person of normal weight whose only weight-related problem is clumps of fat at specific sites such as those listed in the preceding section. Age is not a disqualifier unless it has made your skin significantly less elastic (which means it may not shrink smoothly once fat underneath is removed).

On the other hand, you are probably not a good candidate for liposuction if you have recently had surgery in the area near your fatty spots or if you have

- Diabetes
- Heart disease
- Poor circulation
- Lung disease

How liposuction is done

If you are having liposuction in a small area, your doctor will give you local anesthesia, a shot similar to what you get at the dentist. For larger areas, your doctor may use regional anesthesia, an injection that numbs an entire portion of your body. An epidural block, used during childbirth, is regional anesthesia. If you are having a lot of liposuction and prefer not to be around to hear and watch what's happening, you may get general anesthesia, which puts you to sleep.

Awake or asleep, you won't be watching the surgery, but if you were you would see the doctor:

- Make a tiny incision in the skin.
- Insert a *cannula* (narrow tube) attached to a vacuum pump or large syringe.
- Inject a fluid containing a saline (salt) solution, lidocaine (a local anesthetic), and epinephrine (a drug that makes blood vessels contract).
- Draw out fatty tissue (fat cells).

This won't hurt a bit

Until 1846, the common anesthetics used for surgery were alcohol or herbal narcotic potions (think of Sleeping Beauty's "poison apple," which some folks think was a combination of natural sleepy time herbs such as poppies — opium — mandrake, henbane, or hemlock), hypnosis, or a swift right to the jaw to knock the patient out. Honest.

By the end of the 18th century, though, chemists had discovered nitrous oxide ("laughing gas"). Inhaling it made people cheerful, relaxed, even giddy. Then came ether, which made everybody drowsy. At first, these gases were thought to be remedies for lung ailments. Eventually, a light went on in someone's head: Hel-lo! This can eliminate pain during surgery.

On October 16, 1846, dentists William Morton and Horace Wells, on instructions from their chemist, Charles T. Jackson, used ether while extracting a tooth from a patient who felt no pain, leading Dr. Charles Collins Warren, Professor of Anatomy at Harvard Medical School and one of the nation's leading surgeons, to issue his famous pronouncement: "Gentlemen, this is no humbug."

After which, everyone shouted, "Huzzah," as they carried Morton, Wells, and Jackson around the room on their shoulders, right? No way. For years, the three (and countless others) fought over who had discovered anesthesia first. At the same time, surgeons who had made their reputation by operating through brute force (that right to the jaw) and lightning quickness fought learning how to proceed slowly and deliberately, depending on skill rather than strength. And religionists who considered pain God's punishment for man's wickedness labeled anesthesia blasphemy.

In the end, Wells died in prison, a possible suicide. Morton succumbed to a cerebral hemorrhage some said was brought on by conflict with Jackson — who ended life in an insane asylum. And you? Well, if you want liposuction, a tummy tuck, or gastric surgery, rest assured. It won't hurt a bit.

Some doctors use a special cannula that emits ultrasonic energy, which breaks down the walls of fat cells, making them easier to remove. This technique is called *ultrasound assisted lipoplasty (UAL)*.

The risks and benefits of liposuction

The benefits of well-done, successful liposuction are obvious: a tiny scar where the cannula was inserted but smooth contours that make for a better-looking body after the four to six weeks it takes for swelling to subside.

The risks are less obvious. One definition of minor surgery is surgery that happens to someone else. As with any surgery, liposuction carries a risk of:

✔ Infection

✔ Fat clots or blood clots that can travel to your lungs (a possibly fatal effect)

- Excessive loss of fluids (ditto)
- Excessive fluid accumulation (ditto again)
- Burns from the instrument
- Damaged skin or nerves
- Perforated organs (that cannula moving in and out)
- Adverse reactions to the anesthesia or other drugs

My goodness!

Abdominoplasty

Abdominoplasty is a six-syllable word for tummy tuck, but don't let either the polysyllabic science-talk or the cutesy terminology distract you from the main event: This procedure is serious surgery, an operation under general anesthesia or local anesthesia plus sedatives.

How to do a tummy tuck

If you're awake and hold a mirror over your middle, you will be able to watch your doctor:

- Make an incision across your middle, from hip bone to hip bone, just above your pubic area.
- Peel back the skin — hold on, hold on — to create a large flap that can stretch all the way up to your ribs.
- Tighten the exposed muscles by stitching them into a new, firm position, which gives you a neater, smaller waist.
- Pull the skin flap back down and trim the excess, setting aside your navel for a minute.
- Cut a new hole for the navel (which is still the innie or outie your started with).
- And sew everything back in place.

A few weeks later when all the swelling goes down, your previously flabby middle will be flat as a board. Well, maybe not that flat. But definitely flatter than before.

Who's a candidate for a tummy tuck?

The best candidate for a tummy tuck is pretty much the person who fits the bill for liposuction (see the list in the preceding section). The difference between liposuction and abdominoplasty is the tissue involved. In liposuction, you lose plain old fat. In abdominoplasty, the target is droopy excess skin that:

- Hasn't tightened up after you lost weight.
- Has been stretched by several pregnancies.
- Has lost its elasticity because, sigh, you've gotten older.

Stop! You're not ready for abdominoplasty if:

- You plan to lose more weight (more stretching ahead: better to finish weight loss first).
- You plan to become pregnant again (surgically tightened muscles may stretch during pregnancy).

The risks and benefits

The risks of this surgery are the same as those for liposuction. However, the risk of infection is higher because this surgery involves more cutting, repositioning, and stitching of tissue, and the possibility of an adverse reaction to anesthesia rises because the operation is usually done with general anesthesia.

Bariatric Surgery

Bariatric surgery is not a cosmetic procedure. It does not remove fat tissue or reposition skin or tighten muscles. Instead, this kind of surgery changes the size and position of your stomach and intestines in order to restrict the amount of calories you can consume by limiting the space available for food in your stomach and/or restrict the amount of calories you can absorb by limiting the space available for absorbing nutrients

Who is the candidate for bariatric surgery?

Clearly, this surgery is not meant for casual or minimal weight loss. In fact, the National Institutes of Health 1998 Clinical Guidelines on the Identification, Evaluation, and Treatment of Overweight and Obesity in Adults says you're a candidate for bariatric surgery *only* if:

✔ You have a body mass index (BMI) 40 or higher (about 100 pounds overweight on the MetLife weight tables).

✔ You have a BMI 35 or higher and have serious weight-related health problems such as high blood pressure, high cholesterol, heart disease, diabetes, sleep apnea, or arthritis.

✔ You are morbidly obese, meaning that your risk of dying from your weight-related health problems is greater than your risk of dying from surgery.

✔ You have tried, really tried, other, more conventional weight loss methods — diets, exercise, and behavior modification (more about that in Chapter 17) — but failed miserably.

The risks of bariatric surgery

Check the list of risks for liposuction in the preceding section. They apply here, too. In addition, as with any major surgery, bariatric surgery carries a risk of:

✔ Nausea

✔ Vomiting

✔ Bloating

✔ Heartburn

✔ Wound infection

✔ Adverse reactions to anesthesia and other drugs

And there's more. As many as two of every ten bariatric surgery patients may need follow up surgery to correct tears in the internal tissues or external wound. Other possible postsurgical problems include

✔ Gallstones caused by rapid weight loss, which concentrates cholesterol (a material which comprises some gallstones) in the gall bladder.

✔ Nutritional deficiencies due to your inability to absorb nutrients (easily remedied with supplements).

✔ Problem pregnancy due to an inability to provide enough nutrients for the fetus.

Still interested? The following sections describe the two specific forms of gastric surgery for obesity approved by the National Institutes of Health: gastric bypass and vertical banded gastroplasty (VBG).

Gastric bypass

The current gold standard for bariatric surgery is the 40-year-old procedure called *gastric bypass,* an operation done under general anesthesia. While you're dreaming, your doctor:

- ✔ Makes an incision down your middle.
- ✔ Staples closed a small pouch at the upper part of your stomach.
- ✔ Connects the pouch to your intestines at a place called the Roux limb (more about this a few paragraphs down).
- ✔ Sews you up and sends you off to the recovery room.

Peephole

This is not a weight loss story. Nobody gets thinner or looks trimmer. But this tale testifies to human courage, curiosity, and scientific accomplishment. So read it!

On June 6, 1822, U.S. Army surgeon William Beaumont met up with Alexis St. Martin, an 18-year-old French Canadian fur trader who had been wounded accidentally when his own musket discharged by mistake. St. Martin survived, and the wound in his gut healed. But the edges refused to close. Two years later, when all efforts to close the hole in the belly failed, St. Martin gave Beaumont permission to use the wound as the world's first window on a working human digestive system.

Beaumont's method was simplicity itself. At noon on August 1, 1825, he tied small pieces of food (cooked meat, raw meat, cabbage, bread) to a silk string and inserted the string into the hole in St. Martin's stomach.

An hour later, he pulled the food out to find the cabbage and bread half digested; the meat, untouched. After another hour, he pulled the string out again. This time, only the raw meat remained untouched, and St. Martin, who now had a headache and a queasy stomach, called it quits for the day.

But in more than 230 later trials, Beaumont — with the help of his remarkably compliant patient — discovered that the carbohydrates (veggies and bread) were digested quickly, while the protein and fat foods took hours and hours. Beaumont attributed this to the fact that the carb veggies had been cut into small pieces and the bread was porous; modern nutritionists know that carbohydrates are simply digested faster than proteins and that digesting fats (including those in beef) takes longest of all.

Beaumont and St. Martin separated in 1833 when the patient, now a sergeant in the United States Army, was posted elsewhere, leaving the doctor to write "Experiments and Observations on the Gastric Juice and the Physiology of Digestion." The treatise is now considered a landmark in the understanding of the human digestive system. Now, admit it. Doesn't that story make you feel good all over?

Certainly sounds straightforward, but when I say the surgeon "creates a small pouch," I mean really small. Like, teensy. Your new "stomach" holds about 20 to 30 ml of food, about two or three ounces, just enough to fill a whisky shot glass. As a result, you can't eat very much at one time, one reason gastric bypass enables you to lose weight.

Gastric bypass also cuts back on the amount of calories you absorb from any food you do eat due to the place where your newly tiny stomach is attached to your intestines, an area called the *Roux limb*. (Gastric bypass is also known as *Roux-en-Y,* sort of French for Roux is here.)

Ordinarily, you digest (metabolize) your food throughout your intestine. But the Roux limb can't handle calorie-dense food with lots of sugar and/or fat. If you eat ice cream, for example, your body will rebel, pushing the sugary, fatty food along really fast in a reaction called *dumping syndrome.*

Dumping syndrome ain't dangerous, but believe you me, it's not something you want to experience twice. When your intestine dumps the food, your heart races, your skin turns clammy, you are queasy and nauseated, and you may vomit or develop diarrhea. These yucky moments are a true inducement to watch what you eat, another reason people who have gastric bypass lose weight.

Which they definitely do, beginning right after surgery. One Mayo Clinic study released in 2000 showed bypass patients losing 50 percent of their weight and keeping it off for three years. Other studies show patients' weight stabilizing 18 to 24 months after the operation, at about 30 percent above the standard weights listed on the MetLife weight tables shown in Chapter 2. In the process, previously life-threatening health problems improve dramatically, so for the right patient, this stitch is a blessing.

Other forms of bariatric surgery

NIH's second approved form of bariatric surgery is *vertical banded gastroplasty*. This procedure limits the amount of food you can eat at one time by creating a very small pouch in your otherwise relatively large stomach. Food goes into the pouch from your gullet (okay, esophagus) and then exits directly into your lower stomach and on into your intestines where it is metabolized and nutrients absorbed. True, this operation is less drastic than gastric bypass, but studies show that it may also be less effective at enabling people to maintain weight loss.

Bariatric surgeons have also been experimenting with bypass via laparascopy, the procedure that allows the doctor to pass very small instruments into the body through a small incision in the skin. Another form of laparascopic surgery for obesity is *laparascopic adjustable silastic banding (LASB),* an operation most commonly done in Europe. In this surgery, a doctor slips a small elastic ring around the upper part of the stomach, again creating as small pouch. The ring has an inner lining filled with a saline (salt water) solution. Because the lining is connected to an opening in the patient's skin, the surgeon can make the ring tighter or looser simply by draining or adding liquid.

Currently, the statistics for laparascopic obesity surgery are pretty skimpy. However, it is clear that people who need bariatric surgery have extra weight that puts extra stress on the long incision used in traditional bypass, leading to a higher risk of infection or failure of the wound to heal. Laparoscopy requires a very small incision, which decreases these risks and causes fewer common surgical complications such as breathing problems or blood clots. So you can bet you'll be hearing more about this in the future.

Chapter 16

Gadgets and Gimmicks

● ●

In This Chapter

▶ Describing odd weight loss products

▶ Weighing the risks of gimmicky diet aids

▶ Running down misleading ads

▶ Corresponding with the Federal Trade Commission

● ●

*Y*ou've seen the ads. You've read the headlines: "Lose 10 Pounds in 10 days!" "Lose weight while you sleep!" "Scrub away the pounds!" Your brain knows it won't work, but that hopeful little voice inside whispers, "Hey, maybe this time. . . ." And there you go, spending good money on yet another ineffective product that won't reduce anything but your bank account. Worse yet, the energy you spend trying to sort through the current list of razzle-dazzle weight loss gadgets and gimmicks won't make even a fraction of an ounce disappear from your hips. Thinking hard may make you feel as though you're working up a sweat, but in reality your brain is only using one skinny calorie every four minutes. This chapter can save you money and time. Use the money for the new clothes you'll want when you skinny down. Use the time for real work that benefits your bod. Walk. Jog. Run. Skip. Jump. . . . Hup, two, three, four!

An Alphabetical Tour of Weight Loss Gimmicks

Right now, as you are reading this page, here's a list of some unusual products ab-solutely, de-finitely guaranteed to get rid of excess pounds in unusual ways (in alphabetical order):

✔ Appetite suppressant earrings and earmuffs

✔ Appetite suppressant eyeglasses

✔ Appetite suppressant innersoles

✔ Appetite suppressant skin patches

- Cleansing or detoxifying pills and potions
- Electrical muscle stimulators
- Fat-melting soaps and skin creams
- Loofahs, sponges, and body wrappings
- Slimming finger ring
- Steam baths
- Saunas

Sounds ridiculous? Well, as TV pioneer Jack Paar used to say way, way, way before Dave and Jay and Conan hit the late night screen: "I kid you not." So with a little help from my friends at the Food and Drug Administration and the Federal Trade Commission, I feel it is my duty to tell you if you buy this stuff, the only place you'll lose weight is in your wallet.

Water whirled

Every profession has its hazards. Doctors catch more colds. Secretaries suffer sore wrists. Mountain climbers fall off mountains. And writers? I can't speak for anyone else, but I know that covering nutrition and weight loss can sometimes warp my perceptions. For example, when you hear the nursery rhyme that starts, "Rub-a-dub-dub, three men in a tub," I bet you see these three guys starting out to sea. Me, I imagine them climbing into a sauna to lose weight.

Steam baths, herb baths, saunas, and other watery wonders have been employed for centuries to soothe mind and body. Using them to lose weight is relatively new. So are the extra little touches such as *loofahs* (natural spongers) or soaps or creams or lotions to scrub away fat or seaweed wraps or scented cloths to swaddle you from head to toe and squeeze away the extra pounds.

Does it work? Yes. And no. The "yes" refers to the fact that steaming yourself like a giant wonton makes you perspire, which means you lose water. The more you perspire, the more water you lose. The more water you lose, the less you weigh — and the more water you'll drink to alleviate the discomfort you feel when you're thirsty or dehydrated, which means you gain back what you just lost. That's the "no" part.

As for an opinion on the value of fat-melting soaps and creams and lotions and fat-scrubbing sponges, I defer to that notable weight expert, S. ("Just Call Me Santa") Claus: "Ho. Ho. Ho."

Patches, earrings, earmuffs, eyeglasses, innersoles, and finger rings

Earmuffs? Eyeglasses? Innersoles? A ring that (as reported in *The New York Times,* for heavens' sake) claims to slim your thighs when you where it on your pinky, your stomach when you wear it on your ring finger, your face (your face?) when you wear it on your thumb, and your . . . well, why go on? You get the picture.

The most complimentary thing you can say about these tricky little appurtenances is that the people who came out with them are creative as all get-out.

- ✔ The patches promise to deliver a magic weight-wasting ingredient. Yeah, yeah.

- ✔ The earrings and earmuffs (or cuffs) are custom-made (wow!) to fit your very own ears where they are supposed to stimulate sites that control your appetite. Yes, indeed, that's what it says here in my cheat sheet from the Federal Trade Commission (FTC), an arm of The U.S. Department of Commerce. If I were the punning sort, I'd say it sounds like some sort of ear-cupuncture. Wait! Did I really write that rotten pun? Yup. There it is, printed right on the page. Sorry.

- ✔ The eyeglasses come with colored lenses purported to project an (unspecified) image to your retina that wipes out your desire for food. Well, maybe if you stick on a photo of yourself ten pounds heavier. . . .

- ✔ The ring is supposed to hit acupressure points on your fingers that have the same weight loss effect as "jogging up to six miles a day." (Yes, that's the claim reported in *The New York Times.*) The innersoles are supposed to hit acupressure points on your sole. Well, if they don't work, you can still wear the ring for decoration and use the innersoles to cushion your tootsies on your daily power walk.

Reviewing what you've just read, a smart cookie like you has figured out that these products have two things in common:

- ✔ They're expensive.
- ✔ They probably don't work.

Just to underscore these points, I must point out that practically as soon as a new version of one of these gimmicks goes on sale, FDA and FTC ears perk up, and the agencies are soon on the scene to order the offending device off the market.

Charging ahead

Some people think they can lose weight by plugging themselves into electrical machines that deliver (hopefully) tiny little shocks to their muscles. Some people are wrong. Frankly, it's probably more of a shock to the system to stand naked in front of your bedroom mirror and stare at yourself head on in the mirror. It's also a whale of a lot safer than using some electrical gismo. (By the way: Did you check for the Underwriters Laboratory UL symbol on the package signifying that the product has been safety-tested? Do I need to tell you that with this, as with any other electrical product, no UL symbol means No Sale? I didn't think so!)

You will read more about these devices — known in the trade as *passive exercisers* because it's the machine that moves, not you — in Chapter 18, which describes in tedious detail the indisputable value of exercise for long-term weight control. For now, the short version is that while electrical stimulators have a place in medicine where they help broken bones to heal faster, they have absolutely no raisin d'être (translation: reason to be) in weight control. Why? Because using them doesn't make your muscles move, and if your muscles don't move, you don't lose weight. Worse yet, if you use one of these machines incorrectly, FTC says you might end up with a nasty accidental shock or burn.

Natural miracles and body cleansers

Chapter 14 has the lowdown on the drugs approved for medically supervised weight loss programs plus info on herbal products that promise to help melt away the pounds. This section is about another kind of weight loss product. Its label often carries the words *natural* or *miracle* or *cleansing* or *detoxifying* or some variation or combination thereof.

One kind of supposedly miracle product is a plain old standard dietary supplement: vitamins or vitamins and minerals, or a meal substitute. This product won't do you any harm, but it won't help you lose weight, either.

A second kind of miracle pill or potion contain ingredients alleged to speed up your metabolism or absorb and burn fat or block your absorption of carbohydrates (starches) or fill you up without calories. Oh, please!

A third group of miracle weight loss products is more problematic. This is the totally natural herb or fruit or veggie or fiber-based stuff that promises to cleanse or detoxify your body and thus reduce your weight. Translation: The product contains diuretic or laxative ingredients that make you urinate more frequently or have more frequent bowel movements. The ingredients include (but are not limited to):

- Asparagus

- Birch leaf

- Dandelion (which the French call *pis-en-lit,* meaning — yes — pee in the bed)

- Goldenrod

You can read more about herbal products for weight loss in Chapter 14. If you don't feel like flipping back the pages, all you need to know right here is that using diuretics or laxatives to slim down may lead to Big Trouble such as:

- Dehydration

- Muscle spasms

- Irritation of the intestinal tract

In other words, the best use for herbs and spices is as seasoning that makes your food so tasty your appetite is satisfied with less food and fewer calories. Yum to that!

Policing the Bad Ads

Because you always tell the truth and because you know that it's illegal for an advertisement to promote false claims, you may find it hard to believe that so many weight loss ads are full of so many — how to say this politely? — misrepresentations. Oh, what the heck: Lies.

You are right: Advertising has to be truthful to be legal. But here's the catch: How can you tell an ad is skirting the rules until you actually see it in print or on the air? That's the dilemma facing the Federal Trade Commission.

FTC is the only national agency in this country with broad consumer protection enforcement powers. Their power comes from the Federal Trade Commission Act, which prohibits "unfair or deceptive practices in or affecting commerce." As a result, FTC polices a lot of advertising, including ads that hawk the products listed in the preceding sections. The agency first stuck its toe into the diet ad water in 1927 when it went after a company called McGowan Laboratories, Inc. for advertising a "compound to quickly and permanently dissolve away excess flesh from certain parts of the body."

Since then, FTC has become the dieting consumer's best friend. From 1927 to 1997, the agency issued more than 140 Commission Decisions or Consent Agreements related to deceptive advertising for weight control devices or products. Once cited, the companies FTC targets promise to mend their ways, sometimes nudged along by FTC's levying fines.

To check out the entire list of FTC decisions and agreements on weight loss products from 1927 to 1997, click onto your CD-ROM . Or you may click onto the same list at the Web address www.ftc.gov/opa/1997/9703/dietcase.htm from which you can search out more specific info on each decision on FTC's list of no-goodniks.

Partners in weight control

In addition to its role as the official federal advertising watchdog, FTC is a member of the Partnership for Healthy Weight Management, a coalition of representatives from government, academia, health-care, professional societies, commercial manufacturers, and public interest groups that promotes responsible marketing and advertising of weight loss products. You can find a complete list of the Partnership members on your CD-ROM.

In 2000, the Partnership launched a campaign called Ad Nauseam (get it?), an inelegant name that nonetheless makes the point. To start the campaign off with a bang, the Partnership contacted nine major magazines and newspapers that had carried ads with dubious weight loss claims. The letter asked the zines and papers to explain their current screening policies and urged them to adopt a new policy requiring proof for advertising claims. The letters went to

- *Cosmopolitan*
- *Esquire*
- *McCall's*
- *Redbook*
- *Woman's Day*
- *The Atlanta Constitution*
- *The Rocky Mountain News*
- *USA Today*
- *Smart Source*

Only one publication, *USA Today,* bothered to respond, and even it did not describe its screening policies. Yipes! Undeterred by this boorish behavior, the Partnership plans to press ahead encouraging all mainstream media (and maybe a few rogue publications) to ask for proof of extravagant weight loss claims before accepting weight loss ads.

And guess what: You can help.

Pssssst! Want to see a new pyramid?

The U.S. Departments of Agriculture and Health and Human Services Food Guide Pyramid (you can see a copy in Chapter 5) is so popular that it was only a question of time until other agencies, such as FTC, came up with a pyramid of their own. Figure 16-1 shows the FTC pyramid, which symbolizes the agency's role in consumer protection. As you can plainly see, the FTC pyramid stands on a broad base of education (for consumers) and self-regulation (for companies) with a (hopefully) small peak of enforcement (by FTC) for those nasties who refuse to obey the rules. Neat.

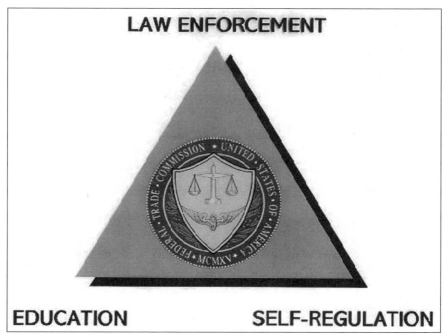

Figure 16-1:
The FTC
Pyramid.

Clearly, consumers like you are a big part of the process. In 1999, FTC received more than 600 complaints from consumers regarding misleading diet ads. Now the Partnership has invited all consumers to collect examples of horrible ads with miracle claims. Send the ads to The Partnership for Healthy Weight Management, Federal Trade Commission, S-4302, 601 Pennsylvania Avenue NW, Washington, D.C. 20580. Or you can dial up FTC's toll-free Hot Line at 1-887-FTC-HELP (1-800-382-4357). Or you can click onto FTC's complaint form at www.ftc.gov/ftc/complaint.htm.

Click on to your CD-ROM for a copy of the complaint form you can print and mail in. The more people who join the effort to watchdog advertising for weight loss products, the more effective the FTC and the Partnership will be in tossing the ads onto the junk heap where they belong and the more certain you can be that what you see advertised actually does what it says it will.

Now that's a goal that's worth working for. Besides all that clicking, and typing, and pasting, and mailing will use up some calories. No, not many. But some.

Part V
Lifelong Weight Control

The 5th Wave   By Rich Tennant

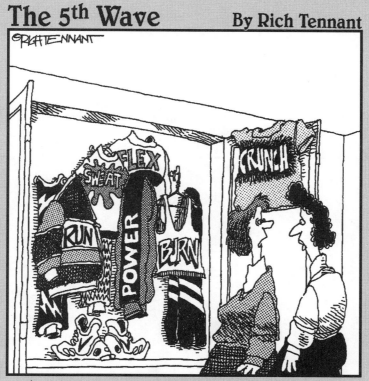

FLEX
SWEAT
CRUNCH
RUN
POWER
BURN

"I'm not sure I can live up to my workout clothes."

In this part . . .

Hooray! You've met your weight loss goals. But what happens now? For most people, it's a yo-yo life — down a few pounds, up a few pounds, bounce, bounce. You can be different. This part lays out strategies for changing your attitudes and changing your body for the rest of your life.

Chapter 17

Changing Your Food Attitudes

• •

In this chapter

▶ Defining behavior modification

▶ Modifying your own behavior

▶ Finding weight loss buddies

▶ Keeping tabs on what you eat

• •

*E*ver since Freud burst upon the human consciousness (unconscious-ness?) with the idea that what happens when you are a child influences the rest of your emotional life, Mom's been taking it on the chin. Hate math? Blame Mom. Can't stand your cousin Kate? Blame Mom? Eat too much? Blame — who else? — Mom! Well, maybe.

True, Mom may have set your first relationship with food, but you're a grown-up now and you can change your attitudes. This chapter lays out one method for doing that. It's called behavior modification, and it can help you skinny down. Read about it. Give Mom a rest. Maybe even send her a box of chocolates.

Behavior and Weight: A Close Couple

When you were an itty-bitty baby, someone close to you — your mother, your grandmother, an older sister or brother — fed you every meal, probably while holding your close and warm. As a result, you learned to associate food with love and comfort.

Naturally, as you got older, you discovered pleasure in other pursuits, such as a challenging job or an enriching hobby, and you found love with other people — although you still love your mom, and a friendly dog is pretty good, too.

My point, of course, is that an infant's view of food as the primary source of warmth and security should turn into an adult's appreciation of what's good to eat as eating habits adjust. Making this transition successfully enables you to keep your food intake within reasonable limits. Yes, you may binge once in a while, gain or lose a pound or two or three. But if food is just one of the good things in life, your weight is likely to stay pretty much within healthy limits.

The problem lies in holding onto the idea that food is an extraordinary source of comfort. I'm not talking here about foodies who enjoy being the first at the newest restaurant or knowing how to identify seven gazillion different mushrooms. And I certainly don't mean food writers or green grocers or butchers or culinary professionals who make their living from food. And let me add that I'm certainly not talking about people who are just plain larger than the rest of us and need more food to stay happily healthy.

No, the people I'm describing still see food as the best reward in the world. Under stress, these guys head for the fridge. If they don't have a full plate, they feel bereft. Denied a second ice cream cone, they sulk. Their behavior regarding food is off-kilter, so no matter how many diets they try or how much weight they lose, they will eventually fall off (onto?) the chuck wagon and gain weight again.

People like this can't control their weight with a New! Miracle! food plan. They must change the way they react to food. One method experts use to bring about that change is called *behavior modification,* a fancy name for the process of altering your reactions to the stimuli in your life.

What behavior modification is

Ordinarily, most people behave according to a pattern that can be translated to the simple mathematical equation 1 + 2 = 3.

- ✔ 1 = A trigger or a cue or a stimulus
- ✔ 2 = Your behavior in response to the cue
- ✔ 3 = The result of your behavior

For example, if you see a red light when you are about to cross the street, you stop.

- ✔ 1 = The trigger = The red light
- ✔ 2 = Your behavior = You stop
- ✔ 3 = The result = You avoid being hit by a car

Because children don't instinctively recognize a red light as a stop signal, parents exercise a kind of behavior modification by teaching them to stop and look at the light before crossing.

The same system works when you're talking about food and excess weight. For example, suppose that you binge when you're under stress.

  ✔ 1 = The trigger = Stress

  ✔ 2 = Your behavior = Binge eating

  ✔ 3 = The result = Excess pounds

It's very hard (sometimes impossible) to change triggers such as stress that make you want to dive into an entire apple pie. But you can alter your behavior and the result by identifying your triggers and changing your response. In other words, when you're under stress, instead of eating, your decide to go for a walk, away from the kitchen, maybe even out of the house. Bingo! You've altered the equation. That's behavior modification.

Why you eat

As a general rule, people eat for one of two reasons. The first is hunger, the second, appetite.

Hunger is

  ✔ The need for food

  ✔ A physical reaction triggered by blood chemistry and hormones

  ✔ An instinctive, protective mechanism that makes sure that your body gets the fuel it requires to function well

Appetite is

  ✔ The desire for food

  ✔ A psychological reaction (looks good! smells good!) that stimulates your brain to send signals that trigger a physical response (your mouth waters, your stomach contracts)

  ✔ A conditioned response to food (When you were a child, your mother gave you strawberry ice cream, and ever since then, just tasting strawberries makes you feel good because it reminds you of Mom.)

In practical terms, the real difference between hunger and appetite is this: When you are hungry, you eat one burger. After that, your appetite may say, "More!" just because the burgers look good and smell good. Or, to be fair, because you are eating so fast that your body has not had time to say, "I'm full."

Appetite, not hunger is what leads you down the garden path in Diet Land. Luckily, your body has a mechanism to counter overeating. It's called *satiety* (pronounced say-tee-uh-tee), a satisfying feel of fullness that lets most people know when they've had enough.

Unfortunately, lots of other people just don't get the message to stop eating. Nobody really knows why this is so, but as the scientific understanding of brain functions have become more sophisticated, some researchers have zeroed in on the *hypothalamus,* a small gland towards the back of the brain on top of the brain stem (the part of the brain that connects to the top of the spinal cord). The hypothalamus seems to be where your *appestat (appetite* plus *statos,* the Greek word for *standing*) lives.

The appestat is not a body part. It is a place, a site in your brain, where bio-chemicals are made, including appetite regulators such as *neuropeptide Y (NPY)* and *peptide YY,* two chemicals that latch on to brain cells, which then send out a signal: More Food! Your brain secretes *urocortin,* a hormone that makes you lose your appetite when you are under stress, and other cells join in making your body say, "I'm full."

The most famous example is the hormone leptin, named for the Greek work meaning *thin.* Leptin is produced under the direction of a gene in your fat cells, body cells where fat is stored. Leptin slows down the hypothalamus' secretion of NPY, the hormone that signals hunger. Mice given leptin eat less food, burn it faster, and slim down really quick. Continuing studies of leptin's activity have led to literally hundreds of news stories suggesting that the hormone may turn out to be the magic chemical that tells your body when you've stored enough fat and don't have to eat any more.

Eventually, researchers hope that following leads such as leptin will enable them to manufacture safe and effective drugs to combat obesity. But that day hasn't yet arrived, so obesity experts are stuck with finding other ways to help you reduce the amount of food you eat in order to reduce your weight.

Do-It-Yourself Behavior Modification

The first step toward changing your behavior with food is to identify the triggers (other than ordinary hunger) that make you head for the fridge. Or the candy counter.

Making a food trigger tracker

One reliable tool in identifying triggers is a food trigger tracker in which you record exactly what you are doing when you feel the sudden need for a snack. Click onto your CD-ROM and print Table 17-1. Print two copies, one for home and one for your purse or pocket. Fill it in for a week. See whether any clues to your personal triggers emerge. Some likely candidates are

✔ Deadline at work

✔ An appointment at the dentist

✔ Being alone or watching TV or waiting for someone who's late

✔ A fight with your Significant Other

✔ Shopping while you're hungry

✔ A buffet table (all that food!)

✔ A really full refrigerator (all that food!)

And that's just the tip of the chocolate cream cake. I am certain that you can list more triggers than I could come up with in a month of Sundays. So do it now.

Table 17-1	A Food Trigger Tracker	
Day	*What I Was Doing When The Hungries Hit*	*What I Ate*
Sunday		
Monday		
Tuesday		
Wednesday		
Thursday		
Friday		
Saturday		

Disarming your food triggers

Once you know what sets off your food feasts, how can you go about changing your behavior? Good question. The following suggestions, adapted from info supplied by the National Heart, Lung, and Blood Institute's Obesity Education Initiative, should simplify your task.

1. **Identify your own food triggers.**

   Once you know what they are, you can counter them. For example, when work gets stressful, get up, and have . . . a drink of water. When you have a fight with someone you love, be first with the "I'm sorry." Don't watch TV or sit around alone. If you have nothing else to do, you can always clean your closet. Eat before you shop for food. Fill your buffet plate to overflowing with low-cal stuff and go back several times for more of the same. Be nice to yourself. You deserve it.

2. When dieting, set reasonable goals.

Every time you try to lose weight, you promise yourself you're going to exercise. Like run a mile a day. When you don't (and you know you won't), you figure you've failed. Which definitely calls for some soothing ice cream.

Forget the marathons. Promise yourself a brisk 30-minute walk each day. As you can see in Chapter 18, that burns 80 calories, which gets rid of 3,500 calories (one pound) in six weeks. Okay, so it's not a world's record, but do it steadily, and at the end of one year, you'll be nine pounds thinner. Good work!

3. Plan to lose weight in stages.

Say that you want to lose ten pounds. Trying to do it all in one week means either using a diet that take off lots of water weight (which comes right back) or — need I spell it out? — f-a-i-l-u-r-e. Boy! Talk about a trigger! The modified way is to set a reasonable time limit for a reasonable start such as two pounds in two weeks. It's do-able without starving yourself, and at the end of two weeks, you'll have a success to celebrate. Doesn't that feel warm and comforting?

4. Keep track of your progress.

Ignore people who tell you not to weigh yourself each day. Yes, it can be depressing to see how long it takes to make the scale drop, but when it starts, it's fun! (Check out Chapter 3 for a guide to using scales.)

Do an instant check of your menu, too, to be sure that when you fill your plate, it's with the "right" foods. Did you have your five fruits and veggies today? Are you actually beginning to like the foods that help you slim down. . . . C'mon now, admit it feels better to be slimming.

5. Give yourself presents.

When you lose the first two pounds, take an extra hour for lunch and stroll around your favorite store, eyeballing the clothes you'll wear when you hit your ten-pound mark. If the boss hollers when you get back, apologize. But inside, make a memo to yourself: Repeat this hour when you lose five pounds. And careful: Don't let the boss' holler upset you. Maybe she should lose some weight, too!

6. Practice feeling full.

If you've never tried this step, it will be a revelation: Eat s-l-o-w-l-y and take sips of water between each bite. What you eat takes a few minutes to slide down your gullet into your tummy. If you give your body time to cooperate, it will. When you feel that fullness, stop. Really, just stop. Try it a couple of times. It will get easier as you go.

Alternatives to keep your mind off food

No, acupuncture, aromatherapy, hypnosis, and meditation don't teach you how to control your calories or help you burn up the ones you consume. But they do tend to calm you down, reduce stress, and maybe even keep your fingers from ferrying food from your plate to your mouth. After all:

✔ Acupuncture relieves pain. Why not food cravings?

✔ Sniffing a wonderful food aroma — vanilla, chocolate, cinnamon-scented apple pie — can sometimes satisfy a craving as well (okay, almost as well) as a fork full of the real stuff.

✔ Hypnosis enables some smokers to kick the habit, so there's no reason to think it cannot do the same for compulsive eaters.

✔ Meditation is the mother of all relaxation techniques. For folks who eat when anxious, it may be an answer to a dieter's prayer.

Unfortunately, nobody seems to have much serious scientific evidence (translation: well-controlled studies) to demonstrate that relaxation actually enhances weight loss. For some people, after all, feeling mellow means chocolate. Lacking proof, you're on your own. That's the bad news. The good news is, these methods are drug-free, have no side effects, and you can stop any time if they don't work.

The Buddy System

Everybody needs a friend from time to time. When you're trying to lose weight, you may need one all the time to help you change your diet and your attitudes toward food and weight.

The different kinds of weight loss programs

In the world of weight control, buddies come in four basic forms:

✔ **Support groups such as Overeaters Anonymous or TOPS (Take Off Pounds Sensibly).** These program do not offer medical advice or formal behavior modification training (although you're likely to talk about beneficial lifestyle changes). There are no exercise regimens or food products or special diets or specific weight loss goals. Instead, these nonprofit, volunteer programs offer support for the weight loss goals set up by you and your own physician. The we're-all-in-this-together experience can be just what the doctor ordered to get you through the rough patches on your way to healthful weight control.

✔ **Meal programs such as Jenny Craig and Nutrisystems.** These commercial programs provide a full line of meals and snacks for people who hate to cook, loathe counting calories, and tend to snack compulsively whenever they walk into the kitchen. Both plans give you nutritionally balanced frozen meals that provide about 800 to 1,000 calories a day based on the Food Guide Pyramid. You are expected to supplement with vitamins/ minerals plus milk, fresh fruits, and vegetables. Each program has an exercise component (Nutrisystem's "virtual exercise instructor" shows you how to do it online) plus information on "lifestyle changes," all expected to help you drop about 1.5 to 2 pounds a week. The meal plans are pricey. Only you can decide whether the results are worth the expense.

✔ **Combination programs such as Weight Watchers.** This true Golden Oldie takes a little bit from Column A (weekly support meetings with weekly weigh-ins) and a little bit from Column B (endorsed products and optional prepacked frozen meals at your local supermarket) to come up with moderate but steady weight loss, which the American Pharmaceutical Association has compared favorably to what you'd expect from a hospital run food-and-exercise program. Because the meal plan is not required, you may also find out how to make your own diet meals.

✔ **Formula food plans known as very low-calorie diets (VLCD).** These programs, which require medical supervision, are definitely not a do-it-yourself project so they don't really belong in this chapter. For more info on formula food, check out Chapter 13. You can find a description of VLCDs in Chapter 5.

Table 17-2 lists the important characteristics of the representative consumer weight loss plans. For contact information, see Appendix B.

Table 17-2	**Some Popular Weight Loss Programs**				
Service	*Jenny Craig*	*Nutri-system*	*Overeaters Anonymous*	*TOPS*	*Weight Watchers*
Date program began	1983	1972	1960	1948	1961
Locations	USA, Canada, Puerto Rico, Australia, New Zealand	On the Web	USA & 50 countries worldwide	USA & 20 foreign countries	USA & 60 foreign countries

Service	Jenny Craig	Nutri-system	Overeaters' Anonymous	TOPS	Weight Watchers
Type of organization	Meal-based	Meal-based	Nonprofit 12-step support group modeled after Alcoholics Anonymous (no fees)	Volunteer-led support group	Support group with optional meals
Diet	Created for individual customer	Lowfat, based on Food Guide Pyramid	Determined by your own physician	Deter-mined by your own physician	Individually assigned, long-term weight loss regimen (based on "points)(for example, food groups)
Scheduled meetings	No	No	Yes	Yes	Yes
Endorsed products	Yes	Yes	No	No	Yes
Prepacked meals	Yes	Yes	No	No	Yes

The five weight loss programs listed in Table 17-1 have been in business long enough for most experts to judge that they are pretty sound, nutrition-wise. But they do differ in some important respects. For example:

- ✔ Overeaters Anonymous and TOPS are no-nonsense paths to long-term weight control, even if (I blush to write this) TOPS has a follow-up support group called KOPS, for "keep off pounds sensibly." Cute!

- ✔ Jenny Craig and Nutrisystems' low-calorie meal plans may work best for quick, short-term weight loss.

- ✔ Weight Watchers' support/food plan combination can lead to steady and sustainable weight loss.

Thinking about cost

In terms of dollars and cents, there's no question that volunteer-led, no-product-endorsements plan such as Overeaters Anonymous and TOPS are clear winners. In January 1998, *Environmental Nutrition Newsletter* estimated that you might spend $1,000 to lose 25 pounds with Nutrisystem versus $38 with TOPS. Whew!

But wait! The fact is that some people do much better when they shell out lots of moola for their purchases and services. So don't make your choice based on false moral judgments. When it comes to weight loss, as long as the program give you nutritionally sound advice and products, what works, works.

That doesn't mean you should add up the costs before you sign on the dotted line. For starters, ask about:

- ✔ Membership costs
- ✔ Weekly fees
- ✔ Food costs
- ✔ The costs of nutritional supplements (if any)
- ✔ Payment schedules
- ✔ Health insurance eligibility
- ✔ Refunds if you're just not happy (or successful)

Then add them all up on your pocket calculator and see whether the price meets your budget. If it doesn't, pass it by.

Asking the right questions

Still need help choosing how to lose? Like how to decide among all those plans I haven't got the space to include here? No problem. This section lists important questions to ask when choosing a program. The questions are adapted from The National Heart, Lung, and Blood Institute's Obesity Education Program. To access the original on the NHLBI site, click onto www.nhlbi.gov and type **weight loss programs** in the search bar.

Ask these questions. Evaluate the answers. Pick a plan. Lose weight. Easy, right? Not so fast. When I say "evaluate," I mean "consider judiciously and weigh all the options." That's a mouthful, but a necessary one. For example, right off the bat, the first question asks whether the program you're considering provides "counseling." Does that mean one-on-one sessions? Then you'd have to rule out Overeaters Anonymous and TOPS, which advise getting professional help from outside professionals. On the other hand, if "counseling" translates to "support," the Overeaters and TOPS guys are back in. See what I mean by "evaluate"? Now the questions:

- ✔ **Does the program provide counseling to help you change your eating activity and personal habits?** As I said, it depends what counseling is.

- ✔ **Is the staff made up of qualified counselors and health professionals such as nutritionists, registered dietitians, doctors, nurses, psychologists, and exercise physiologists?** Of course, some programs train their own volunteers. In that case, the trainers should be credentialed and capable of tossing out ineffective volunteers. Evaluate, evaluate!

- ✔ **Is training available on how to deal with times when you slip back to old habits?** Is there someone available to talk you through the tough times, à la Alcoholics Anonymous?

- ✔ **Does the program have plans to help keep weight off long-term? How long?** For some people, learning how to handle food does the trick. Others may require life-long maintenance. Once again, what works, works. The question is, does a specific program have what works for you?

- ✔ **Do you get nutritious, palatable food?** Whether you cook up your own food or order it prepacked, nutrition counts, and so does choice. You don't want to add a nutritional deficiency to your woes, and you certainly don't want food choices so boring they send you right back to . . . whatever.

- ✔ **Who sets your personal weight goals? You or the program?** Your weight goal should be one you can live with for the rest of your life. Set it too low, and you'll bounce back; set it too high, and . . . why bother? This goal is such an important choice that it should be undertaken by your and you doctor, not dictated by a group or someone who hasn't got your full medical and personal history at hand.

Chapter 18

Exercise: The Essential Extra

. . . .

. . . .

*L*osing weight is easy. Keeping it off is hard. One way to maintain a slimmed-down body is to rethink your attitudes toward food. The aim is to eat light and healthy all the time, not just in the desperate lose-ten-pounds-interludes between pigging out. To find out how to change you mind while changing your body, turn back to Chapter 17.

This chapter describes a second way to maintain your new weight: exercise. After all, moving your body uses up calories, builds muscles, and helps you feel fit and trim. What a wonderful idea!

Yes! It's Time to Exercise

About three weeks into your weight loss plan, just as everything is trending nicely downward, something horrible happens.

Days go by. A week goes by. You're eating less but the scale is stuck on the same number. What's happening? You've hit the dreaded "Plateau."

Plateauing may sound like a fast ride downhill on a skateboard, but it's not. In fact, in weight loss terms, when you plateau, you're not moving an inch (off your waistline, that is). The problem is that your body can't tell a weight loss plan from starvation. The only thing your body knows is that it's getting less food and less energy than usual. So without even asking your permission, it cannily slows down its activity to conserve energy for what it perceives to be rough times ahead.

If you were actually starving, you would welcome this defensive action because you would be able to survive longer on minimal rations. But when you want to lose weight, plateauing is a plain pain in the — you fill in the blank.

It's not the only one.

Another annoying occurrence for dieters is something I call "The Climb," the moment when you start to gain back pounds you thought you'd lost forever. This nasty moment comes some time after you stop dieting. Suddenly, without warning — well, okay, so you had a hot fudge sundae yesterday, three chocolate cookies today, and so on (and on) — the scale indicator begins to creep up again.

Sad to say, The Climb is no surprise. No matter how successful the initial weight loss program, within one to three years, most dieters gain back the weight they worked so hard to lose.

The question is, how can you get yourself moving again?

The answer is, get yourself moving.

The Basic Benefits of Exercise

Regular exercise is so important that for the first time it is a whole separate entry in the USDA/HHS Dietary Guidelines for Americans.

The authors of the 2000 edition of the guidelines write, "Be physically active each day" in the No. 2 spot right after "Aim for a healthy weight." You can read the "Recommendations for a New Guideline" (on exercise), which is on the CD-ROM that accompanies this book. Or you can run your finger down this list to read the short version, which is that literally dozens of studies in the last decade have shown that moderate exercise for 30 minutes a day does the following:

✔ Helps control obesity

✔ Builds lean body mass, also known as muscle

✔ Strengthens bones

✔ Improves heart health

✔ Lowers blood pressure

✔ Reduces the risk of diabetes and certain forms of cancer

Exercise and calories

According to experts, such as the American Society of Bariatric Physicians — from the Greek words *baros* (weight) and *iateria* (treatment) — the No. 1 predictor for long-term weight stability is exercise. True, you can lose weight by cutting calories, but as the Bariatricians explain, you'll lose pounds faster and keep them off longer if you exercise.

As you have heard a zillion times or more, your body measures energy from food in terms of calories. If you take in more calories from food than you use for your *resting energy expenditure (REE),* the amount of calories/energy it takes to run your own body factory — heart, lungs, brain, and so on — and all the other "work" you do each day, you will store the excess calories as fat. In short: Move less, use less, gain weight.

On the other hand, if you spend more energy on body work and daily work than you take in as food, you will pull the extra energy you need out of stored fat. Ergo: Move more, use more, lose weight.

This is not an empty promise. Chapter 5 explains in really tedious detail exactly how many calories you can take in each day without gaining weight. Table 5-1 shows the calculations for your REE. Table 5-2 shows the REE multiple, a number you use to factor in the calories you need for work to get your estimated total daily allowance. Table 5-3 shows the National Research Council's average recommended daily calorie allowances. You may want to put your finger in this page and flip back just to see what they look like.

Okay, here's the important point. No matter what the numbers in the charts say, exercising regularly will enable you to up the totals, eating more food while still losing weight or maintaining a weight loss.

For example, the REE for a 30-year-old man who weighs 130 pounds (I know, I know, it sounds ridiculously low, but it's easy to work with, so just go with it) is 1,563 calories. Obviously, this man also needs calories to do his normal day's "work" such as walking to the bus to get to his office and so on; so multiply 1,563 calories by 1.60, the REE multiple in Table 5-2. This guy can consume 2,500 calories in a normal day without gaining weight.

Being even mildly active increases the number of calories this 30-year-old man can eat without piling on the pounds. Of course, the more strenuous your exercise regimen is, the more plentiful your calorie allowance will be. According to the National Research Council:

- ✔ Mild activity such as carpentry or housecleaning increases the number of calories he can take in without gaining weight to 2,643.

- ✔ Moderate activity such as walking briskly at up to 4 miles per hour raises the total number of allowable calories to 2,808.

- ✔ Strenuous activity like playing a football game or digging ditches pushes the amount of calories all the way up to 3,469.

In other words, this lucky man can add 826 calories to his diet every day without gaining weight just by stepping up the energy he spends in physical work. By the way, 826 calories just happens to be almost exactly the number of calories in a McDonald's hamburger, small fries, and lowfat chocolate milkshake. Aren't you glad you read this paragraph?

Exercise and your muscles

Regular exercise increases the amount of muscle in your body while reducing the amount of fatty tissue. This is a good thing because muscle tissue is active tissue. Muscle tissue uses more calories than fatty tissue even when you're asleep. The more muscle you have, the more efficiently you burn calories — meaning that you use more calories for work and store fewer calories as fat. This explains why men, who have proportionately more muscle than fat, can take in about 10 percent more calories than women (who have proportionately more fat than muscle) without gaining weight.

Just about the only drawback to making muscles is that you may end up looking slimmer but weighing more because, as I explain in Chapter 2, muscle tissue weighs more than fat tissue. But a recent study from the U.S. Department of Agriculture Grand Forks (North Dakota) Human Nutritional Research Center says that the higher muscle-to-fat ratio is healthier and more important in the long run than their actual weight in pounds. Exercise that changes your body's ratio of muscle to fat gives you a leg up in the longevity race. So forget the scale and enjoy how you look.

Exercise and your heart

Your heart is a muscle, so all the good stuff exercise does for other muscles applies here, too.

Not only does exercise strengthen the heart muscle, it also:

- ✔ Increases oxygen flow into the body
- ✔ Relaxes blood vessels and reduces the risk of high blood pressure
- ✔ Lowers total cholesterol levels
- ✔ Raises the level of high density lipoprotiens (HDLs), the good fat and protein particles that carry cholesterol out of your body

And guess what? Exercise can change your body shape. Not just by making your muscles bulge, but by switching you from an apple to a healthier fruit shape.

One way to describe body shape is to say that a person is either an apple (fat around the middle) or a pear (fat around the hips). Or maybe a banana, a category I just invented to describe people who are plain slim up and down the trunk. To find out which one you are, check out Chapter 2.

More men than women are apples, and more apples than pears are at risk of heart disease and high blood pressure. Fat around the middle seems to be a serious warning sign of trouble ahead. This is an interesting fact since more women than men diet to lose weight.

An apple will always be likely to pick up pounds around the center, while a pear will always have broader hips. But adding exercise to your diet can help get rid of the basketball sticking out of your middle, thus lowering the risk of heart disease. (Fat around the hips may not be chic, but it's not unhealthy — and it's really hard to remove without surgery, which you can read about in Chapter 15.)

Exercise and your bones

Like all the tissue in your body, the cells in your bones are constantly being replaced as old cells are broken down (resorbed) and new ones are made. This wonderful process is started by specialized bone cells called *osteoclasts* that bore tiny holes into solid bone so that other specialized cells called *osteoblasts* can refill the open spaces with fresh bone.

This cycle is controlled by sex hormones, principally testosterone (the male sex hormone), which builds bigger, stronger bones, and estrogen (the female sex hormone), which prevents excess resorption of bone cells. Because men have proportionately more testosterone, the average man almost always has larger, stronger bones than the average woman. Even in early adulthood, when her bones are at peak density, a woman has about one-third less bone mass than a man. As she grows older and her estrogen secretion declines, she conserves less bone tissue and loses more bone density than he does.

In the first five years after menopause, a woman may lose as much as 2 percent of her total bone mass. After that, she is likely to lose about 1 percent a year for the rest of her life. At the end, she may have lost as much as half of her *trabecular bone* (the spongy bone in her vertebrae and at the rounded ends of the long bones in her arms and legs) plus 35 percent of her *cortical bone* (the denser bone in the middle of the long bones). In the same time period, the average man will lose only 25 percent of both his trabecular and his cortical bone combined.

As a result, women are far more likely than men to develop osteoporosis, literally, "bones full of holes." Women are also more likely to suffer bone fractures. Right now in the United States, 15 to 20 million people are living with osteoporosis, and an estimated 1.5 million have suffered a hip fracture, adding about $18 billion in cost to the health-care system. Of every seven people with a broken hip, six are women.

Is thinking hard work?

Does thinking about this use up energy? Yes, but not as much as you might imagine. To solve a crossword puzzle — or write a chapter of this book — the average brain uses about one calorie every four minutes. That's only one-third the amount needed to keep a 60-watt bulb burning for the same length of time. Does that mean that even really smart people are pretty dim bulbs? Sorry, I couldn't resist that one.

The good news is that exercising strengthens muscles that support bones. The better news is that exercise can actually slow, stop, or even reverse bone loss, producing a significant reduction in the risk of bone fractures and a lower risk of potentially fatal complications, such as pneumonia caused by being confined to bed.

Exercise and your brain

You know that aerobic exercise increases the flow of oxygen to the heart. Well, it also increases the flow of oxygen to the brain so that you think faster and clearer. This happens even in the middle of the night, when you've been up for hours cramming for an exam or rushing to get through a sales report for your boss (who always shows up promptly at 7:45 a.m., no excuses). In the wee small hours of the morning, natural body rhythms tell you to cool down for sleep. A break for some push-ups or stretches or walking about the room or running in place can zip up your metabolism, raise your body temp, increase blood circulation, and send more oxygen into your sleepy brain.

You also feel better because exercise increases your brain's production of *endorphins,* natural chemicals that make you calm and happy. Making lots of endorphins is what produces an "exercise high" during long-distance exercising.

Hup, two, three, four. Get you butt out the door. Or simply off the floor. Now!

Creating an Exercise Program

Did you wake up this morning and decide it's time to exercise?

Well, don't just do something. Sit there! Yes, you heard me right. Untie your running shoes. Unzip your warm-up jacket. Brew yourself a cup of tea or coffee or whatever and relax in your favorite armchair while you carefully consider how to put together an exercise program that fits your personal needs. That means

✔ Determining your fitness for exercise

✔ Setting your exercise goals

✔ Choosing exercise that fits your lifestyle

✔ Coming up with a way to keep track of your exercise program and the results it produces

Take it one step at a time.

Step 1: Check with your doctor

No matter what your reason is for wanting to exercise, your first step is to check with your doctor. You need to make sure that you are fit to start a new exercise program if you've recently gained weight, or you've been overweight for a long time, or you haven't lifted a finger in a while (except to ferry your fork to your mouth), or you are older than 40, or you have a chronic medical condition, or you've just started taking new medication, or you have a medical problem I missed.

And here's a real red flag: If you skipped Step 1 and headed straight for the health club even though I told you to wait, check out of any gym that lets you in without checking out your vital signs first. Even if you are (or think you are) a healthy young person, this is one time when safe beats sorry six ways to Tuesday. Exercise is hard work, and you want to be sure that your body can handle it.

Step 2: Set reasonable goals

You've been checked out and deemed ready to rumble. Don't move yet. Sit there a little longer and consider this rule, "Moderation in all things." That's the ancient Greek approach to life. It's a pretty good idea for modern exercise programs, too.

Your goal for an exercise program should be to help you lose weight at a reasonable pace while toning your body without stress or strain. Luckily, even a moderate increase in activity can get rid of a serious number of calories. For example:

✔ Slouching on the couch to watch other people play football on TV uses about 20 calories in 15 minutes or 80 calories in one hour, the equivalent of one 2.5-inch apple or a slice of bread.

✔ Getting up and walking at a brisk 3 to 4 mph to the field to watch the game in person doubles your energy (calorie) expenditure to 40 calories in 15 minutes or 160 calories in one hour, which equals two small or 1¼ large (3.5 inch) apples or two slices of bread.

✔ Moving into the action on the field triples your energy (calorie) output to 60 calories in 15 minutes or 240 calories in one hour. Now you're burning 4 small or 2 large apples or 3 slices of bread. Or whatever.

What does this mean for your goal of weight loss or weight control? Good stuff. Stick to the moderate middle choice (walking one hour a day at 3 to 4 mph) and you burn 160 calories a day — 4,800 calories in a 30-day month. To lose one pound, you must cut back 3,500 calories, either by eating less or exercising more. So, just by walking an hour a day, you can lose 1.4 pounds a month or a whopping 16.8 pounds in one year. Even cutting all these numbers in half — a half-hour walk rather than a full hour — will carve more than 8 pounds off your frame in one year. That's what I call a thoroughly reasonable goal.

Keep in mind that your exercise goal is to burn some calories, not wear yourself to a frazzle in an unsuccessful attempt to qualify for the U.S. Olympics Weight Loss Exercise Team — which doesn't exist yet. In other words, it's okay to settle for the wonderful warm and competent sense of well being you get by stretching your muscles while walking a mile or jogging a while. "No pain, no gain" is an outmoded, never-was-right slogan that should be buried right alongside that other Golden Oldie, "calories don't count." (They do, of course, as you can see in Chapter 5.) If your exercising leaves you hobbling, you're doing something wrong and need to seek guidance from a professional trainer or check out *Fitness For Dummies* (written by Suzanne Schlosberg and Liz Neporent and published by Hungry Minds, Inc.) — which also lays out rules for finding a trainer. What a super two-fer bargain!

Step 3: Choose exercise that fits your lifestyle

Okay, so you hate football, loathe jogging, despise aerobics, and can't stand to get your hair wet in a pool. Any exercise program that includes those won't last long in your life, so find something else, a kind of movement you'd actually enjoy. Or at least one that fits into your normal daily routine.

Remember, exercise is anything that moves your muscles, which includes everything from brushing your teeth in the morning to hoeing a row of petunias in the garden or working out in the gym. The best program for non-professionals — you and me, kid — is a consistent regimen of moderate intensity movement 30 minutes to 40 minutes a day, five days a week.

No, you don't have to do it all at once; you can break it into smaller periods of exercise during the day. No, you don't have to turn yourself into a painful pretzel. Like a ship at sea, your best course is steady as she goes. Of course, the easiest course is plain old walking. As you can see from the example in Step 2, walking works. And boy is it easy to integrate into your daily routine. For example:

✔ If you now drive to work, park 15 minutes away and walk the final distance.

✔ If you use public transportation, get off a few stops (15 minutes' worth) early and walk.

Back and forth, there's 30 minutes a day. You would be amazed at how quickly these effortless short periods of exercise will translate into chunks of calories burned and pounds lost. Of course, you may prefer riding a stationary bike in front of the TV set or jogging a mile before or after work or mowing the lawn seven times a week. They're all good, too.

Run your finger down Table 18-1, Table 18-2, and Table 18-3 to pick the exercise you are most likely to enjoy (and thus most likely to do). Table 18-1 shows you how many calories you use in an hour at different levels of exercise. Table 18-2 defines the energy level of various common activities. Table 18-3 estimates the number of calories you burn in 15 minutes or in one hour at various kinds of exercises. By the way, the numbers in Table 18-3 clearly indicate that you can choose something you enjoy — say you choose tennis doubles rather than tennis singles — and still burn up calories while having a good time.

Table 18-1	Counting Activity Calories
Level of Activity	*Calories Used in One Hour*
Resting	80–100
Very light	80–100
Light	80–100
Moderate	170–240
Heavy	250–350
Exceptional	350 and up

Source: "Food and Your Weight," U.S. Department of Agriculture Home and Garden Bulletin, 74.

Table 18-2	How Active Are You When You're Active?
Activity Level	*Type of Activity*
Very light	Seated and standing activities, painting trades, driving, laboratory work, typing, sewing, ironing, cooking, playing cards, playing a musical instrument
Light	Walking on a level surface at 2.5 to 3 mph, garage work, electrical trades, carpentry, restaurant trades, housecleaning, child care, golf, sailing, table tennis

(continued)

Table 18-2 *(continued)*

Activity Level	Type of Activity
Moderate	Walking 3.5 to 4 mph, weeding and hoeing, cycling, skiing, tennis, dancing
Heavy	Walking with load of laundry uphill, tree felling, heavy manual digging, basketball, climbing, football, soccer

Source: Adapted with permission from The National Research Council, Recommended Dietary Allowances. (Washington, D.C.: National Academy Press, 1989).

Table 18-3   Estimated Calories Burned per 15 Minutes or 1 Hour of Exercise

Exercise	Calories (15 Minutes)	Calories (1 hour)
Aerobic dance	171	684
Bicycling (12 mph)	142	566
Downhill skiing	105	420
Golf (no caddy!)	87	348
Jumping rope (60–80 skips/minute)	143	572
Rowing machine	104	415
Running (10-minute mile)	183	731
Swimming (freestyle 35 yards/min)	124	497
Tennis (singles)	116	464
Tennis (doubles)	43	170
Walking (20-minute mile, flat ground)	60	240
Walking (20-minute mile, hills)	81	324
Water aerobics	70	280

Source: Fitness For Dummies.

Step 4: Make a chart

This is the fun part. Table 18-4 is a daily exercise chart and is on the CD-ROM that accompanies that book. So feel free to print as many copies as you want. Then fill in the blanks to make sure that you do something physical each day. Enter your weight on Sunday morning, as this table shows. After a few weeks, as long as you keep your diet steady, you should see a downward trend.

By the way, the Old Wives' Tale that exercising makes you eat more and gain weight is just that, an Old Wives' Tale. Yes, people who exercise regularly are likely to have a healthy (normal) appetite, but they're rarely hungry right after exercising because exercise pulls stored energy (glucose) out of body tissues, keeping blood-sugar levels steady and hunger down. It also slows the passage of food through the digestive tract so that you feel fuller longer, and it reduces stress, which, for many people, means less desire to reach for a snack.

Table 18-4	Daily Exercise Chart		
Day	*Exercise*	*Time*	*Calories*
Sunday	walking	30 minutes	80 calories
My Weight Today:			
Monday			
My Weight Today:			
Tuesday			
My Weight Today:			
Wednesday			
My Weight Today:			
Thursday			
My Weight Today:			
Friday			
My Weight Today:			
Saturday			
My Weight Today:			

Too much of a good thing

Some people can't stop dieting. As they get skinnier and skinner, they eat less and less. The image they see in the mirror — which looks positively skeletal to others — looks fat to them.

Some people do the same thing with exercise. Where you and I are content to run a little here, walk a little there, jump up and down a couple of times, and call it a well-spent hour or so, these guys just can't seem to stop. Like a person who can't give up ciggies or someone who gets high on seven cups of coffee a day, exercise addicts get their kicks from excessive work outs.

Experts call this behavior *obligatory exercise.* It is most commonly linked to running, a logical choice because even healthy runners are expected to spend so much time at their sport.

But exercise addicts don't just run (or whatever). As the experts at Anorexia Nervosa and Related Eating Disorders, Inc. — ANRED, for short — explain, for addicts working out is no longer a free choice or a pleasurable part of life. It is an obligation, or as ANRED puts it, "a top priority to which everything else is subordinate."

Exercise addicts keep detailed records. They may observe a rigid diet. They focus completely on improving their performance. They feel euphoric when they're working out, perhaps because they have forced their bodies to produce excessive amounts of endorphins, natural substances similar to morphine. When they don't exercise to excess, they feel guilty or anxious. Either way, their conversation, and their life, is all about their sport, their training, and inevitably, their injuries.

How can you tell if you or someone you love is tipping over from sensible exercise to exercise addiction? One clear sign is that exercise is no longer fun; it's a job. A second sign is a swelling chorus of worried comments from friends and acquaintances concerned about the amount of time devoted to the exercise. A third possible sign is turning to drugs, such as steroid products, to increase muscle bulk.

At this point, ANRED says, people who are in control will stop and step back to reassess their activities. Exercise addicts, like people suffering from eating disorders (more about those in Chapter 4), ignore all warnings and continue their destructive behavior.

And boy, is it destructive. Obsessive exercise may cause injuries that get worse because they don't get time to heal, which means that injuries may result in permanent damage to muscle or bone. In addition, the psychological damage inflicted by addictive exercise can ruin a person's grades, damage his career, and shortcut personal relationships.

Because compulsive exercising has not yet been codified as a psychological or medical disorder, ANRED has no definitive stats to show how many people are affected. But if you or someone you know fits the bill, you can go to ANRED's Web site at www.anred.com.html for more info and more sources of medical assistance.

Part VI
The Part of Tens

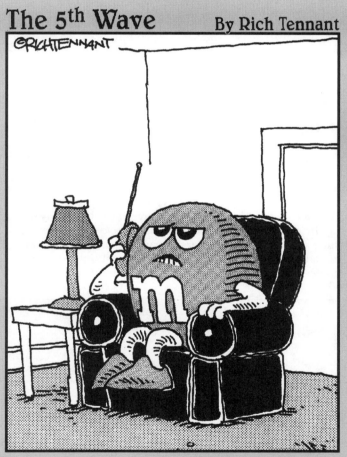

"My body type? I'm an 'M.' But I'd like to get down to an 'N,' maybe an 'H.'"

In this part . . .

Have you ever read a *For Dummies* book? Then you know what to expect here: useful lists of ten special factoids that you can use to improve your weight loss program (not to mention your cocktail conversation!).

If this is your first expedition into the *For Dummies* territory, welcome to the part that makes a *For Dummies* book a *For Dummies* book. This Part of Tens gives you the skinny on myths about losing weight, Web sites packed with diet info, super-special foods any person trying to lose weight can learn to love, and, wonder of wonder! healthful low-cal choices at your favorite fast food emporium. Yum!

Chapter 19

Ten Diet Myths

*T*his chapter is a short but valuable collection of diet myths. I'd bet you already know that what you read here isn't true, but it helps to hear it one more time. For more diet myths, check out *Dieting For Dummies* (Hungry Minds, Inc.) by Jane Kirby, R.D., for The American Dietetic Association. The more you know about the diet tricks that never work, the better your chances of sticking with the solid nutritional regimens that do.

Calories Don't Count

Oh, yes, they do. Calories are the energy on which your body runs. For weight control, the magic number is 3,500, the number of calories it takes to add (or subtract) one pound of body fat. If you reduce your intake by 500 calories a day, even without stepping up your work (read: activity and/or exercise), you'll be one pound lighter one week later. On the other hand, if you increase your intake by 500 calories a day without increasing your work (activity and/or exercise, again), one week later you'll be one pound heavier.

And when I say work, I mean physical exercise. Sweating over a report for your prof or your boss uses some calories, but not enough to make a difference. To solve a marketing puzzle or figure out whether Shakespeare really wrote his plays takes about one-quarter calorie a minute, less than one-third the amount of energy needed to keep a 60-watt bulb burning for the same length of time. Not that you're a dim bulb. Just that to lose the weight, you have to watch the calories, 3,500 per pound. That formula is carved in stone. So memorize it!

People Who Eat Fast Gain Weight Faster Than People Who Eat Slow

Only if they eat more food, a distinct possibility when a person is shoveling grub into his mouth as fast as his little arms can move. To see what I mean, just watch those TV shots of hot dog eating contests with guys cramming buns and — horrors! — swallowing without chewing. I always wonder how these people manage to keep from choking, one good reason not to eat really fast.

A second, weight-related reason to slow down is that eating slowly allows the food you put into your mouth time enough to move down into your tummy, where it settles for a while, giving you that lovely feeling of fullness that enables you to say, "No more, thank you." I don't mean you have to chew your food 100 times before swallowing, a practice once mistakenly thought to help "get the nutrients out." But maintaining a reasonable pace really can help you control what you eat, which means, control what you weigh. By the way, so can taking a few bites of something a half hour before the meal.

Sticking to One — Okay, Maybe Two — Foods Guarantees Weight Loss

New versions of this form of weight loss program pop up every five years or so. The Grapefruit Diet. The Cabbage Soup Diet. The Ice Cream Diet. The Who-Knows-What's-Next-On-The List Diet. If this kind of restrictive eating works, the real reason is fewer calories and more boredom. After all, how many grapefruits or cabbages or ice cream scoops or who-knows-what can a human being eat without going gaga? I make it a safe bet that you can't stick to any one-or-two-food diet long enough to lose the weight you want. And when you stop? Bam! The pounds are back.

You Can Jump-Start Your Daily Weight Loss by Skipping Breakfast

Forget it. When you miss a meal, your body moves into low gear to make up for lost energy by conserving what you've already given it. Your metabolism slows; you digest food more slowly; you get hungrier than usual; and you tend to pig out when you finally do get to the table. Boring though the facts may be, study after study has shown that the best way to control your appetite is to keep yourself from getting so hungry that you eat everything in sight. Nutrition researchers usually agree that you can accomplish this most easily by *grazing,* a term for eating several small meals throughout the day: breakfast, snack, lunch, "tea," dinner, snack. Keep the meals small, and the pounds will come off. Imagine: Losing weight by eating more often.

Cutting Back on Fluids Helps You Lose Weight

Absolutely — right up to the minute you fall flat on your face from the effects of dehydration. Your body needs water for so many essential functions that I wouldn't have space to list them all even if I started on page one of this book and continued right through to the end (there's an abbreviated list in Chapter 21 under, what else? Water). But I have room enough to give you the basic facts about water. First off, the average adult body needs about 2,500 milliliters a day (30 milliliters = 1 ounce; 2,500 milliliters = 83 ounces). When you cut back on fluids, your body goes right along eliminating water as urine or sweat or perspiration or breath. Eventually, without taking in sufficient new water, you lose water weight. (You don't need to drink all this water; much comes from your foods. For example, fruit and vegetables may be 90 percent water.)

But your body doesn't care that you want to lose weight. Its only concern is to stay alive, so when you stop drinking enough water, your body starts pulling liquid out of its own tissues. Your blood thickens. You lack the fluid needed to conduct electrical signals between cells, which means your movement and your thinking slow. And, then . . . why spell out the horrible details? Just drink your water. Now!

P.S. A subsidiary myth, that taking *water pills* — diuretic drugs — can help you lose weight faster is potentially dangerous. Diuretics make you urinate more copiously and may increase your risk of dehydration. Besides, as soon as you stop the pills and get your normal amount of water, back come the pounds. I repeat what I said earlier: Drink your water. Now!

Eating Two Kinds of Food at One Time Makes You Gain Weight

The theory here is that because your body must secrete different kinds of enzymes to digest proteins, fats, and carbohydrates, tossing in two kinds of food — say, a salmon steak (protein) plus a potato (carbohydrate) — makes the process less efficient and you absorb more (or is it less) food, which means you gain weight. Huh? If you had a hard time figuring out that last sentence, you are not alone. Serious nutritionists consider it pure twaddle.

You were truly designed to be an omnivore. Nature made your digestive enzymes and your stomach acid strong enough to chew through virtually anything short of wood, glass, or nails (the metal kind, not your fingernails). Besides, some food combinations are more nutritious than either food alone. A good example is a peanut butter sandwich. Ordinarily, the proteins in peanuts and the proteins in bread are labeled "limited" or "incomplete" because they contain less than optimal amounts of some *amino acids* (the building blocks of proteins). But put them together, and they complement each other to produce "complete" proteins, a process explained in detail in *Nutrition For Dummies*. In other words, your body loves all kinds of food.

To lose weight, don't lose the foods, cut the portions. Or here's a thought: Choose smaller dishes and create the illusion of a full plate or meal.

Carbs Are More Fattening than Proteins

If you're watching calories, you should know that carbs and proteins both have 4 calories per gram. However, because animal protein foods, like meat, come with naturally occurring fat (9 calories per gram), a serving of plain meat, even the lean kind, almost always has more calories than a similar serving of naked bread or pasta.

And I can prove it: According to USDA stats, 3.5 ounces (100 grams) lean broiled sirloin with all the visible fat cut off has 212 calories, while 3.5 ounces (100 grams) al dente, naked linguini has 141. Enough said.

As for the second part of the equation, by cutting back on carbs to lose weight, you're eliminating not only bread and pasta, but also fruit and veggies, which are also high-carb foods. Who's kidding whom?

The Only Exercise That Takes Off Weight Is Exercise That Works Up a Sweat

No. Non. Nyet. Any time you increase your body's "work" (see Chapter 5 and Chapter 18), you use up more calories. True, you won't use as many calories on a brisk walk through town as you do on a treadmill, but studies have shown that even minimal effort, every other day can pay off. For example, in university studies, a 150-pound person who walks at a pace of four miles an hour for 45 minutes every other day (!) uses up enough calories to get rid of nearly 20 pounds in one year without changing his or her diet. Why are you still sitting here?

Some Nutrients or Nutritional Supplements Burn Off Fat

The theory is that some special, maybe even secret, nutrients rev up your metabolism, which means you burn more calories and lose the fat. The usual candidate is a really tart food like grapefruit (have you noticed how often it pops up on magic diets?) or some new and slightly mysterious nutrient that worked for, oh, the Pharaohs, and has just been rediscovered by a diet guru sailing down the Ganges who saw it eat through body fat like a hot knife through butter. (Butter? Butter? Where is the . .) If only it were true. It isn't. What revs up your metabolism to burn fat is exercise. So as I said a few sections ago, why are you still sitting here?

Eating Foods High in Sugar Makes You Hungry

The idea (as spelled out in excruciating detail in Chapter 8) is that eating sugars stimulates your body to release *insulin,* a hormone required to digest carbs, and that insulin increases your appetite. Yes to the first (you need insulin to digest sugars). No to the second. In fact, eating a small amount of something sweet about a half hour before meal time may actually decrease your appetite.

Chapter 20

Ten Sensible Weight Control Web Sites

Remember what life was like before the Internet? Remember having to get up, get dressed, pack your legal pad and pencil, and trundle off to the library to search for info on whatever? Every time I think about it, I offer up a silent thank-you to the silicons who laid down their lives so that I could have chips that let me do my research without leaving the apartment.

Take diet, for example. The ten diet Web sites listed here provide reliable nutritional guidelines, medical news, interactive pages, directories, and more and more and more. And it's only a start. When I wrote the Part of Tens for *Nutrition For Dummies,* I said that if Hungry Minds called it The Part of 100, I could have easily met that goal. Ditto here. Cyber space is big, really BIG. Asking me to choose among sites is like asking a Mom to choose a favorite child. Each site listed here has something special to offer.

Tufts University Nutrition Navigator

`navigator.tufts.edu`

Stop! Before you read another word, eyeball that Web site address. See something unusual? Right: Navigator has no www in front of its name. Remember, no www. Okay, now I'll talk about the site.

Nutrition Navigator is the mother of all online nutrition guides. The Navigator rates hundreds of nutrition Web sites on a 25-point scale that measures nutrition accuracy (1 to 10 points), depth of nutrition information (1 to 7 points), site updating (1 to 3 points), and ease of use (1 to 5 points). Based on total score, Web sites are described as Among The Best (22-25 points), Better Than Most (17-21 points), Average (13-16 points), or Not Recommended (below 13 points).

To use the Navigator:

1. **Click the bright red apple at General Nutrition on the home page.**

2. **When the screen changes, run down the column on the left until you come to Search; click here.**

   On the next screen, you see a write-in box.

3. **In the write-in box, check next to Tufts, then type in** weight loss, **and click Seek.**

   Enjoy your reading!

When I last used this site on August 3, 2000, I got a list of 837 results. If you think that's heavy, how about this: Checking Internet rather than Tufts brought up 1,282,783 sites. Talk about information overload!

Can you find all these sites on your own? Maybe. But the Navigator's virtue is its ability to save precious time while steering you to a safe harbor through seas of information. Oh, heck, forget the watery metaphors. The simple truth is that I love this site. And so will you.

The U.S. Department of Agriculture Nutrient Database

www.nal.usda.gov/fnic/cgi-bin/nut_search.pl

This site is the ultimate calorie chart, with nutrient info on several thousand foods in various size portions and different kinds of preparation (for example., boiled, broiled, fried, and so on). Each entry on the list is a snapshot of a specific food serving ("raw apple with skin") that shows you how much the serving weighs and lists the amount of

- Water (as a percentage of the serving's weight)
- Food energy (calories)
- Protein
- Fat

- Saturated, monounsaturated, and polyunsaturated fat
- Cholesterol
- Carbohydrates
- Dietary fiber
- Calcium
- Phosphorus
- Iron
- Potassium
- Magnesium
- Sodium
- Vitamin A
- Thiamin (vitamin B1)
- Riboflavin (vitamin B2)
- Niacin
- Vitamin B6
- Folate
- Vitamin B12
- Vitamin C

When you click on to this site, the first page that comes up is headlined Search the USDA Nutrient Database for Standard Reference. To find the food you're looking for:

1. **Type the name of the food you're looking for — apple, for example — into the empty box and then press Enter.**

   That will bring up a list of possibilities such as "Babyfood, juice, apple and grape" or "Babyfood, apple and turkey strained."

2. **Ignore the fancy stuff and scroll down to something basic such as "Apples, raw, with skin" and click onto it.**

   A new screen pops up listing various forms of raw apple such as "100 grams edible portion" or "1 cup, quartered or chopped" or "1 small (2-1/2"dia) (approx 4 per pound)."

3. **Put an "x" in the box in front of the serving you prefer, click the button marked "report," and — bingo!**

   There you are — calories and nutrients for one small apple. Neat!

Food and Nutrition Information Center (FNIC)

```
www.nal.usda.gov/fnic
```

FNIC has something in common with the Nutrient Database listed in the preceding section: The agency is one of several information centers at the U.S. Department of Agriculture's National Agricultural Library. To use this site:

1. **Open the home page and click FNIC Resources List, the first button in a stack on the right side of the page.**

   Your click brings up a long list of possibilities, starting with eating disorders and ending with weight control.

2. **Pick your category, such as weight control, to display another long list.**

   If you chose weight control for example, your list includes guidelines, weight control programs, plus more Web sites and resource list. Go ahead. Graze. No calories here!

National Heart, Lung, and Blood Institute (NHLBI)

```
www.nhlbi.nih.gov
```

If you want to find out what a healthy weight is for your body, you're in luck. The first thing you see at the NHLBI site is a list on the right hand side of the page under the heading Highlights. Under that, click Aim for Healthy Weight. On that page, click Information for Patients and General Public. Now your screen shows a whole list of things under a familiar heading (Aim for a Healthy Weight). Click Key Recommendations and then follow the directions to continue. The information here is basic, but solid — and it works. I expect it will take you about 30 minutes to wind you way through it — longer, if you decide to print things out. When you are done, click the Back button until you get back to the NHLBI home page.

This page has something you don't usually run into in a diet book or on a nutrition site, a heading for Studies Seeking Patients. You know that before a new medicine or treatment method is approved by the Food and Drug Administration, it must have proof that it is "safe and efficacious." (Translation: It won't kill you, and it does work.) Much of this information comes from government-sponsored trials. This page lists some current ones. If you're interested in joining, here's your chance.

Weight Control Information Network (WIN)

www.niddk.nih.gov/health/nutrit/win.htm

WIN was created in 1994 by the National Institutes of Health (NIH) and the National Institute of Diabetes and Digestive and Kidney Diseases (NIDDK) to give consumers and health professionals easy access to science-based info on obesity, weight control, and nutrition. You can reach this site either through NIDDK (www.niddk/nih.gov) or through its very own address, listed in this section. Either way, you should move your mouse halfway down the home page to click onto the address for the Combined Health Information Database (chid.nih.gov). Open that, and you find an armful of abstracts, science-speak for short takes on articles, books, and audio-visual and education material. Start reading. You could lose weight just lifting this pile of stuff!

Mayo Clinic Health Oasis

www.mayohealth.org

If you have any question about weight loss topics, then you'll find the Mayo Clinic Health Oasis page helpful. When you bring up the Health Oasis home page, run your finger down the list of Centers on the right hand side of the page and click Nutrition. At the Nutrition Center page, click Ask the Mayo Dietitian. Now go down the screen; click the last line (weight management) under Ask the Mayo Dietitian. This action triggers a five-page list of topics. Scroll through to the last page where you will find weight management topics. Want to add to the info? Press your Back button until your come to the page with the nutritionist's picture. The last line says, "Send us your question." Go ahead: Do it!

The American Society of Bariatric Physicians (ASBP)

www.asbp.org

I'll start with a definition. The word *bariatric* comes from the Greek words *baros* (weight) and *itareia* (treatment). A *bariatric physician* is a doctor specializing in the medical treatment of obesity.

Now to the site. This Web site has two important tools for dieters. Scroll down to the bottom of the home page. Your first good choice is Obesity. Click Obesity, and you get an excellent definition of what obesity is, some serious facts about the prevalence of obesity, a chart showing how to figure out your Body Mass Index (BMI), an explanation of what the number means to your health, and a list of weight loss treatment options.

The second good choice is Locate A Physician. Click this button, and you pull up a page with four easy choices. You can either click onto your state to get a list of doctors by city, with phone numbers; you can fax a request, which ASBP promises to answer by return fax in about five minutes; you can call for names; or you can e-mail. The doctors on the ASBP list are society members who have pledged to follow the ASBP guidelines for sensible weight loss.

The American Dietetic Association

www.eatright.org

ADA (which shares initials with the American Diabetes Association) is the world's largest membership association of nutrition professionals. Its Web site is jam-packed with food and diet tips, guidelines, research, policy, and stats. The ADA home page displays nine choices. Member Services, Classifieds, and Government Affairs are designed primarily for association members. Press Room is fun if you're addicted to press releases or enjoy browsing through the ADA Journal. Nutrition Resources has daily diet tips. Marketplace is an online shopping guide to ADA publications. Gateway to related sites is, well, self-explanatory.

The most useful choice is Find A Dietitian. Click that, and you get a hot line for recorded nutrition messages or referral to a registered dietitian in your area (1-800-366-1655), an e-mail address (hotline@eatright.org), and — my personal favorite — an on-screen questionnaire you can fill out to find an R.D. practically in your own neighborhood.

If you can bend your brain around the much-too-adorable Net address (eatright? give me a break!), you'll find this site a true treasure. And golly gee, who wouldn't love having a personal dietitian to lead the way through the maze of conflicting weight loss advice?

The American Heart Association (AHA)

www.americanheart.org

AHA's user-friendly approach makes this site a must-stop on any diet tour of the Web. True, most of the info here is geared to reducing the obesity-related risk of heart disease. However, AHA also dishes up solid advice for anyone looking for diet advice.

But boy, oh, boy, do they make you work to get to it!

1. **Start at the AHA home page.**
2. **Run your mouse down the left side of the page and click Family Health.**

   Underneath is a listing for Nutrition.
3. **Click Nutrition to bring up a page headed Diet And Nutrition.**

   This page includes a category called Dietary Recommendations.
4. **Click Dietary Recommendations to get to Fit Forever.**

   Now give your clicking finger a rest; you're where you want to be.

The Fit Forever section of the AHA site has factoids (your genes count, but some people just eat too much) and advice, which AHA calls "tips, tricks, and motivational secrets."

Once you've worked your way through Fit Forever, you can go back to the Nutrition heading, and check out AHA's diet recommendations, sample recipes from AHA cookbooks, AHA nutrition facts, food certification program, or the AHA eating plan, a clear explanation of how to use food and diet to reduce your risk of heart disease. Factoid fans will groove on Nutrition Facts, a list of short takes on 33 different aspects of nutrition and heart disease, including what to do with that nasty high-fat, high-cholesterol chicken skin (toss it out).

CyberDiet and eDiets

www.CyberDiet.com

www.eDiets.com

Shhhh! This entry has an extra Web site, so you're really getting 11 sites for the price of ten. Wow. What a bargain.

Unlike the other sites listed here, these two are thoroughly commercial. Nonetheless, Nutrition Navigator scores CyberDiet at 24, one point higher than the American Dietetic Association site, while eDiets gets 18.

eDiets is by far the most aggressive, sales-wise. Within a day of my checking into the site, I got the first of multiple e-mails offering services and other goodies. Ignore the products. Stick to the diet advice. You'll do fine.

Chapter 21

Ten Diet-Friendly Foods

*Y*es, you're right. Eating lots of low-calorie foods when you want to lose weight is a no-brainer. But low-cal is not enough. Your body also needs specific nutrients: vitamins, minerals, proteins, carbs, and *phytochemicals* (the newly identified compounds in plants that seem to protect against heart disease, certain kinds of cancer, and who knows what else).

Every food on this diet friendly list meets this standard. But so do lots of other good choices. Which is lucky, since seven days of tomatoes and cantaloupe could get pretty boring.

Water

You can live for weeks without food, drawing energy from stored body fat or even digesting your own muscles if you have to. But without water, it's good-bye Charlie in a matter of days. Water carries nutrients and other materials such as blood cells to every nook and cranny of your body. It moves food and waste through your intestines. It is the place where biological reactions occur and the medium through which cells transmit electrical messages that power your muscles and organs. It lubricates your moving parts and regulates your body temperature.

Water may provide minerals such as sodium, calcium, phosphorus, potassium, iron, copper, and others acquired as it runs through the ground or pipes to your faucet. The exact mineral content of your tap water depends on what's in the ground or in the pipes. Ditto for most bottled water. The exception is *distilled water,* which is water that's been boiled to produce steam, which is collected and condensed, leaving all the mineral matter behind.

An average adult body requires about 2,500 milliliters (ml) water a day. One ounce of water equals 30 ml, so the traditional daily recommendation of eight 8-ounce (240 ml) glasses is pretty much on the mark.

By the way, you get some water from food. For example, one medium apple has about 4 ounces of water; 1 cup of cooked pasta, about 3 ounces; one hard-boiled egg, about 1 ounce; and 3 ounces baked salmon, about 2 ounces.

Wait: Did I mention that water has no calories? But you knew that.

Skim Milk

Lots of people take calcium supplements to prevent osteoporosis, but nutritionists say cow juice is the better bargain. In addition to calcium, it provides protein, B vitamins, bone-building phosphorous and magnesium, and vitamin D, the nutrient that enables your body to absorb calcium.

The best choice for dieters is clearly skim milk, a.k.a. fat-free or no-fat milk. Less fat means fewer calories and more room for calcium. For example, 1 cup regular milk has 149 calories, 8 grams total fat, 5.1 grams saturated fat, and 290 mg calcium; 1 cup fat-free skim milk has only 85 calories, 1 gram total fat, 0.3 grams saturated fat, and 301 mg calcium. Three 8-ounce glasses of skim milk or three 8-ounce containers of yogurt made from skim milk provide 903 mg calcium, within a whisker of the RDA (1,000).

And did I mention you can take your skim milk as plain lowfat yogurt (413 mg calcium per cup) or plain nonfat yogurt (454 mg calcium per cup)? Both kinds of yogurt give you more calcium per ounce than plain skim milk. Low- or nonfat frozen yogurt? Maybe, but be sure to read the label carefully, with calculator in hand. Sometimes the yummy treat passes muster; more often it has more calories (from sugar) and less calcium per ounce than either skim milk or plain yogurts.

Cantaloupe

At 24 calories per half cup, cantaloupe is a sweet treat that serves up 114 to 157 percent of the RDA for vitamin A, 80 to 100 percent of the RDA for vitamin C, and more than 15 percent of the RDA for that old heart-helper, folate. Cantaloupe also packs a plateful of antioxidant pigments, including beta carotene. The American Cancer Society says eating foods rich in beta carotene and other yellow pigments may lower your risk of cancer of the larynx, esophagus, and lungs.

Given the American propensity for popping pills, you might ask why you need melon when you can get your carotenes from supplements. Tsk. Tsk. Supplements do not provide the same benefits as real cantaloupe. In fact, one study actually showed a higher rate of lung cancer among smokers taking beta carotene pills.

P.S. A hollowed-out half melon makes a neat bowl for other fruits or veggies including cold bean, fish, or poultry salads. Try it, you'll like it.

Tomato

He says "to-may-to." She says "to-mah-to." But it's really *xitomatle,* which is what Mexican Indians called the round red globe that captivated 17th-century Spanish conquistadors at the court of Montezuma. In Italy, the tomato was renamed *pomo d'oro* ("golden apple") or *pomei dei mori* ("apple of the Moors," a reference to those Spanish sailors). The French heard that as *pomme d'amour,* the "apple of love," a felicitous misperception that led to the fruit's once being considered an aphrodisiac.

Nutritionally, tomatoes are top-drawer, at 25 calories for a 2.5-inch fruit. Tomatoes have vitamin C (mostly in the jellied stuff around the seeds), folate, potassium, and vitamin A. In the future, they're to have even more A. As you read this chapter, research scientists at USDA's Vegetable Laboratory in Beltsville, Maryland, are toiling away to make tomatoes with more *beta carotene,* the pigment your body changes to vitamin A. Right now, ordinary tomatoes have 2 to 5 micrograms of beta carotene per gram; USDA's new power globes will average 55.5 to 57.6 micrograms per gram.

The tomato's special contribution to your diet is *lycopene,* the red antioxidant pigment newly identified as a cancer fighter and heart protector. In one 1995 Harvard study, men who ate tomato-based foods four to seven times a week lowered their risk of prostate cancer by 20 percent; ten or more times a week, 45 percent. And a 1997 700-man European review showed fewer heart attacks among men eating lots of tomatoes.

The redder the tomato and the longer it ripens on the vine, the higher its lycopene content.

Lettuce

How do leaves improve your diet? Lettuce count the ways.

First, lettuce is loaded with vitamin A drawn from cancer-fighting deep yellow carotene pigments hidden under its green chlorophyll. Second, lettuce is a great source of *folate,* a heart-protective B vitamin that also lowers the risk of birth defects. Third, lettuce serves up vitamin C, plus small amounts of iron, calcium, and copper. Fourth, you get all this goodness at a mere 3 to 5 calories per ½ cup shredded leaves.

While all lettuce is good, USDA nutrition stats show that romaine is better than most. Ounce for ounce, romaine has three times as much vitamin A as butterhead (a.k.a. Boston or Bibb) and a whopping eight times as much as iceberg — not to mention twice as much folate as iceberg or butterhead and six times as much vitamin C as iceberg. One half cup of romaine provides 15 to 18 percent of the RDA for vitamin A, 19 to 21 percent of the RDA for folate, 7 to 9 percent of the RDA for vitamin C, and 3 percent of the RDA for iron.

Just about the only drawback to lettuce is its vitamin K, a blood-clotting nutrient made naturally by friendly residents living in your gut. The extra vitamin from the lettuce may make *blood thinners* such as warfarin (a.k.a. Coumadin) less effective. If you are taking this kind of medication, check with your doctor before digging into a salad.

Onions

Onions? A basic diet-friendly food? You bet. They're low in calories and high in vitamin C and the heart healthy B vitamin folate, plus they've got that zippy flavor to dress up those other low-cal standards, the grains and chicken breast below.

The Oxford Companion to Food says human beings have been eating onions since the days of the cave men (and women). The first reports of onion cultivation comes from the ancient civilization of Ur, another name for Sumer, the Biblical city of Abraham's birth. Can that be the source of the 1920s admonition to "know Ur onions"? Okay, okay, I apologize for the terrible pun.

The onion family has lots of attractive branches, including yellow onions, white onions, red onions, and immature onions — called *scallions,* if picked before the bulbs develop, and *green onions* or *spring onions,* if picked later. Scallions have small amounts of vitamin A from yellow carotenes masked under the green chlorophyll (the pigments in red, white, and yellow onions have no vitamin A activity). One half cup yellow, white, or red onions has 30 calories and up to 6 percent of the RDA for vitamin C and 20 percent of the RDA for folate. One half cup dehydrated onion flakes has a whopping 45 calories and up to 13 percent of the RDA for C and 30 of the RDA for folate.

Grains

The USDA/HHS Food Guide Pyramid is built on a base of up to 11 servings of lowfat whole-grain bread, cereal, rice, or pasta a day. It's easy to see why.

Whole grains are high in dietary fiber, both the soluble kind that appears to lower cholesterol levels and the insoluble kind that prevents constipation. They are packed with B vitamins. Their proteins — labeled *incomplete* because they have limited amounts of some essential amino acids — can be made perfect just by serving the grain foods with beans (including peanut butter) or with a high-quality protein food such as milk, meat, chicken, or fish. And grains have bulk; they are filling. ***Note:*** For more about protein and dietary fiber, check out Chapters 6 and 7.

By the way, common wisdom to the contrary, commercial whole-wheat bread is not necessarily more nutritious than commercial white bread. Want proof? Next time you go to the supermarket, line up several comparable loaves of bread (preferably from the same manufacturer) with the Nutrition Facts Label facing out. Now read the numbers. See? The funny little secret of American commercial baking is that all yeast breads are pretty much the same in nutritional value, with similar amounts of calories, fat, dietary fiber, and protein.

Chicken Breast

The skinless chicken breast is queen of the diet dinner table. Broil it, boil it, roast it, grill it, chill it, eat it whole, or slice it into a salad or sandwich. It's one great nutrition bargain with a mere 141 calories, 27 grams protein, 0.9 grams sat fat, and 73 mg cholesterol per naked roast chicken breast. By comparison, a 3-ounce serving of roast turkey breast is a close second with 133 calories, 26 grams protein, 3 grams fat, 0.9 grams sat fat, and 59 mg cholesterol per serving. The same size serving of lean roast beef has 204 calories, 23 grams protein, 12 grams fat, 5 grams sat fat, and 69 mg cholesterol. Any questions?

Tuna Fish

I'm talking here about those handy little cans of white meat tuna in spring water, which are lower in fat and calories than tuna packed in oil. The fish is low-cal, but plumb full of omega-3 fatty acids, polyunsaturates credited with lowering your risk of heart disease.

Your body converts omega-3s to anti-inflammatory hormone-like substances called eicosapentaenoic acid (EPA) and docosahexaenoic acid (DHA). The Arthritis Foundation says that omega-3s relieve joint inflammation in people with rheumatoid arthritis. Nutrition researchers at Purdue University say that they also prevent the natural breakdown of bone tissue and increase new bone formation in laboratory animals.

Fish oils also contain *calciferol,* a naturally occurring form of vitamin D, the nutrient that enables your body to absorb bone-building calcium. Finally, the soft edible bones in omega-3 rich canned salmon (No, no, no! You can't eat the bones in cooked fresh salmon!) give you fluoride and calcium, two more bone builders. But tuna still holds the edge in calories, 19 calories less per 3-ounce serving than canned salmon. Go fish!

Chocolate

Chocolate belongs on every diet. It's a soul-satisfying treat that says, "I've been good, and I deserve this." Of course, it has to be the right kind of chocolate.

Contrary to popular wisdom, dark chocolate is not an empty-calorie food. Like other beans, the cocoa bean has protein, B vitamins, and minerals (iron, magnesium, copper). It has small amounts of caffeine (an average 18 mg per cup of cocoa versus 130 mg per 5-ounce cup of drip brewed coffee), and theobromine (a muscle stimulant). And it's got *flavonoids* and *catechins,* the newly identified, naturally occurring chemicals credited with making grapes, wine, and tea heart healthy.

Cocoa beans and dark chocolate have no cholesterol, and food techs have done a swell job creating chocolate products without cocoa butter, an artery-clogging sat fat. The crowning glory is chocolate sorbet, a superstar substitute for chocolate ice cream. Some sorbets, such as Haagen Daaz, are totally fat-free with up to 2 grams fiber per ½ cup serving. Drizzle on some fat-free chocolate syrup. Top it with a sliced medium banana, which adds 1 gram of fat but contributes 3 grams dietary fiber and morphs what would otherwise be pure indulgence into one of the five daily servings of fruit and veggies advocated by the Dietary Guidelines for Americans. Gloriosky!

Part VII
Appendixes

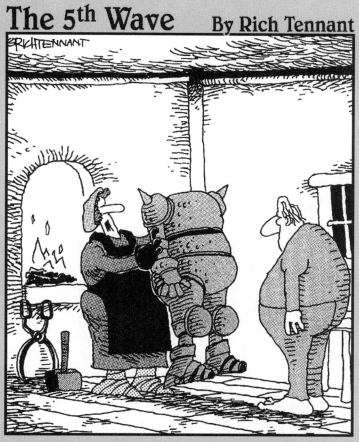

The 5th Wave   By Rich Tennant

ⒸRICHTENNANT

"Okay, Sir Loungealot, I was able to pound out another inch in the waist, but you're gonna have to start taking care of yourself or buy a new suit of armor."

In this part . . .

What a bonus! Three useful appendixes, one to show the nutrients in common foods, a second to provide a weight loss "help list," and a third to explain what's on the spiffy CD-ROM.

Appendix A

The Calories and Other Nutrients in Food

For *Dummies* books are special because they are (a) accessible and (b) complete. Really complete. Really, really complete.

This appendix is about as good as it gets. You get a printed chart showing the important nutrients in several hundred every day foods. You also get instructions on how to access and use the totally wonderful 5,976 food entry U.S. Department of Agriculture Nutrient Database, the (shhhh!) secret source of every nutrition expert's info on foods. Yes, this is the same Web site listed in Chapter 20, but frankly the material is so good that the Web site merits mentioning twice. Maybe even three times. In each case, we use a large fresh apple, with the high fiber skin, to illustrate the info source.

The Nutrient Chart

The really long chart shows a standard set of nutrients for several hundred common foods. The abbreviations used in this chart (and in all nutrient descriptions) are

* g = gram
* mg = milligram
* mcg = micrograms
* IU = International Units

The listing for the large apple (skin on), with numbers rounded off, looks like this:

Description and Serving	
Apple, 1 large, raw	3 1/2″ diameter
Grams	212
Water [gm]	178
Calories	125
Protein [gm]	0.4
Carbohydrates [gm]	32
Fiber [gm]	5.7
Calcium [mg	14.8
Phosphorus [mg]	14.8
Iron [mg	0.4
Sodium [mg]	0.0
Potassium [mg]	243.8
Magnesium [mg]	10.6
Zinc [mg]	0.1
Copper [mg]	0.1
Vitamin A [IU]	112.4
Thiamin [mg]	0.04
Riboflavin [mg]	0.03
Niacin [mg]	0.2
Vitamin B6 [mg]	0.1
Folate [mcg]	5.9
Vitamin B12 [mcg]	0.0
Vitamin C [mg]	12.1
Fat (total) [gm]	0.8
Fat (saturated) [gm]	0.1
Fat (monounsaturated) [gm]	0.0
Fat (polyunsaturated) [gm]	0.2
Cholesterol [gm]	0.0

The order of the nutrients shown in this chart does not match the order on the complete USDA Nutrient Database, but it's sensible in grouping the fats together and putting potassium right next to calcium.

The USDA Nutrient Database

The USDA nutrient database is the nutritional equivalent of the River Nile, the source from which our nutrient information flows. Accessing the database begins with an address:

```
www.nal.usda.gov/fnic/cgi-bin/nut_search.pl
```

Click here, and you are in nutrition heaven — surrounded by bits and bytes of data for 5,976 foods and servings, each listed by its exact name and size.

You can thumb back to Chapter 20 for directions on how to use this site. Or you can simply follow the on-screen prompts. When you connect to the entry you want, the chart that pops up on the screen will look like the one you find printed, for Apple, raw, with skin, in five different varieties, including an old favorite, 1 large (3-1/4" dia) (approx.2 per lb):

NDB#	Description & Serving	Grams	Water	Calories	Protein	Carbohydrates	Fiber	Calcium	Phosphorus	Iron	Sodium	Potassium	Magnesium
		gm	kcal	gm	gm	gm	mg	mg	mg	mg	mg	mg

Beans (legumes) and bean products

NDB#	Description & Serving	Grams	Water	Calories	Protein	Carbohydrates	Fiber	Calcium	Phosphorus	Iron	Sodium	Potassium	Magnesium
16015	Black beans, cooked, boiled, wo/salt												
	1 cup	172	113.07	227.04	15.24	40.78	14.96	46.44	240.8	3.61	1.72	610.6	120.4
16053	Broadbeans (fava beans), cooked, boiled, wo/salt												
	1 cup	170	121.62	187	12.92	33.41	9.18	61.2	212.5	2.55	8.5	455.6	73.1
16058	Chickpeas (garbanzo beans, bengal gm), seeds, canned												
	1 cup	240	167.26	285.6	11.88	54.29	10.56	76.8	216	3.24	717.6	412.8	69.6
16025	Great northern beans, cooked, boiled, wo/salt												
	1 cup	177	122.13	208.86	14.74	37.33	12.39	120.36	292.05	3.77	3.54	692.07	88.5
16028	Kidney beans, all types, cooked, boiled, wo/salt												
	1 cup	177	118.48	224.79	15.35	40.37	11.33	49.56	251.34	5.2	3.54	713.31	79.65
16070	Lentils, cooked, boiled, wo/salt												
	1 cup	198	137.89	229.68	17.86	39.88	15.64	37.62	356.4	6.59	3.96	730.62	71.28
16072	Lima beans, lrg, cooked, boiled, wo/salt												
	1 cup	188	131.21	216.2	14.66	39.27	13.16	31.96	208.68	4.49	3.76	955.04	80.84
16038	Navy beans, cooked, boiled, wo/salt												
	1 cup	182	114.99	258.44	15.83	47.88	11.65	127.4	285.74	4.51	1.82	669.76	107.38
16086	Peas, split, cooked, boiled, wo/salt												
	1 cup	196	136.2	231.28	16.35	41.38	16.27	27.44	194.04	2.53	3.92	709.52	70.56
16090	Peanuts, all types, dry-roasted, w/salt												
	1 oz	28.35	0.44	165.85	6.71	6.1	2.27	15.31	101.49	0.64	230.49	186.54	49.9
16097	Peanut butter, chunk style, w/salt												
	2 tablespoons	32	0.36	188.48	7.7	6.91	2.11	13.12	101.44	0.61	155.52	239.04	50.88
16098	Peanut butter, smooth style, w/salt												
	2 tablespoons	32	0.39	189.76	8.07	6.17	1.89	12.16	118.08	0.59	149.44	214.08	50.88
16109	Soybeans, cooked, boiled, wo/salt												
	1 cup	172	107.59	297.56	28.62	17.06	10.32	175.44	421.4	8.84	1.72	885.8	147.92
16120	Soy milk, fluid												
	1 cup	245	228.51	80.85	6.74	4.43	3.19	9.8	120.05	1.42	29.4	345.45	46.55
16123	Soy sauce made from soy & wheat (shoyu)												
	1 tablespoon	16	11.37	8.48	0.83	1.36	0.13	2.72	17.6	0.32	914.4	28.8	5.44
16124	Soy sauce made from soy (tamari)												
	1 tablespoon	18	11.88	10.8	1.89	1	0.14	3.6	23.4	0.43	1005.48	38.16	7.2
16114	Tempeh												
	1 cup	166	91.22	330.34	31.46	28.27	0	154.38	341.96	3.75	9.96	609.22	116.2
16127	Tofu, raw, regular												
	1 cup (1/2" cubes)	248	209.68	188.48	20.04	4.66	2.98	260.4	240.56	13.29	17.36	300.08	255.44
16046	White beans, small, cooked, boiled, wo/salt												
	1 cup	179	113.2	254.18	16.06	46.2	18.62	130.67	302.51	5.08	3.58	828.77	121.72

Beverages

Alcohol beverages

NDB#	Description & Serving	Grams	Water	Calories	Protein	Carbohydrates	Fiber	Calcium	Phosphorus	Iron	Sodium	Potassium	Magnesium
14037	Alcoholic bev, distilled, all (gin, rum, vodka, whiskey) 80 proof												
	1 fl oz	27.8	18.51	64.22	0	0	0	0	1.11	0.01	0.28	0.56	0
14550	Alcoholic bev (gin, rum, vodka, whiskey) 86 proof												
	1 fl oz	27.8	17.76	69.5	0	0.03	0	0	1.11	0.01	0.28	0.56	0
14533	Alcoholic bev, distilled, all 100 proof												
	1 fl oz	27.8	15.99	82.01	0	0	0	0	1.11	0.01	0.28	0.56	0

NDB#	Zinc	Copper	Vitamin A	Thiamin	Riboflavin	Niacin	Vitamin B6	Folate	Vitamin B12	Vitamin C	Fat	Fat: Saturated	Fat: Monounsaturated	Fat: Polyunsaturated	Cholesterol
	mg	mg	IU	mg	mg	mg	mg	mcg	mcg	mg	gm	gm	gm	gm	mg
Beans (legumes) and bean products															
16015	1.93	0.36	10.32	0.42	0.1	0.87	0.12	255.94	0	0	0.93	0.24	0.08	0.4	0
16053	1.72	0.44	25.5	0.16	0.15	1.21	0.12	176.97	0	0.51	0.68	0.11	0.13	0.28	0
16058	2.54	0.42	57.6	0.07	0.08	0.33	1.14	160.32	0	9.12	2.74	0.28	0.62	1.22	0
16025	1.56	0.44	1.77	0.28	0.1	1.21	0.21	180.89	0	2.3	0.8	0.25	0.04	0.33	0
16028	1.89	0.43	0	0.28	0.1	1.02	0.21	229.39	0	2.12	0.89	0.13	0.07	0.49	0
16070	2.51	0.5	15.84	0.33	0.14	2.1	0.35	357.98	0	2.97	0.75	0.1	0.13	0.35	0
16072	1.79	0.44	0	0.3	0.1	0.79	0.3	156.23	0	0	0.71	0.17	0.06	0.32	0
16038	1.93	0.54	3.64	0.37	0.11	0.97	0.3	254.62	0	1.64	1.04	0.27	0.09	0.45	0
16086	1.96	0.35	13.72	0.37	0.11	1.74	0.09	127.2	0	0.78	0.76	0.11	0.16	0.32	0
16090	0.94	0.19	0	0.12	0.03	3.83	0.07	41.19	0	0	14.08	1.95	6.99	4.45	0
16097	0.89	0.16	0	0.04	0.04	4.38	0.14	29.44	0	0	15.98	3.07	7.54	4.53	0
16098	0.93	0.04	0	0.03	0.03	4.29	0.15	23.68	0	0	16.33	3.31	7.77	4.41	0
16109	1.98	0.7	15.48	0.27	0.49	0.69	0.4	92.54	0	2.92	15.43	2.23	3.41	8.71	0
16120	0.56	0.29	78.4	0.39	0.17	0.36	0.1	3.68	0	0	4.68	0.52	0.8	2.04	0
16123	0.06	0.02	0	0.01	0.02	0.54	0.03	2.48	0	0	0.01	0	0	0.01	0
16124	0.08	0.02	0	0.01	0.03	0.71	0.04	3.28	0	0	0.02	0	0	0.01	0
16114	3	1.11	1138.76	0.22	0.18	7.69	0.5	86.32	1.66	0	12.75	1.84	2.81	7.19	0
16127	1.98	0.48	210.8	0.2	0.13	0.48	0.12	37.2	0	0.25	11.85	1.71	2.62	6.69	0
16046	1.95	0.27	0	0.42	0.11	0.49	0.23	245.05	0	0	1.15	0.3	0.1	0.49	0
Beverages															
Alcohol beverages															
14037	0.01	0.01	0	0	0	0	0	0	0	0	0	0	0	0	0
14550	0.01	0.01	0	0	0	0	0	0	0	0	0	0	0	0	0
14533	0.01	0.01	0	0	0	0	0	0	0	0	0	0	0	0	0

NDB#	Description & Serving	Grams	Water	Calories	Protein	Carbohydrates	Fiber	Calcium	Phosphorus	Iron	Sodium	Potassium	Magnesium
			gm	kcal	gm	gm	gm	mg	mg	mg	mg	mg	mg
14003	Beer, reg 1 can (12 fl oz)	356	328.59	145.96	1.07	13.17	0.71	17.8	42.72	0.11	17.8	89	21.36
14006	Beer, light 1 can (12 fl oz)	354	337.01	99.12	0.71	4.6	0	17.7	42.48	0.14	10.62	63.72	17.7
14096	Wine, red 1 wine glass (3.5 fl oz)	103	91.16	74.16	0.21	1.75	0	8.24	14.42	0.44	5.15	115.36	13.39
14104	Wine, rosé 1 wine glass (3.5 fl oz)	103	91.57	73.13	0.21	1.44	0	8.24	15.45	0.39	5.15	101.97	10.3
14106	Wine, white 1 wine glass (3.5 fl oz)	103	92.29	70.04	0.1	0.82	0	9.27	14.42	0.33	5.15	82.4	10.3
	Carbonated beverages												
14121	Club soda 1 can (16 fl oz)	474	473.53	0	0	0	0	23.7	0	0.05	99.54	9.48	4.74
14400	Cola 1 can (16 fl oz)	492	439.85	201.72	0	51.17	0	14.76	59.04	0.15	19.68	4.92	4.92
14416	Cola, lo cal, w/asprt 1 can (16 fl oz)	474	473.05	4.74	0.47	0.47	0	18.96	42.66	0.14	28.44	0	4.74
14166	Cola, lo cal, or pepper-types, w/saccharin 1 can (16 fl oz)	474	473.05	0	0	0.47	0	18.96	52.14	0.19	75.84	9.48	4.74
14136	Ginger ale 1 can (16 fl oz)	488	445.06	165.92	0	42.46	0	14.64	0	0.88	34.16	4.88	4.88
14155	Tonic water 1 bottle (11 fl oz)	336	306.1	114.24	0	29.57	0	3.36	0	0.03	13.44	0	0
	Coffee and tea												
14209	Coffee, brewed, prep w/tap water 1 cup (8 fl oz)	237	235.34	4.74	0.24	0.95	0	4.74	2.37	0.12	4.74	127.98	11.85
14215	Coffee, instant, reg, prep w/water 6 fl oz	179	177.21	3.58	0.18	0.72	0	5.37	5.37	0.09	5.37	64.44	7.16
14219	Coffee, instant, decaffeinated, pdr, prep w/water 1 cup (6 fl oz)	179	177.21	3.58	0.18	0.72	0	5.37	5.37	0.07	5.37	62.65	7.16
14237	Coffee sub, crl grain bev, prep w/water 1 cup (8 fl oz)	240	236.88	12	0.24	2.4	0	7.2	16.8	0.14	9.6	57.6	9.6
14355	Tea, brewed, prep w/tap water 1 cup (8 fl oz)	237	236.29	2.37	0	0.71	0	0	2.37	0.05	7.11	87.69	7.11
14381	Tea, herb, other than chamomile, brewed 1 cup (8 fl oz)	178	177.47	1.78	0	0.36	0	3.56	0	0.14	1.78	16.02	1.78
14545	Tea, herb, chamomile, brewed 1 cup (8 fl oz)	237	236.29	2.37	0	0.47	0	4.74	0	0.19	2.37	21.33	2.37
Dairy products													
	Butter												
01145	Butter, without salt 1 tablespoon	14.2	2.55	101.81	0.12	0.01	0	3.34	3.24	0.02	1.56	3.69	0.28
	Cheese												
01004	Blue 1 oz	28.35	12.02	100.09	6.07	0.66	0	149.57	109.83	0.09	395.57	72.66	6.5

NDB#	Zinc	Copper	Vitamin A	Thiamin	Riboflavin	Niacin	Vitamin B6	Folate	Vitamin B12	Vitamin C	Fat	Fat Saturated	Fat Monounsaturated	Fat Polyunsaturated	Cholesterol
	mg	mg	IU	mg	mg	mg	mg	mcg	mcg	mg	gm	gm	gm	gm	mg
14003	0.07	0.03	0	0.02	0.09	1.61	0.18	21.36	0.07	0	0	0	0	0	0
14006	0.11	0.08	0	0.03	0.11	1.39	0.12	14.51	0.04	0	0	0	0	0	0
14096	0.09	0.02	0	0.01	0.03	0.08	0.04	2.06	0.01	0	0	0	0	0	0
14104	0.06	0.05	0	0	0.02	0.08	0.02	1.13	0.01	0	0	0	0	0	0
14106	0.07	0.02	0	0	0.01	0.07	0.01	0.21	0	0	0	0	0	0	0
Carbonated beverages															
14121	0.47	0.03	0	0	0	0	0	0	0	0	0	0	0	0	0
14400	0.05	0.05	0	0	0	0	0	0	0	0	0	0	0	0	0
14416	0.38	0.05	0	0.02	0.11	0	0	0	0	0	0	0	0	0	0
14166	0.24	0.12	0	0	0	0	0	0	0	0	0	0	0	0	0
14136	0.24	0.09	0	0	0	0	0	0	0	0	0	0	0	0	0
14155	0.34	0.02	0	0	0	0	0	0	0	0	0	0	0	0	0
Coffee and tea															
14209	0.05	0.02	0	0	0	0.53	0	0.24	0	0	0	0	0	0	0
14215	0.05	0.01	0	0	0	0.51	0	0	0	0	0	0	0	0	0
14219	0.05	0.01	0	0	0.03	0.5	0	0	0	0	0	0	0	0	0
14237	0.07	0.02	0	0.02	0	0.52	0.03	0.72	0	0	0	0.02	0.01	0.05	0
14355	0.05	0.02	0	0	0.03	0	0	12.32	0	0	0	0	0	0.01	0
14381	0.07	0.03	0	0.02	0.01	0	0	1.07	0	0	0	0	0	0.01	0
14545	0.09	0.04	47.4	0.02	0.01	0	0	1.42	0	0	0	0	0	0.01	0
Dairy products															
Butter															
01145	0.01	0	434.24	0	0	0.01	0	0.4	0.02	0	11.52	7.17	3.33	0.43	31.08
Cheese															
01004	0.75	0.01	204.4	0.01	0.11	0.29	0.05	10.32	0.35	0	8.15	5.29	2.21	0.23	21.32

NDB#	Description & Serving	Grams	Water	Calories	Protein	Carbohydrates	Fiber	Calcium	Phosphorus	Iron	Sodium	Potassium	Magnesium
			gm	kcal	gm	gm	gm	mg	mg	mg	mg	mg	mg
01007	**Camembert** 1 wedge	38	19.68	113.83	7.52	0.18	0	147.29	131.7	0.13	319.85	70.9	7.59
01009	**Cheddar** 1 cup, diced	132	48.51	531.4	32.87	1.69	0	952.12	675.97	0.9	819.06	129.89	36.67
01011	**Colby** 1 cup, diced	132	50.42	519.62	31.36	3.39	0	903.67	602.58	1	797.54	166.98	34.08
01012	**Cottage cheese, creamed, lrg curd** 1 cup (not packed, large curd)	210	165.82	217.03	26.23	5.63	0	126	276.78	0.29	850.08	177.03	11.05
01014	**Cottage cheese, uncrmd, dry, lrg or sml curd** 1 cup (not packed)	145	115.67	122.66	25.04	2.68	0	45.97	150.8	0.33	18.56	46.98	5.71
01015	**Cottage cheese, 2% fat** 1 cup (not packed)	226	179.24	202.68	31.05	8.2	0	154.81	340.13	0.36	917.56	217.41	13.56
01016	**Cottage cheese, 1% fat** 1 cup (not packed)	226	186.4	163.62	28	6.15	0	137.63	302.39	0.32	917.56	193.23	12.07
01017	**Cream cheese** 1 tablespoon	14.5	7.79	50.61	1.09	0.39	0	11.59	15.14	0.17	42.85	17.31	0.93
01186	**Cream cheese, fat free** 100 grams	100	75.53	96	14.41	5.8	0	185	434	0.18	545	163	14
01018	**Edam** 1 oz	28.35	11.78	101.1	7.08	0.41	0	207.24	151.84	0.12	273.58	53.21	8.44
01019	**Feta** 1 oz	28.35	15.65	74.72	4.03	1.16	0	139.62	95.6	0.18	316.41	17.52	5.45
01157	**Goat cheese, semisoft type** 1 oz	28.35	12.9	103.19	6.12	0.72	0	84.48	106.31	0.46	146	44.79	8.22
01022	**Gouda** 1 oz	28.35	11.75	101.01	7.07	0.63	0	198.39	154.88	0.07	232.27	34.16	8.22
01023	**Gruyere** 1 cup, diced	132	43.81	545.09	39.35	0.48	0	1334.52	799	0.22	443.52	106.92	47.4
01024	**Limburger** 1 oz	28.35	13.73	92.71	5.68	0.14	0	140.81	111.42	0.04	226.8	36.29	5.95
01025	**Monterey** 1 cup, diced	132	54.13	492.79	32.31	0.9	0	985.25	586.08	0.95	707.92	106.52	35.65
01026	**Mozzarella, whole milk** 1 oz	28.35	15.35	79.77	5.51	0.63	0	146.57	105.09	0.05	105.77	19.02	5.27
01028	**Mozzarella, part skim milk** 1 oz	28.35	15.25	72.08	6.88	0.79	0	183.06	131.26	0.06	132.11	23.73	6.58
01030	**Muenster** 1 cup, diced	132	55.14	486.22	30.9	1.48	0	946.84	617.36	0.54	828.56	177.41	36.1
01031	**Neufchatel** 1 oz	28.35	17.64	73.67	2.82	0.83	0	21.35	38.64	0.08	113.23	32.35	2.15
01032	**Parmesan, grated** 1 tablespoon	5	0.88	22.79	2.08	0.19	0	68.79	40.36	0.05	93.08	5.36	2.54
01034	**Port de salut** 1 cup, diced	132	59.99	464.14	31.39	0.75	0	857.74	475.2	0.57	704.88	179.26	32.1
01035	**Provolone** 1 oz	28.35	11.61	99.65	7.25	0.61	0	214.3	140.64	0.15	248.2	39.21	7.82
01036	**Ricotta, whole milk** 1/2 cup	124	88.91	215.68	13.96	3.77	0	256.68	196.04	0.47	104.28	129.7	14.01

NDB#	Zinc	Copper	Vitamin A	Thiamin	Riboflavin	Niacin	Vitamin B6	Folate	Vitamin B12	Vitamin C	Fat	Fat: Saturated	Fat: Monounsaturated	Fat: Polyunsaturated	Cholesterol
	mg	mg	IU	mg	mg	mg	mg	mcg	mcg	mg	gm	gm	gm	gm	mg
01007	0.9	0.01	350.74	0.01	0.19	0.24	0.09	23.63	0.49	0	9.21	5.8	2.67	0.28	27.36
01009	4.11	0.04	1397.88	0.04	0.5	0.11	0.1	24.02	1.09	0	43.74	27.84	12.4	1.24	138.47
01011	4.05	0.06	1364.88	0.02	0.5	0.12	0.1	24.02	1.09	0	42.39	26.69	12.25	1.26	125.27
01012	0.78	0.06	342.3	0.04	0.34	0.26	0.14	25.62	1.31	0	9.47	5.99	2.7	0.29	31.29
01014	0.68	0.04	43.5	0.04	0.21	0.22	0.12	21.46	1.2	0	0.61	0.4	0.16	0.02	9.72
01015	0.95	0.06	158.2	0.05	0.42	0.33	0.17	29.61	1.61	0	4.36	2.76	1.24	0.13	18.98
01016	0.86	0.06	83.62	0.05	0.37	0.29	0.15	28.02	1.43	0	2.31	1.46	0.66	0.07	9.94
01017	0.08	0	206.92	0	0.03	0.01	0.01	1.91	0.06	0	5.06	3.19	1.43	0.18	15.91
01186	0.88	0.05	930	0.05	0.17	0.16	0.05	37	0.55	0	1.36	0.9	0.33	0.06	8
01018	1.06	0.01	259.69	0.01	0.11	0.02	0.02	4.59	0.44	0	7.88	4.98	2.3	0.19	25.29
01019	0.82	0.01	126.72	0.04	0.24	0.28	0.12	9.07	0.48	0	6.03	4.24	1.31	0.17	25.23
01157	0.19	0.16	378.19	0.02	0.19	0.33	0.02	0.57	0.06	0	8.46	5.85	1.93	0.2	22.4
01022	1.11	0.01	182.57	0.01	0.09	0.02	0.02	5.93	0.44	0	7.78	4.99	2.2	0.19	32.32
01023	5.15	0.04	1609.08	0.08	0.37	0.14	0.11	13.73	2.11	0	42.69	24.97	13.26	2.29	145.2
01024	0.6	0.01	363.16	0.02	0.14	0.04	0.02	16.3	0.29	0	7.73	4.75	2.44	0.14	25.52
01025	3.96	0.04	1254	0.02	0.51	0.12	0.1	24.02	1.09	0	39.97	25.17	11.55	1.19	117.48
01026	0.63	0.01	224.53	0	0.07	0.02	0.02	1.98	0.19	0	6.12	3.73	1.86	0.22	22.23
01028	0.78	0.01	165.56	0.01	0.09	0.03	0.02	2.49	0.23	0	4.51	2.87	1.28	0.13	16.39
01030	3.71	0.04	1478.4	0.02	0.42	0.14	0.07	15.97	1.94	0	39.65	25.23	11.5	0.87	126.19
01031	0.15	0	321.49	0	0.06	0.04	0.01	3.2	0.07	0	6.64	4.19	1.92	0.18	21.57
01032	0.16	0	35.05	0	0.02	0.02	0.01	0.4	0.07	0	1.5	0.95	0.44	0.03	3.94
01034	3.43	0.03	1759.56	0.02	0.32	0.08	0.07	24.02	1.98	0	37.22	22.03	12.33	0.96	162.36
01035	0.92	0.01	231.05	0.01	0.09	0.04	0.02	2.95	0.41	0	7.55	4.84	2.1	0.22	19.53
01036	1.44	0.03	607.6	0.02	0.24	0.13	0.05	15.13	0.42	0	16.1	10.29	4.5	0.48	62.74

NDB#	Description & Serving	Grams	Water	Calories	Protein	Carbohydrates	Fiber	Calcium	Phosphorus	Iron	Sodium	Potassium	Magnesium
			gm	kcal	gm	gm	gm	mg	mg	mg	mg	mg	mg
01037	Ricotta, part skim milk 1 cup	246	183.05	339.62	28.02	12.64	0	669.12	449.2	1.08	306.76	307.5	36.33
01038	Romano 1 oz	28.35	8.76	109.61	9.02	1.03	0	301.59	215.46	0.22	340.2	24.47	11.6
01039	Roquefort 1 oz	28.35	11.16	104.62	6.11	0.57	0	187.62	111.16	0.16	512.85	25.71	8.37
01040	Swiss 1 cup, diced	132	49.12	496.01	37.53	4.46	0	1268.39	798.07	0.22	343.2	146.12	47.4
Eggs													
01123	Egg, whole, raw, fresh 1 extra large	58	43.69	86.42	7.24	0.71	0	28.42	103.24	0.84	73.08	70.18	5.8
01124	Egg, white, raw, fresh 1 large egg white	33.4	29.33	16.7	3.51	0.34	0	2	4.34	0.01	54.78	47.76	3.67
01125	Egg, yolk, raw, fresh 1 large egg yolk	16.6	8.1	59.43	2.78	0.3	0	22.74	81.01	0.59	7.14	15.6	1.49
Milk and cream													
Milk													
01077	Milk, whole, 3.3% fat 1 cup	244	214.7	149.92	8.03	11.37	0	291.34	227.9	0.12	119.56	369.66	32.79
01079	Milk, lofat, 2% fat, w/ vit A 1 cup	244	217.67	121.2	8.13	11.71	0	296.7	232.04	0.12	121.76	376.74	33.35
01082	Milk, lofat, 1% fat, w/ vit A 1 cup	244	219.8	102.15	8.03	11.66	0	300.12	234.73	0.12	123.22	380.88	33.72
01085	Milk, skim, w/ vit A 1 cup	245	222.46	85.53	8.35	11.88	0	302.33	247.21	0.1	126.18	405.72	27.83
01088	Milk, bttrmlk, cultured, from skim milk 1 cup	245	220.82	98.99	8.11	11.74	0	285.18	218.54	0.12	257.01	370.69	26.83
01154	Milk, dry, skim, non-fat sol, reg, w/ vit A 1 cup	120	3.79	434.8	43.39	62.38	0	1508.28	1161.84	0.38	642.36	2152.92	132
01090	Milk, dry, whole 1 cup	128	3.16	634.69	33.69	49.18	0	1167.87	992.64	0.6	475.26	1702.27	108.17
01095	Milk, canned, cond, swtnd 1 cup	306	83.11	981.58	24.2	166.46	0	867.51	775.1	0.58	388.62	1136.48	78.49
01153	Milk, canned, evap, whole, w/ vit A 1 fl oz	31.5	23.32	42.33	2.15	3.16	0	82.15	63.79	0.06	33.33	95.48	7.62
01097	Milk, canned, evap, skim 1 cup	256	203.26	199.48	19.33	29.06	0	741.12	498.94	0.74	294.4	848.64	69.12
01106	Milk, goat 1 cup	244	212.35	167.9	8.69	10.86	0	325.74	270.11	0.12	121.51	498.74	34.09
Cream													
01049	Cream, half and half 1 tablespoon	15	12.09	19.55	0.44	0.65	0	15.74	14.28	0.01	6.11	19.44	1.53
01052	Cream, light whipping 1 cup, fluid (yields 2 cups whipped)	239	151.77	698.88	5.19	7.07	0	165.87	146.03	0.07	81.98	231.35	17.28

NDB#	Zinc	Copper	Vitamin A	Thiamin	Riboflavin	Niacin	Vitamin B6	Folate	Vitamin B12	Vitamin C	Fat	Fat: Saturated	Fat: Monounsaturated	Fat: Polyunsaturated	Cholesterol
	mg	mg	IU	mg	mg	mg	mg	mcg	mcg	mg	gm	gm	gm	gm	mg
01037	3.3	0.08	1062.72	0.05	0.46	0.19	0.05	32.23	0.72	0	19.46	12.12	5.69	0.64	75.77
01038	0.73	0.01	161.88	0.01	0.1	0.02	0.02	1.93	0.32	0	7.64	4.85	2.22	0.17	29.48
01039	0.59	0.01	296.82	0.01	0.17	0.21	0.04	13.89	0.18	0	8.69	5.46	2.4	0.37	25.52
01040	5.15	0.04	1115.4	0.03	0.48	0.12	0.11	8.45	2.21	0	36.23	23.47	9.6	1.28	121.04
Eggs															
01123	0.64	0.01	368.3	0.04	0.29	0.04	0.08	27.26	0.58	0	5.81	1.8	2.21	0.79	246.5
01124	0	0	0	0	0.15	0.03	0	1	0.07	0	0	0	0	0	0
01125	0.52	0	322.87	0.03	0.11	0	0.07	24.24	0.52	0	5.12	1.59	1.95	0.7	212.65
Milk and cream															
Milk															
01077	0.93	0.02	307.44	0.09	0.4	0.2	0.1	12.2	0.87	2.29	8.15	5.07	2.35	0.3	33.18
01079	0.95	0.02	500.2	0.1	0.4	0.21	0.1	12.44	0.89	2.32	4.68	2.92	1.35	0.17	18.3
01082	0.95	0.02	500.2	0.1	0.41	0.21	0.1	12.44	0.9	2.37	2.59	1.61	0.75	0.1	9.76
01085	0.98	0.03	499.8	0.09	0.34	0.22	0.1	12.74	0.93	2.4	0.44	0.29	0.12	0.02	4.41
01088	1.03	0.03	80.85	0.08	0.38	0.14	0.08	12.25	0.54	2.4	2.16	1.34	0.62	0.08	8.58
01154	4.9	0.05	2637.6	0.5	1.86	1.14	0.43	60	4.84	8.11	0.92	0.6	0.24	0.04	23.52
01090	4.28	0.1	1180.16	0.36	1.54	0.83	0.39	47.36	4.16	11.06	34.19	21.43	10.14	0.85	124.29
01095	2.88	0.05	1003.68	0.28	1.27	0.64	0.16	34.27	1.36	7.96	26.62	16.79	7.43	1.03	103.73
01153	0.24	0.01	125.06	0.01	0.1	0.06	0.02	2.49	0.05	0.59	2.38	1.45	0.74	0.08	9.26
01097	2.3	0.04	1003.52	0.12	0.79	0.45	0.14	22.02	0.61	3.17	0.51	0.31	0.16	0.02	9.22
01106	0.73	0.11	451.4	0.12	0.34	0.68	0.11	1.46	0.16	3.15	10.1	6.51	2.71	0.36	27.82
Cream															
01049	0.08	0	65.1	0.01	0.02	0.01	0.01	0.38	0.05	0.13	1.73	1.07	0.5	0.06	5.54
01052	0.6	0.02	2693.53	0.06	0.3	0.1	0.07	8.84	0.47	1.46	73.87	46.22	21.73	2.11	265.29

NDB#	Description & Serving	Grams	Water	Calories	Protein	Carbohydrates	Fiber	Calcium	Phosphorus	Iron	Sodium	Potassium	Magnesium
			gm	kcal	gm	gm	gm	mg	mg	mg	mg	mg	mg
01053	Cream, heavy whipping 1 cup, fluid (yields 2 cups whipped)	238	137.35	820.58	4.88	6.64	0	153.75	148.51	0.07	89.49	179.45	16.73
01053	Cream, heavy whipping 1 tablespoon	15	10.28	36.56	0.37	0.52	0	13.53	10.59	0.01	5.55	17.18	1.26
01056	Cream, sour, cultured 1 cup	230	163.19	492.79	7.27	9.82	0	267.72	195.27	0.14	122.59	331.2	25.83
01056	Cream, sour, cultured 1 tablespoon	12	8.51	25.71	0.38	0.51	0	13.97	10.19	0.01	6.4	17.28	1.35
01074	Cream, sour, imitation, cultured 1 cup	230	163.65	479.46	5.52	15.25	0	5.75	102.35	0.9	234.6	369.15	14.67
Ice cream, ice milk													
19270	Ice cream, chocolate 1/2 cup (4 fl oz)	66	36.76	142.56	2.51	18.61	0.79	71.94	70.62	0.61	50.16	164.34	19.14
19271	Ice cream, strawberry 1/2 cup (4 fl oz)	66	39.6	126.72	2.11	18.22	0.2	79.2	66	0.14	39.6	124.08	9.24
19095	Ice cream, vanilla 1/2 cup (4 fl oz)	66	40.26	132.66	2.31	15.58	0	84.48	69.3	0.06	52.8	131.34	9.24
19088	Ice milk, vanilla 1/2 cup (4 fl oz)	66	45.01	91.74	2.51	14.98	0	91.74	71.94	0.07	56.1	139.26	9.9
Yogurt													
01116	Yogurt, plain, whole milk 1 cup (8 fl oz)	245	215.36	150.48	8.5	11.42	0	295.72	232.51	0.12	113.68	378.77	28.37
01117	Yogurt, plain, lofat 1 cup (8 fl oz)	245	208.42	155.05	12.86	17.25	0	447.37	351.58	0.2	171.99	572.81	42.75
01118	Yogurt, plain, skim milk 1 cup (8 fl oz)	245	208.81	136.64	14.04	18.82	0	487.8	383.43	0.22	187.43	624.51	46.8
Fats and oils													
Fats													
04542	Chicken fat 1 tablespoon	12.8	0.03	115.25	0	0	0	0	0	0	0	0	0
04002	Lard 1 tablespoon	12.8	0	115.46	0	0	0	0.01	0	0	0	0	0
04071	Margarine, reg, hard, corn (hydr) 1 teaspoon	4.7	0.74	33.78	0.04	0.04	0	1.41	1.08	0	44.34	1.99	0.12
04092	Margarine, soft, corn (hydr & reg) 1 teaspoon	4.7	0.76	33.67	0.04	0.02	0	1.25	0.95	0	50.7	1.77	0.11
04585	Margarine blend, 60% corn oil & 40% butter 1 tablespoon	14.2	2.24	101.96	0.12	0.09	0	3.98	3.27	0.01	127.37	5.11	0.28
Oils													
04529	Almond oil 1 tablespoon	13.6	0	120.22	0	0	0	0	0	0	0	0	0
04582	Canola oil 1 tablespoon	14	0	123.76	0	0	0	0	0	0	0	0	0
04518	Corn, salad or cooking oil 1 tablespoon	13.6	0	120.22	0	0	0	0	0	0	0	0	0

NDB#	Zinc	Copper	Vitamin A	Thiamin	Riboflavin	Niacin	Vitamin B6	Folate	Vitamin B12	Vitamin C	Fat	Fat-Saturated	Fat-Monounsaturated	Fat-Polyunsaturated	Cholesterol
	mg	mg	IU	mg	mg	mg	mg	mcg	mcg	mg	gm	gm	gm	gm	mg
01053	0.55	0.01	3498.6	0.05	0.26	0.09	0.06	8.81	0.43	1.38	88.06	54.82	25.43	3.27	326.3
01053	0.04	0	141.3	0	0.02	0.01	0	0.35	0.03	0.11	3.75	2.33	1.08	0.14	13.13
01056	0.62	0.04	1817	0.08	0.34	0.15	0.04	24.84	0.69	1.98	48.21	30.01	13.92	1.79	102.12
01056	0.03	0	94.8	0	0.02	0.01	0	1.3	0.04	0.1	2.52	1.57	0.73	0.09	5.33
01074	2.71	0.13	0	0	0	0	0	0	0	0	44.9	40.92	1.35	0.13	0
Ice cream, ice milk															
19270	0.38	0.09	274.56	0.03	0.13	0.15	0.04	10.56	0.19	0.46	7.26	4.49	2.12	0.27	22.44
19271	0.22	0.02	211.2	0.03	0.17	0.11	0.03	7.92	0.2	5.08	5.54	3.43	0	0	19.14
19095	0.46	0.02	269.94	0.03	0.16	0.08	0.03	3.3	0.26	0.4	7.26	4.48	2.09	0.27	29.04
19088	0.29	0.01	108.9	0.04	0.17	0.06	0.04	3.96	0.44	0.53	2.84	1.74	0.81	0.11	9.24
Yogurt															
01116	1.45	0.02	301.35	0.07	0.35	0.18	0.08	18.13	0.91	1.3	7.96	5.14	2.19	0.23	31.12
01117	2.18	0.03	161.7	0.11	0.52	0.28	0.12	27.44	1.38	1.96	3.8	2.45	1.04	0.11	14.95
01118	2.38	0.04	17.15	0.12	0.57	0.3	0.13	29.89	1.5	2.13	0.44	0.28	0.12	0.01	4.41
Fats and oils															
Fats															
04542	0	0	0	0	0	0	0	0	0	0	12.77	3.81	5.72	2.68	10.88
04002	0.01	0	0	0	0	0	0	0	0	0	12.8	5.02	5.77	1.43	12.16
04071	0	0	167.84	0	0	0	0	0.06	0	0.01	3.78	0.62	2.15	0.85	0
04092	0	0	167.84	0	0	0	0	0.05	0	0.01	3.78	0.66	1.49	1.47	0
04585	0	0	507.08	0	0	0	0	0.28	0.01	0.01	11.46	4.04	4.65	2.26	12.5
Oils															
04529	0	0	0	0	0	0	0	0	0	0	13.6	1.12	9.51	2.37	0
04582	0	0	0	0	0	0	0	0	0	0	14	0.99	8.25	4.14	0
04518	0	0	0	0	0	0	0	0	0	0	13.6	1.73	3.29	7.98	0

NDB #	Description & Serving	Grams	Water	Calories	Protein	Carbohydrates	Fiber	Calcium	Phosphorus	Iron	Sodium	Potassium	Magnesium
		gm	gm	kcal	gm	gm	gm	mg	mg	mg	mg	mg	mg
04053	Olive, salad or cooking oil 1 tablespoon	13.5	0	119.34	0	0	0	0.02	0.16	0.05	0.01	0	0
04042	Peanut, salad or cooking oil 1 tablespoon	13.5	0	119.34	0	0	0	0.01	0	0	0.01	0	0.01
04058	Sesame, salad or cooking oil 1 tablespoon	13.6	0	120.22	0	0	0	0	0	0	0	0	0
04044	Soybean, salad or cooking oil (hydrognated) 1 tablespoon	13.6	0	120.22	0	0	0	0.01	0.03	0	0	0	0
04038	Wheat germ oil 1 tablespoon	13.6	0	120.22	0	0	0	0	0	0	0	0	0
Fruits and fruit juices													
09003	Apples, raw, with skin 3 1/2 "diameter	212	178	125	0.4	32	5.7	14.8	14.8	0.4	0	243.8	10.6
09011	Apples, dried, sulfured, uncooked 1 cup	86	27.31	208.98	0.8	56.67	7.48	12.04	32.68	1.2	74.82	387	13.76
09400	Apple juice, canned or bottled, unsweetened, w/ vit C 1 cup	248	218.07	116.56	0.15	28.97	0.25	17.36	17.36	0.92	7.44	295.12	7.44
09021	Apricots, raw 1 cup, halves	155	133.84	74.4	2.17	17.24	3.72	21.7	29.45	0.84	1.55	458.8	12.4
09024	Apricots, canned, juice pk, w/skin, sol & liquids 1 cup, halves	244	211.35	117.12	1.54	30.11	3.9	29.28	48.8	0.73	9.76	402.6	24.4
09032	Apricots, dried, sulfured, uncooked 1 half	3.5	1.09	8.33	0.13	2.16	0.32	1.58	4.1	0.16	0.35	48.23	1.65
09403	Apricot nectar, canned, w/ vit C 1 cup	251	213.02	140.56	0.93	36.12	1.51	17.57	22.59	0.95	7.53	286.14	12.55
09038	Avocados, raw, California 1 fruit, without skin and seeds	173	125.53	306.21	3.65	11.95	8.48	19.03	72.66	2.04	20.76	1096.82	70.93
09039	Avocados, raw, Florida 1 fruit, without skin and seeds	304	242.38	340.48	4.83	27.09	16.11	33.44	118.56	1.61	15.2	1483.52	103.36
09040	Bananas, raw 1 cup, sliced	150	111.39	138	1.55	35.15	3.6	9	30	0.47	1.5	594	43.5
09042	Blackberries, raw 1 cup	144	123.32	74.88	1.04	18.37	7.63	46.08	30.24	0.82	0	282.24	28.8
09050	Blueberries, raw 1 pint, as purchased, yields	402	340.13	225.12	2.69	56.8	10.85	24.12	40.2	0.68	24.12	357.78	20.1
09063	Cherries, sour, red, raw 1 cup with pits	103	0	0	0	0	0	0	0	0	0	0	0
09070	Cherries, sweet, raw 1 cup, with pits	117	94.49	84.24	1.4	19.36	2.69	17.55	22.23	0.46	0	262.08	12.87
09083	Currants, european black, raw 1 cup	112	91.8	70.56	1.57	17.23	0	61.6	66.08	1.72	2.24	360.64	26.88
09085	Currants, zante, dried 1 cup	144	27.66	407.52	5.88	106.68	9.79	123.84	180	4.69	11.52	1284.48	59.04
09087	Dates, domestic, nat & dry 1 cup, pitted, chopped	178	40.05	489.5	3.51	130.85	13.35	56.96	71.2	2.05	5.34	1160.56	62.3
09088	Elderberries, raw 1 cup	145	115.71	105.85	0.96	26.68	10.15	55.1	56.55	2.32	8.7	406	7.25

NDB#	Zinc	Copper	Vitamin A	Thiamin	Riboflavin	Niacin	Vitamin B6	Folate	Vitamin B12	Vitamin C	Fat	Fat: Saturated	Fat: Monounsaturated	Fat: Polyunsaturated	Cholesterol
	mg	mg	IU	mg	mg	mg	mg	mcg	mcg	mg	gm	gm	gm	gm	mg
04053	0.01	0	0	0	0	0	0	0	0	0	13.5	1.82	9.95	1.13	0
04042	0	0	0	0	0	0	0	0	0	0	13.5	2.28	6.24	4.32	0
04058	0	0	0	0	0	0	0	0	0	0	13.6	1.93	5.4	5.67	0
04044	0	0	0	0	0	0	0	0	0	0	13.6	1.96	3.17	7.87	0
04038	0	0	0	0	0	0	0	0	0	0	13.6	2.56	2.05	8.39	0

Fruits and fruit juices

NDB#	Zinc	Copper	Vitamin A	Thiamin	Riboflavin	Niacin	Vitamin B6	Folate	Vitamin B12	Vitamin C	Fat	Fat: Saturated	Fat: Monounsaturated	Fat: Polyunsaturated	Cholesterol
09003	0.1	0.1	112.4	0.04	0.03	0.2	0.1	5.9	0	12.1	0.8	0.1	0	0.2	0
09011	0.17	0.16	0	0	0.14	0.8	0.11	0	0	3.35	0.28	0.04	0.01	0.08	0
09400	0.07	0.05	2.48	0.05	0.04	0	0.07	0.25	0	103.17	0.27	0.05	0.01	0.08	0
09021	0.4	0.14	4048.6	0.05	0.06	0.93	0.08	13.33	0	15.5	0.6	0.04	0.26	0.12	0
09024	0.27	0.13	4126.04	0.04	0.05	0.84	0.13	4.15	0	11.96	0.1	0.01	0.04	0.02	0
09032	0.03	0.02	253.4	0	0.01	0.1	0.01	0.36	0	0.08	0.02	0	0.01	0	0
09403	0.23	0.18	3303.16	0.02	0.04	0.65	0.06	3.26	0	136.54	0.23	0.02	0.1	0.04	0
09038	0.73	0.46	1058.76	0.19	0.21	3.32	0.48	113.32	0	13.67	29.98	4.48	19.4	3.53	0
09039	1.28	0.76	1860.48	0.33	0.37	5.84	0.85	162.03	0	24.02	26.96	5.34	14.8	4.5	0
09040	0.24	0.16	121.5	0.07	0.15	0.81	0.87	28.65	0	13.65	0.72	0.28	0.06	0.13	0
09042	0.39	0.2	237.6	0.04	0.06	0.58	0.08	48.96	0	30.24	0.56	0.02	0.05	0.32	0
09050	0.44	0.25	402	0.19	0.2	1.44	0.14	25.73	0	52.26	1.53	0.13	0.22	0.67	0
09063	0	0	0	0	0	0	0	0	0	0	0	0	0	0	0
09070	0.07	0.11	250.38	0.06	0.07	0.47	0.04	4.91	0	8.19	1.12	0.25	0.31	0.34	0
09083	0.3	0.1	257.6	0.06	0.06	0.34	0.07	0	0	202.72	0.46	0.04	0.06	0.2	0
09085	0.95	0.67	105.12	0.23	0.2	2.33	0.43	14.69	0	6.77	0.39	0.04	0.07	0.26	0
09087	0.52	0.51	89	0.16	0.18	3.92	0.34	22.43	0	0	0.8	0.34	0.27	0.06	0
09088	0.16	0.09	870	0.1	0.09	0.73	0.33	8.7	0	52.2	0.73	0.03	0.12	0.36	0

NDB#	Description & Serving	Grams	Water	Calories	Protein	Carbohydrates	Fiber	Calcium	Phosphorus	Iron	Sodium	Potassium	Magnesium
		gm	gm	kcal	gm	gm	gm	mg	mg	mg	mg	mg	mg
09094	**Figs, dried, uncooked** 1 fig	19	5.4	48.45	0.58	12.42	1.77	27.36	12.92	0.42	2.09	135.28	11.21
09109	**Gooseberries, canned, light syrup pk, sol & liquids** 1 cup	252	201.85	183.96	1.64	47.25	6.05	40.32	17.64	0.83	5.04	194.04	15.12
09111	**Grapefruit, raw, pink & red & white, all areas** 1 cup sections with juice	230	209.05	73.6	1.45	18.58	2.53	27.6	18.4	0.21	0	319.7	18.4
09123	**Grapefruit juice, canned, unsweetened** 1 cup	247	222.55	93.86	1.28	22.13	0.25	17.29	27.17	0.49	2.47	377.91	24.7
09131	**Grapes, American type (slip skin), raw** 1 cup	92	74.8	57.96	0.58	15.78	0.92	12.88	9.2	0.27	1.84	175.72	4.6
09132	**Grapes, European type (adherent skin), raw** 1 cup, seedless	160	128.9	113.6	1.06	28.43	1.6	17.6	20.8	0.42	3.2	296	9.6
09135	**Grape juice, canned or bottled, unsweetened, wo/ vit C** 1 cup	253	212.82	154.33	1.42	37.85	0.25	22.77	27.83	0.61	7.59	333.96	25.3
09139	**Guavas, common, raw** 1 cup, strawberry	244	210.08	124.44	2	28.99	13.18	48.8	61	0.76	7.32	692.96	24.4
09148	**Kiwi fruit, (Chinese gooseberries), fresh, raw** 1 large fruit, without skin	91	75.58	55.51	0.9	13.54	3.09	23.66	36.4	0.37	4.55	302.12	27.3
09149	**Kumquats, raw** 1 fruit, without refuse	19	15.52	11.97	0.17	3.12	1.25	8.36	3.61	0.07	1.14	37.05	2.47
09152	**Lemon juice, raw** 1 fl oz	30.5	27.67	7.63	0.12	2.63	0.12	2.14	1.83	0.01	0.31	37.82	1.83
09160	**Lime juice, raw** 1 fl oz	30.8	27.78	8.32	0.14	2.78	0.12	2.77	2.16	0.01	0.31	33.57	1.85
09176	**Mangos, raw** 1 fruit, without refuse	207	169.14	134.55	1.06	35.19	3.73	20.7	22.77	0.27	4.14	322.92	18.63
09181	**Melons, cantaloupe, raw** 1 cup, balls	177	158.91	61.95	1.56	14.8	1.42	19.47	30.09	0.37	15.93	546.93	19.47
09184	**Melons, honeydew, raw** 1 cup, diced (approx 20 pieces per cup)	170	152.42	59.5	0.78	15.61	1.02	10.2	17	0.12	17	460.7	11.9
09191	**Nectarines, raw** 1 fruit (2-1/2" dia)	136	117.34	66.64	1.28	16.02	2.18	6.8	21.76	0.2	0	288.32	10.88
09193	**Olives, ripe, canned (small-extra lrg)** 1 large	4.4	3.52	5.06	0.04	0.28	0.14	3.87	0.13	0.15	38.37	0.35	0.18
09194	**Olives, ripe, canned (jumbo-super colossal)** 1 jumbo	8.3	7	6.72	0.08	0.47	0.21	7.8	0.25	0.28	74.53	0.75	0.33
09201	**Oranges, raw, California, Valencias** 1 fruit (2-5/8" dia, sphere)	121	104.47	59.29	1.26	14.39	3.03	48.4	20.57	0.11	0	216.59	12.1
09202	**Oranges, raw, California, navels** 1 fruit (2-7/8" dia)	140	121.53	64.4	1.44	16.28	3.36	56	26.6	0.17	1.4	249.2	14
09203	**Oranges, raw, Florida** 1 fruit (2-5/8" dia, sphere)	141	122.87	64.86	0.99	16.27	3.38	60.63	16.92	0.13	0	238.29	14.1
09206	**Orange juice, raw** 1 cup	248	218.98	111.6	1.74	25.79	0.5	27.28	42.16	0.5	2.48	496	27.28

NDB#	Zinc	Copper	Vitamin A	Thiamin	Riboflavin	Niacin	Vitamin B6	Folate	Vitamin B12	Vitamin C	Fat	Fat-Saturated	Fat-Monounsaturated	Fat-Polyunsaturated	Cholesterol
	mg	mg	IU	mg	mg	mg	mg	mcg	mcg	mg	gm	gm	gm	gm	mg
09094	0.1	0.06	25.27	0.01	0.02	0.13	0.04	1.43	0	0.15	0.22	0.04	0.05	0.11	0
09109	0.28	0.55	347.76	0.05	0.13	0.39	0.03	8.06	0	25.2	0.5	0.03	0.05	0.28	0
09111	0.16	0.11	285.2	0.08	0.05	0.58	0.1	23.46	0	79.12	0.23	0.03	0.03	0.06	0
09123	0.22	0.09	17.29	0.1	0.05	0.57	0.05	25.69	0	72.12	0.25	0.03	0.03	0.06	0
09131	0.04	0.04	92	0.08	0.05	0.28	0.1	3.59	0	3.68	0.32	0.1	0.01	0.09	0
09132	0.08	0.14	116.8	0.15	0.09	0.48	0.18	6.24	0	17.28	0.93	0.3	0.04	0.27	0
09135	0.13	0.07	20.24	0.07	0.09	0.66	0.16	6.58	0	0.25	0.2	0.06	0.01	0.06	0
09139	0.56	0.25	1932.48	0.12	0.12	2.93	0.35	34.16	0	447.74	1.46	0.42	0.13	0.62	0
09148	0.15	0.14	159.25	0.02	0.05	0.46	0.08	34.58	0	89.18	0.4	0.03	0.04	0.22	0
09149	0.02	0.02	57.38	0.02	0.02	0.1	0.01	3.04	0	7.11	0.02	0	0	0	0
09152	0.02	0.01	6.1	0.01	0	0.03	0.02	3.93	0	14.03	0	0	0	0	0
09160	0.02	0.01	3.08	0.01	0	0.03	0.01	2.53	0	9.02	0.03	0	0	0.01	0
09176	0.08	0.23	8060.58	0.12	0.12	1.21	0.28	28.98	0	57.34	0.56	0.14	0.21	0.11	0
09181	0.28	0.07	5706.48	0.06	0.04	1.02	0.2	30.09	0	74.69	0.5	0.13	0.01	0.19	0
09184	0.12	0.07	68	0.13	0.03	1.02	0.1	10.2	0	42.16	0.17	0.04	0	0.07	0
09191	0.12	0.1	1000.96	0.02	0.06	1.35	0.03	5.03	0	7.34	0.63	0.07	0.24	0.31	0
09193	0.01	0.01	17.73	0	0	0	0	0	0	0.04	0.47	0.06	0.35	0.04	0
09194	0.02	0.02	28.72	0	0	0	0	0	0	0.12	0.57	0.08	0.42	0.05	0
09201	0.07	0.04	278.3	0.11	0.05	0.33	0.08	46.71	0	58.69	0.36	0.04	0.07	0.07	0
09202	0.08	0.08	256.2	0.12	0.06	0.41	0.1	47.18	0	80.22	0.13	0.02	0.02	0.03	0
09203	0.11	0.05	282	0.14	0.06	0.56	0.07	24.39	0	63.45	0.3	0.04	0.05	0.06	0
09206	0.12	0.11	496	0.22	0.07	0.99	0.1	75.14	0	124	0.5	0.06	0.09	0.1	0

NDB#	Description & Serving	Grams	Water	Calories	Protein	Carbohydrates	Fiber	Calcium	Phosphorus	Iron	Sodium	Potassium	Magnesium
		gm	gm	kcal	gm	gm	gm	mg	mg	mg	mg	mg	mg
09218	Tangerines (mandarin oranges), raw 1 large (2-1/2" dia)	98	85.85	43.12	0.62	10.97	2.25	13.72	9.8	0.1	0.98	153.86	11.76
09219	Tangerines (mandarin oranges), canned, juice pk 1 cup	249	222.88	92.13	1.54	23.83	1.74	27.39	24.9	0.67	12.45	331.17	27.39
09226	Papayas, raw 1 cup, cubes	140	124.36	54.6	0.85	13.73	2.52	33.6	7	0.14	4.2	359.8	14
09229	Papaya nectar, canned 1 cup	250	212.55	142.5	0.43	36.28	1.5	25	0	0.85	12.5	77.5	7.5
09231	Passion-fruit (granadilla), purple, raw 1 fruit, without refuse	18	13.13	17.46	0.4	4.21	1.87	2.16	12.24	0.29	5.04	62.64	5.22
09236	Peaches, raw 1 large (2-3/4" dia) (approx 2 1/2 per lb)	157	137.63	67.51	1.1	17.43	3.14	7.85	18.84	0.17	0	309.29	10.99
09246	Peaches, dried, sulfured, uncooked 1 half	13	4.13	31.07	0.47	7.97	1.07	3.64	15.47	0.53	0.91	129.48	5.46
09251	Peach nectar, canned, wo/ vit C 1 cup	249	213.24	134.46	0.67	34.66	1.49	12.45	14.94	0.47	17.43	99.6	9.96
09252	Pears, raw 1 medium (approx 2 1/2 per lb)	166	139.12	97.94	0.65	25.08	3.98	18.26	18.26	0.42	0	207.5	9.96
09259	Pears, dried, sulfured, uncooked 1 half with liquid	76	20.28	199.12	1.42	52.97	5.7	25.84	44.84	1.6	4.56	405.08	25.08
09265	Persimmons, native, raw 1 fruit, without refuse	25	16.1	31.75	0.2	8.38	0	6.75	6.5	0.63	0.25	77.5	0
09266	Pineapple, raw 1 cup, diced	155	134.08	75.95	0.6	19.2	1.86	10.85	10.85	0.57	1.55	175.15	21.7
09273	Pineapple juice, canned, unsweetened, wo/ vit C 1 cup	250	213.83	140	0.8	34.45	0.5	42.5	20	0.65	2.5	335	32.5
09278	Plantains, cooked 1 cup, slices	154	103.64	178.64	1.22	47.97	3.54	3.08	43.12	0.89	7.7	716.1	49.28
09279	Plums, raw 1 fruit (2-1/8" dia)	66	56.23	36.3	0.52	8.59	0.99	2.64	6.6	0.07	0	113.52	4.62
09286	Pomegranates, raw 1 pomegranate (3-3/8" dia)	154	124.69	104.72	1.46	26.44	0.92	4.62	12.32	0.46	4.62	398.86	4.62
09287	Prickly pears, raw 1 fruit	103	90.18	42.23	0.75	9.86	3.71	57.68	24.72	0.31	5.15	226.6	87.55
09291	Prunes, dried, uncooked 1 prune	8.4	2.72	20.08	0.22	5.27	0.6	4.28	6.64	0.21	0.34	62.58	3.78
09294	Prune juice, canned 1 cup	256	207.97	181.76	1.56	44.67	2.56	30.72	64	3.02	10.24	706.56	35.84
09296	Quinces, raw 1 fruit, without refuse	92	77.1	52.44	0.37	14.08	1.75	10.12	15.64	0.64	3.68	181.24	7.36
09298	Raisins, seedless 1 cup, packed	165	25.44	495	5.31	130.56	6.6	80.85	160.05	3.43	19.8	1239.15	54.45
09302	Raspberries, raw 1 cup	123	106.48	60.27	1.12	14.23	8.36	27.06	14.76	0.7	0	186.96	22.14
09309	Rhubarb, frozen, uncooked 1 cup, diced	137	128.11	28.77	0.75	6.99	2.47	265.78	16.44	0.4	2.74	147.96	24.66

NDB#	Zinc	Copper	Vitamin A	Thiamin	Riboflavin	Niacin	Vitamin B6	Folate	Vitamin B12	Vitamin C	Fat	Fat: Saturated	Fat: Monounsaturated	Fat: Polyunsaturated	Cholesterol
	mg	mg	IU	mg	mg	mg	mg	mcg	mcg	mg	gm	gm	gm	gm	mg
09218	0.24	0.03	901.6	0.1	0.02	0.16	0.07	19.99	0	30.18	0.19	0.02	0.03	0.04	0
09219	1.27	0.08	2121.48	0.2	0.07	1.11	0.1	11.45	0	85.16	0.07	0.01	0.01	0.01	0
09226	0.1	0.02	397.6	0.04	0.04	0.47	0.03	53.2	0	86.52	0.2	0.06	0.05	0.04	0
09229	0.38	0.03	277.5	0.02	0.01	0.38	0.02	5.25	0	7.5	0.38	0.12	0.1	0.09	0
09231	0.02	0.02	126	0	0.02	0.27	0.02	2.52	0	5.4	0.13	0.01	0.02	0.07	0
09236	0.22	0.11	839.95	0.03	0.06	1.55	0.03	5.34	0	10.36	0.14	0.02	0.05	0.07	0
09246	0.07	0.05	281.19	0	0.03	0.57	0.01	0.04	0	0.62	0.1	0.01	0.04	0.05	0
09251	0.2	0.17	642.42	0.01	0.03	0.72	0.02	3.49	0	13.2	0.05	0	0.02	0.03	0
09252	0.2	0.18	33.2	0.03	0.07	0.17	0.03	12.12	0	6.64	0.66	0.04	0.14	0.16	0
09259	0.3	0.28	2.28	0.01	0.11	1.04	0.05	0	0	5.32	0.48	0.03	0.1	0.11	0
09265	0	0	0	0	0	0	0	0	0	16.5	0.1	0	0	0	0
09266	0.12	0.17	35.65	0.14	0.06	0.65	0.13	16.43	0	23.87	0.67	0.05	0.07	0.23	0
09273	0.28	0.23	12.5	0.14	0.06	0.64	0.24	57.75	0	26.75	0.2	0.01	0.02	0.07	0
09278	0.2	0.1	1399.86	0.07	0.08	1.16	0.37	40.04	0	16.79	0.28	0.11	0.02	0.05	0
09279	0.07	0.03	213.18	0.03	0.06	0.33	0.05	1.45	0	6.27	0.41	0.03	0.27	0.09	0
09286	0.18	0.11	0	0.05	0.05	0.46	0.16	9.24	0	9.39	0.46	0.06	0.07	0.1	0
09287	0.12	0.08	52.53	0.01	0.06	0.47	0.06	6.18	0	14.42	0.53	0.07	0.08	0.22	0
09291	0.04	0.04	166.91	0.01	0.01	0.16	0.02	0.31	0	0.28	0.04	0	0.03	0.01	0
09294	0.54	0.17	7.68	0.04	0.18	2.01	0.56	1.02	0	10.5	0.08	0.01	0.05	0.02	0
09296	0.04	0.12	36.8	0.02	0.03	0.18	0.04	2.76	0	13.8	0.09	0.01	0.03	0.05	0
09298	0.45	0.51	13.2	0.26	0.15	1.35	0.41	5.45	0	5.45	0.76	0.25	0.03	0.22	0
09302	0.57	0.09	159.9	0.04	0.11	1.11	0.07	31.98	0	30.75	0.68	0.02	0.07	0.38	0
09309	0.14	0.03	146.59	0.04	0.04	0.28	0.03	11.23	0	6.58	0.15	0.04	0.03	0.07	0

NDB#	Description & Serving	Grams	Water	Calories	Protein	Carbohydrates	Fiber	Calcium	Phosphorus	Iron	Sodium	Potassium	Magnesium
		gm	gm	kcal	gm	gm	gm	mg	mg	mg	mg	mg	mg
09316	Strawberries, raw 1 cup, halves	152	139.19	45.6	0.93	10.67	3.5	21.28	28.88	0.58	1.52	252.32	15.2
09326	Watermelon, raw 1 cup, balls	154	140.93	49.28	0.95	11.06	0.77	12.32	13.86	0.26	3.08	178.64	16.94
Grain products													
Breads													
18001	Bagels, plain, enriched, w/ca prop (incl onion, poppy, sesame) 1 bagel (3" dia)	57	18.58	156.75	5.99	30.44	1.31	42.18	54.72	2.03	304.38	57.57	16.53
18007	Bagels, oat bran 1 bagel (3" dia)	57	18.75	145.35	6.1	30.38	2.05	6.84	94.05	1.76	288.99	116.28	32.49
18079	Bread crumbs, dry, grated, plain 1 cup	108	6.7	426.6	13.5	78.3	2.59	245.16	158.76	6.61	930.96	238.68	49.68
18080	Breadsticks, plain 1 small stick (approx 4-1/4" long)	5	0.31	20.6	0.6	3.42	0.15	1.1	6.05	0.21	32.85	6.2	1.6
18347	Dinner rolls, wheat 1 roll (1 oz)	28.35	10.49	77.4	2.44	13.04	1.07	49.9	33.45	1.01	96.39	37.71	11.91
18258	English muffins, plain, enriched, w/ca prop (incl sourdough) 1 muffin	57	24	133.95	4.39	26.22	1.54	99.18	75.81	1.43	264.48	74.67	11.97
18266	English muffins, whole-wheat 1 muffin	66	30.16	133.98	5.81	26.66	4.42	174.9	186.12	1.62	420.42	138.6	46.86
18349	French rolls 1 roll	38	13.22	105.26	3.27	19.08	1.22	34.58	31.92	1.03	231.42	43.32	7.6
18029	French or vienna bread (incl sourdough) 1 large slice (5" x 2-1/2" x 1")	35	12.01	95.9	3.08	18.17	1.05	26.25	36.75	0.89	213.15	39.55	9.45
18350	Hamburger or hotdog, plain rolls 1 roll	43	14.62	122.98	3.66	21.63	1.16	59.77	37.84	1.36	240.8	60.63	8.6
18353	Hard (incl kaiser) rolls 1 roll (3-1/2" dia)	57	17.67	167.01	5.64	30.04	1.31	54.15	57	1.87	310.08	61.56	15.39
18033	Italian bread 1 large slice (4-1/2" x 3-1/4" x 3/4")	30	10.71	81.3	2.64	15	0.81	23.4	30.9	0.88	175.2	33	8.1
18035	Mixed-grain (incl whole-grain, 7-grain) bread 1 large slice	32	12.06	80	3.2	14.85	2.05	29.12	56.32	1.11	155.84	65.28	16.96
18041	Pita, white, enriched bread 1 large pita (6-1/2" dia)	60	19.26	165	5.46	33.42	1.32	51.6	58.2	1.57	321.6	72	15.6
18042	Pita, whole-wheat bread 1 large pita (6-1/2" dia)	64	19.58	170.24	6.27	35.2	4.74	9.6	115.2	1.85	340.48	108.8	44.16
18044	Pumpernickel bread 1 regular slice	26	9.85	65	2.26	12.35	1.69	17.68	46.28	0.75	174.46	54.08	14.04
18047	Raisin, enriched bread 1 large slice	32	10.75	87.68	2.53	16.74	1.38	21.12	34.88	0.93	124.8	72.64	8.32
18060	Rye bread 1 slice	32	11.94	82.88	2.72	15.46	1.86	23.36	40	0.91	211.2	53.12	12.8
18064	Wheat (incl wheat berry) bread 1 slice	25	9.28	65	2.28	11.8	1.08	26.25	37.5	0.83	132.5	50.25	11.5
18069	White bread, commly prep (incl soft bread crumbs) 1 cup, crumbs	45	16.52	120.15	3.69	22.28	1.04	48.6	42.3	1.36	242.1	53.55	10.8

NDB #	Zinc	Copper	Vitamin A	Thiamin	Riboflavin	Niacin	Vitamin B6	Folate	Vitamin B12	Vitamin C	Fat	Fat: Saturated	Fat: Monounsaturated	Fat: Polyunsaturated	Cholesterol
	mg	mg	IU	mg	mg	mg	mg	mcg	mcg	mg	gm	gm	gm	gm	mg
09316	0.2	0.07	41.04	0.03	0.1	0.35	0.09	26.9	0	86.18	0.56	0.03	0.08	0.28	0
09326	0.11	0.05	563.64	0.12	0.03	0.31	0.22	3.39	0	14.78	0.66	0.07	0.16	0.22	0

Grain products

Breads

NDB #	Zinc	Copper	Vitamin A	Thiamin	Riboflavin	Niacin	Vitamin B6	Folate	Vitamin B12	Vitamin C	Fat	Fat: Saturated	Fat: Monounsaturated	Fat: Polyunsaturated	Cholesterol
18001	0.5	0.09	0	0.31	0.18	2.6	0.03	12.54	0	0	0.91	0.13	0.07	0.4	0
18007	1.19	0.07	2.28	0.19	0.19	1.69	0.12	26.22	0	0.11	0.68	0.11	0.14	0.28	0
18079	1.32	0.18	1.08	0.83	0.47	7.4	0.11	27	0.02	0	5.83	1.36	2.26	1.68	0
18080	0.04	0.01	0	0.03	0.03	0.26	0	1.5	0	0	0.48	0.07	0.19	0.18	0
18347	0.29	0.04	0	0.12	0.08	1.15	0.02	4.25	0	0	1.79	0.43	0.92	0.3	0
18258	0.4	0.07	0	0.25	0.16	2.21	0.02	21.09	0.02	0.06	1.03	0.15	0.17	0.51	0
18266	1.06	0.14	0	0.2	0.09	2.25	0.11	32.34	0	0	1.39	0.22	0.34	0.55	0
18349	0.29	0.07	1.52	0.2	0.11	1.65	0.02	12.54	0	0	1.63	0.37	0.75	0.32	0
18029	0.3	0.07	0	0.18	0.12	1.66	0.02	10.85	0	0	1.05	0.22	0.43	0.24	0
18350	0.27	0.05	0	0.21	0.13	1.69	0.02	11.61	0.01	0	2.19	0.51	1.07	0.39	0
18353	0.54	0.09	0	0.27	0.19	2.42	0.03	8.55	0	0	2.45	0.35	0.65	0.98	0
18033	0.26	0.06	0	0.14	0.09	1.31	0.01	9	0	0	1.05	0.26	0.24	0.42	0
18035	0.41	0.08	0	0.13	0.11	1.4	0.11	15.36	0.02	0.1	1.22	0.26	0.49	0.3	0
18041	0.5	0.1	0	0.36	0.2	2.78	0.02	14.4	0	0	0.72	0.1	0.06	0.32	0
18042	0.97	0.18	0	0.22	0.05	1.82	0.15	22.4	0	0	1.66	0.26	0.22	0.68	0
18044	0.38	0.07	0	0.09	0.08	0.8	0.03	8.84	0	0	0.81	0.11	0.24	0.32	0
18047	0.23	0.06	0.64	0.11	0.13	1.11	0.02	10.88	0	0.16	1.41	0.35	0.73	0.22	0
18060	0.36	0.06	1.28	0.14	0.11	1.22	0.02	16.32	0	0.06	1.06	0.2	0.42	0.26	0
18064	0.26	0.05	0	0.1	0.07	1.03	0.02	10.25	0	0	1.03	0.22	0.43	0.23	0
18069	0.28	0.06	0	0.21	0.15	1.79	0.03	15.3	0.01	0	1.62	0.36	0.73	0.33	0.45

NDB#	Description & Serving	Grams	Water	Calories	Protein	Carbohydrates	Fiber	Calcium	Phosphorus	Iron	Sodium	Potassium	Magnesium
			gm	kcal	gm	gm	gm	mg	mg	mg	mg	mg	mg
18360	Taco shells, baked 1 large (6-1/2" dia)	21	1.26	98.28	1.51	13.1	1.58	33.6	52.08	0.53	77.07	37.59	22.05
18363	Tortillas, rtb or -fry, corn 1 medium tortilla (approx 6" dia)	26	11.47	57.72	1.48	12.12	1.35	45.5	81.64	0.36	41.86	40.04	16.9
18364	Tortillas, rtb or -fry, flour 1 medium tortilla (approx 6" dia)	32	8.58	104	2.78	17.79	1.06	40	39.68	1.06	152.96	41.92	8.32
	Crackers												
18214	Cheese, regular 1 cup, bite size	62	1.92	311.86	6.26	36.08	1.49	93.62	135.16	2.96	616.9	89.9	22.32
18215	Cheese, sandwich-type w/pnut butter filling 1 sandwich	7	0.27	33.74	0.88	3.99	0.2	5.53	22.68	0.2	69.44	17.15	4.06
18216	Crispbread, rye 1 crispbread or cracker	10	0.61	36.6	0.79	8.22	1.65	3.1	26.9	0.24	26.4	31.9	7.8
18217	Matzoh, plain 1 matzoh	28.35	1.22	111.98	2.84	23.73	0.85	3.69	25.23	0.9	0.57	31.75	7.09
18220	Melba toast, plain 1 cup, pieces	30	1.53	117	3.63	22.98	1.89	27.9	58.8	1.11	248.7	60.6	17.7
18226	Rye, wafers, plain 1 cracker (4-1/2" x 2-1/2" x 1/8")	11	0.55	36.74	1.06	8.84	2.52	4.4	36.74	0.65	87.34	54.45	13.31
18228	Saltines (incl oyster, soda, soup) 1 cup, oyster crackers	45	1.85	195.3	4.14	32.18	1.35	53.55	47.25	2.43	585.9	57.6	12.15
18232	Wheat, regular 1 euphrates	4	0.12	18.92	0.34	2.6	0.18	1.96	8.8	0.18	31.8	7.32	2.48
	Flours and meals												
20011	Buckwheat flour, whole-groat 1 cup	120	13.38	402	15.14	84.71	12	49.2	404.4	4.87	13.2	692.4	301.2
20322	Cornmeal, degermed, enriched, white 1 cup	138	15.99	505.08	11.7	107.2	10.21	6.9	115.92	5.7	4.14	223.56	55.2
20022	Cornmeal, degermed, enriched, yellow 1 cup	138	15.99	505.08	11.7	107.2	10.21	6.9	115.92	5.7	4.14	223.56	55.2
20320	Cornmeal, whole-grain, white 1 cup	122	12.52	441.64	9.91	93.81	8.91	7.32	294.02	4.21	42.7	350.14	154.94
20020	Cornmeal, whole-grain, yellow 1 cup	122	12.52	441.64	9.91	93.81	8.91	7.32	294.02	4.21	42.7	350.14	154.94
18236	Cracker meal 1 cup	115	8.74	440.45	10.7	93.04	2.94	26.45	119.6	5.34	32.2	132.25	27.6
20090	Rice flour, brown 1 cup	158	18.91	573.54	11.42	120.84	7.27	17.38	532.46	3.13	12.64	456.62	176.96
20061	Rice flour, white 1 cup	158	18.79	578.28	9.4	126.61	3.79	15.8	154.84	0.55	0	120.08	55.3
20063	Rye flour, dark 1 cup	128	14.17	414.72	17.96	87.99	28.93	71.68	808.96	8.26	1.28	934.4	317.44
20064	Rye flour, medium 1 cup	102	10.05	361.08	9.58	79.04	14.89	24.48	211.14	2.16	3.06	346.8	76.5
20065	Rye flour, light 1 cup	102	8.96	374.34	8.56	81.83	14.89	21.42	197.88	1.84	2.04	237.66	71.4
20076	Wheat flour, durum 1 cup	192	21	650.88	26.27	136.57	0	65.28	975.36	6.76	3.84	827.52	276.48

NDB#	Zinc	Copper	Vitamin A	Thiamin	Riboflavin	Niacin	Vitamin B6	Folate	Vitamin B12	Vitamin C	Fat	Fat-Saturated	Fat-Monounsaturated	Fat-Polyunsaturated	Cholesterol
	mg	mg	IU	mg	mg	mg	mg	mcg	mcg	mg	gm	gm	gm	gm	mg
18360	0.29	0.03	73.5	0.05	0.01	0.28	0.08	1.26	0	0	4.75	0.7	1.99	1.81	0
18363	0.24	0.04	62.92	0.03	0.02	0.39	0.06	3.9	0	0	0.65	0.09	0.17	0.29	0
18364	0.23	0.09	0	0.17	0.09	1.14	0.02	3.84	0	0	2.27	0.35	0.92	0.89	0
Crackers															
18214	0.7	0.13	100.44	0.35	0.27	2.9	0.34	15.5	0.29	0	15.69	5.81	5.58	3	8.06
18215	0.08	0.02	22.33	0.03	0.02	0.46	0.1	1.75	0	0	1.62	0.36	0.85	0.31	0.35
18216	0.24	0.03	0	0.02	0.01	0.1	0.02	2.2	0	0	0.13	0.01	0.02	0.06	0
18217	0.19	0.02	0	0.11	0.08	1.1	0.03	3.97	0	0	0.4	0.06	0.04	0.17	0
18220	0.6	0.09	0	0.12	0.08	1.23	0.03	7.8	0	0	0.96	0.13	0.23	0.38	0
18226	0.31	0.05	2.53	0.05	0.03	0.17	0.03	4.95	0	0.01	0.1	0.01	0.02	0.04	0
18228	0.35	0.09	0	0.25	0.21	2.36	0.02	13.95	0	0	5.31	0.95	2.91	0.83	0
18232	0.06	0.01	0	0.02	0.01	0.2	0.01	0.72	0	0	0.82	0.15	0.47	0.12	0
Flours and meals															
20011	3.74	0.62	0	0.5	0.23	7.38	0.7	64.8	0	0	3.72	0.81	1.14	1.14	0
20322	0.99	0.11	0	0.99	0.56	6.95	0.35	66.24	0	0	2.28	0.31	0.57	0.98	0
20022	0.99	0.11	569.94	0.99	0.56	6.95	0.35	66.24	0	0	2.28	0.31	0.57	0.98	0
20320	2.22	0.24	0	0.47	0.25	4.43	0.37	30.99	0	0	4.38	0.62	1.16	2	0
20020	2.22	0.24	572.18	0.47	0.25	4.43	0.37	30.99	0	0	4.38	0.62	1.16	2	0
18236	0.79	0.26	0	0.8	0.54	6.56	0.04	25.3	0	0	1.96	0.31	0.17	0.83	0
20090	3.87	0.36	0	0.7	0.13	10.02	1.16	25.28	0	0	4.39	0.88	1.59	1.57	0
20061	1.26	0.21	0	0.22	0.03	4.09	0.69	6.32	0	0	2.24	0.61	0.7	0.6	0
20063	7.19	0.96	0	0.4	0.32	5.47	0.57	76.8	0	0	3.44	0.4	0.42	1.54	0
20064	2.03	0.29	0	0.29	0.12	1.76	0.27	19.38	0	0	1.81	0.2	0.21	0.78	0
20065	1.79	0.26	0	0.34	0.09	0.82	0.24	22.44	0	0	1.39	0.15	0.16	0.58	0
20076	7.99	1.06	0	0.8	0.23	12.94	0.8	83.14	0	0	4.74	0.87	0.66	1.88	0

NDB#	Description & Serving	Grams	Water	Calories	Protein	Carbohydrates	Fiber	Calcium	Phosphorus	Iron	Sodium	Potassium	Magnesium
			gm	kcal	gm	gm	gm	mg	mg	mg	mg	mg	mg
20080	Wheat flour, whole-grain 1 cup	120	12.32	406.8	16.44	87.08	14.64	40.8	415.2	4.66	6	486	165.6
20081	Wheat flour, white, all-purpose, enriched, bleached 1 cup	125	14.9	455	12.91	95.39	3.38	18.75	135	5.8	2.5	133.75	27.5
20581	Wheat flour, white, all-purpose, enriched, unbleached 1 cup	125	14.9	455	12.91	95.39	3.38	18.75	135	5.8	2.5	133.75	27.5
	Grains and cereals												
20006	Barley, pearled, cooked 1 cup	157	108.02	193.11	3.55	44.31	5.97	17.27	84.78	2.09	4.71	146.01	34.54
20010	Buckwheat groats, roasted, cooked 1 cup	168	127.06	154.56	5.68	33.5	4.54	11.76	117.6	1.34	6.72	147.84	85.68
20013	Bulgur, cooked 1 cup	182	141.52	151.06	5.61	33.82	8.19	18.2	72.8	1.75	9.1	123.76	58.24
08161	Corn grits, white, regquick, enriched, cooked w/water, w/salt 1 cup	242	206.43	145.2	3.39	31.46	0.48	0	29.04	1.55	539.66	53.24	9.68
08164	Corn grits, yellow, regquick, enriched, cooked w/water, wo/salt (corn) 1 cup	242	206.43	145.2	3.39	31.46	0.48	0	29.04	1.55	0	53.24	9.68
20029	Couscous, cooked 1 cup, cooked	157	113.93	175.84	5.95	36.46	2.2	12.56	34.54	0.6	7.85	91.06	12.56
08174	Farina, unenr, cooked w/water, wo/salt, (wheat) 1 cup	233	204.81	116.5	3.26	24.7	3.26	4.66	27.96	0.05	0	30.29	4.66
20030	Hominy, canned, white 1 cup	165	136.17	118.8	2.44	23.53	4.13	16.5	57.75	1.02	346.5	14.85	26.4
20330	Hominy, canned, yellow 1 cup	160	132.05	115.2	2.37	22.82	4	16	56	0.99	336	14.4	25.6
20032	Millet, cooked 1 cup	240	171.38	285.6	8.42	56.81	3.12	7.2	240	1.51	4.8	148.8	105.6
20034	Oat bran, cooked 1 cup	219	183.96	87.6	7.03	25.05	5.69	21.9	260.61	1.93	2.19	201.48	87.6
08121	Oats, reg & quick & instant, wo/fort, cooked w/water, wo/salt (oats) 1 cup	234	199.6	145.08	6.08	25.27	3.98	18.72	177.84	1.59	2.34	131.04	56.16
08123	Oats, instant, fort, plain, prep w/water (oats) 1 cup, cooked	234	200.07	138.06	5.85	23.87	3.98	215.28	175.5	8.33	376.74	131.04	56.16
20037	Rice, brown, long-grain, cooked 1 cup	195	142.53	216.45	5.03	44.77	3.51	19.5	161.85	0.82	9.75	83.85	83.85
20041	Rice, brown, medium-grain, cooked 1 cup	195	142.27	218.4	4.52	45.84	3.51	19.5	150.15	1.03	1.95	154.05	85.8
20345	Rice, white, long-grain, reg, cooked, enriched, w/salt 1 cup	158	108.14	205.4	4.25	44.51	0.63	15.8	67.94	1.9	603.56	55.3	18.96
20055	Rice, white, glutinous, cooked 1 cup, cooked	174	133.34	168.78	3.51	36.7	1.74	3.48	13.92	0.24	8.7	17.4	8.7
20066	Semolina, enriched 1 cup	167	21.16	601.2	21.18	121.63	6.51	28.39	227.12	7.28	1.67	310.62	78.49
20067	Sorghum 1 cup	192	17.66	650.88	21.7	143.29	0	53.76	551.04	8.45	11.52	672	0
08084	Wheat germ, toasted, plain 1 cup	113	6.33	431.66	32.88	56.05	14.58	50.85	1294.98	10.27	4.52	1070.11	361.6

NDB #	Zinc	Copper	Vitamin A	Thiamin	Riboflavin	Niacin	Vitamin B6	Folate	Vitamin B12	Vitamin C	Fat	Fat-Saturated	Fat-Monounsaturated	Fat-Polyunsaturated	Cholesterol
	mg	mg	IU	mg	mg	mg	mg	mcg	mcg	mg	gm	gm	gm	gm	mg
20080	3.52	0.46	0	0.54	0.26	7.64	0.41	52.8	0	0	2.24	0.39	0.28	0.93	0
20081	0.88	0.18	0	0.98	0.62	7.38	0.06	32.5	0	0	1.23	0.19	0.11	0.52	0
20581	0.88	0.18	0	0.98	0.62	7.38	0.06	32.5	0	0	1.23	0.19	0.11	0.52	0
Grains and cereals															
20006	1.29	0.16	10.99	0.13	0.1	3.24	0.18	25.12	0	0	0.69	0.15	0.09	0.34	0
20010	1.02	0.25	0	0.07	0.07	1.58	0.13	23.52	0	0	1.04	0.23	0.32	0.32	0
20013	1.04	0.14	0	0.1	0.05	1.82	0.15	32.76	0	0	0.44	0.08	0.06	0.18	0
08161	0.17	0.03	0	0.24	0.15	1.96	0.06	2.42	0	0	0.48	0.07	0.12	0.19	0
08164	0.17	0.03	145.2	0.24	0.15	1.96	0.06	2.42	0	0	0.48	0.07	0.12	0.19	0
20029	1.37	0.22	0	0.33	0.14	5.19	0.27	79.2	0	0	0.84	0.15	0.12	0.34	0
08174	0.16	0.03	0	0.02	0.02	0.23	0.02	4.66	0	0	0.23	0.02	0.02	0.07	0
20030	1.73	0.05	0	0	0.01	0.05	0.01	1.65	0	0	1.45	0.2	0.38	0.66	0
20330	1.68	0.05	176	0	0.01	0.05	0.01	1.6	0	0	1.41	0.2	0.37	0.64	0
20032	2.18	0.39	0	0.25	0.2	3.19	0.26	45.6	0	0	2.4	0.41	0.44	1.22	0
20034	1.16	0.14	0	0.35	0.07	0.32	0.05	13.14	0	0	1.88	0.36	0.64	0.74	0
08121	1.15	0.13	37.44	0.26	0.05	0.3	0.05	9.36	0	0	2.34	0.42	0.75	0.87	0
08123	1.15	0.13	1996.02	0.7	0.37	7.23	0.98	198.9	0	0	2.34	0.42	0.75	0.87	0
20037	1.23	0.2	0	0.19	0.05	2.98	0.28	7.8	0	0	1.76	0.35	0.64	0.63	0
20041	1.21	0.16	0	0.2	0.02	2.59	0.29	7.8	0	0	1.62	0.32	0.59	0.58	0
20345	0.77	0.11	0	0.26	0.02	2.33	0.15	4.74	0	0	0.44	0.12	0.14	0.12	0
20055	0.71	0.09	0	0.03	0.02	0.5	0.05	1.74	0	0	0.33	0.07	0.12	0.12	0
20066	1.75	0.32	0	1.35	0.95	10	0.17	120.24	0	0	1.75	0.25	0.21	0.72	0
20067	0	0	0	0.46	0.27	5.62	0	0	0	0	6.34	0.88	1.91	2.63	0
08084	18.84	0.7	0	1.89	0.93	6.32	1.11	397.76	0	6.78	12.09	2.07	1.7	7.48	0

NDB#	Description & Serving	Grams	Water	Calories	Protein	Carbohydrates	Fiber	Calcium	Phosphorus	Iron	Sodium	Potassium	Magnesium
		gm	gm	kcal	gm	gm	gm	mg	mg	mg	mg	mg	mg
08084	Wheat germ, toasted, plain												
	1 oz	28.35	1.59	108.3	8.25	14.06	3.66	12.76	324.89	2.58	1.13	268.47	90.72
08145	Whole wheat hot nat crl, cooked w/water, wo/salt, (wheat)												
	1 cup	242	202.31	150.04	4.84	33.15	3.87	16.94	166.98	1.5	0	171.82	53.24
20089	Wild rice, cooked												
	1 cup	164	121.25	165.64	6.54	35	2.95	4.92	134.48	0.98	4.92	165.64	52.48
Pasta													
20100	Macaroni, cooked, enriched												
	1 cup elbow shaped	140	92.39	197.4	6.68	39.68	1.82	9.8	75.6	1.96	1.4	43.4	25.2
20108	Macaroni, whole-wheat, cooked												
	1 cup elbow shaped	140	94.01	173.6	7.46	37.16	3.92	21	124.6	1.48	4.2	61.6	42
20110	Noodles, egg, cooked, enriched												
	1 cup	160	109.92	212.8	7.6	39.74	1.76	19.2	110.4	2.54	11.2	44.8	30.4
20112	Noodles, egg, spinach, cooked, enriched												
	1 cup	160	109.63	211.2	8.06	38.8	3.68	30.4	91.2	1.74	19.2	59.2	38.4
20113	Noodles, chinese, chow mein												
	1 cup	45	0.33	237.15	3.77	25.89	1.76	9	72.45	2.13	197.55	54	23.4
20115	Noodles, japanese, soba, cooked												
	1 cup	114	83.23	112.86	5.77	24.44	0	4.56	28.5	0.55	68.4	39.9	10.26
20121	Spaghetti, cooked, enriched, wo/ salt												
	1 cup	140	92.39	197.4	6.68	39.68	2.38	9.8	75.6	1.96	1.4	43.4	25.2
20127	Spaghetti, spinach, cooked												
	1 cup	140	95.4	182	6.41	36.61	0	42	151.2	1.46	19.6	81.2	86.8
20125	Spaghetti, whole-wheat, cooked												
	1 cup	140	94.01	173.6	7.46	37.16	6.3	21	124.6	1.48	4.2	61.6	42
Herbs, spices, and condiments													
02001	Allspice, ground												
	1 teaspoon	1.9	0.16	4.99	0.12	1.37	0.41	12.55	2.15	0.13	1.46	19.84	2.56
02002	Anise seed												
	1 teaspoon	2.1	0.2	7.08	0.37	1.05	0.31	13.56	9.24	0.78	0.33	30.26	3.57
02003	Basil, ground												
	1 teaspoon	1.4	0.09	3.52	0.2	0.85	0.57	29.59	6.86	0.59	0.48	48.06	5.91
02004	Bay leaf, crumbled												
	1 teaspoon	0.6	0.03	1.88	0.05	0.45	0.16	5.01	0.68	0.26	0.14	3.18	0.72
02005	Caraway seed												
	1 teaspoon	2.1	0.21	6.99	0.42	1.05	0.8	14.47	11.93	0.34	0.36	28.37	5.42
02006	Cardamon, ground												
	1 teaspoon	2	0.17	6.23	0.22	1.37	0.56	7.66	3.55	0.28	0.37	22.38	4.57
11935	Catsup												
	1 tablespoon	15	9.99	15.6	0.23	4.09	0.2	2.85	5.85	0.11	177.9	72.15	3.3
02007	Celery seed												
	1 teaspoon	2	0.12	7.84	0.36	0.83	0.24	35.33	10.93	0.9	3.2	28	8.8
02008	Chervil, dried												
	1 teaspoon	0.6	0.04	1.42	0.14	0.29	0.07	8.08	2.7	0.19	0.5	28.44	0.78
02009	Chili powder												
	1 teaspoon	2.6	0.2	8.16	0.32	1.42	0.89	7.23	7.88	0.37	26.26	49.82	4.42
11615	Chives, freeze-dried												
	1 tablespoon	0.2	0	0.62	0.04	0.13	0.05	1.63	1.04	0.04	0.14	5.92	1.28

NDB #	Zinc	Copper	Vitamin A	Thiamin	Riboflavin	Niacin	Vitamin B6	Folate	Vitamin B12	Vitamin C	Fat	Fat: Saturated	Fat: Monounsaturated	Fat: Polyunsaturated	Cholesterol
	mg	mg	IU	mg	mg	mg	mg	mcg	mcg	mg	gm	gm	gm	gm	mg
08084	4.73	0.18	0	0.47	0.23	1.58	0.28	99.79	0	1.7	3.03	0.52	0.43	1.88	0
08145	1.16	0.2	0	0.17	0.12	2.15	0.18	26.62	0	0	0.97	0.15	0.14	0.49	0
20089	2.2	0.2	0	0.09	0.14	2.11	0.22	42.64	0	0	0.56	0.08	0.08	0.35	0
Pasta															
20100	0.74	0.14	0	0.29	0.14	2.34	0.05	9.8	0	0	0.94	0.13	0.11	0.38	0
20108	1.13	0.23	0	0.15	0.06	0.99	0.11	7	0	0	0.76	0.14	0.11	0.3	0
20110	0.99	0.14	32	0.3	0.13	2.38	0.06	11.2	0.14	0	2.35	0.5	0.69	0.65	52.8
20112	1.01	0.13	164.8	0.39	0.2	2.36	0.18	33.6	0.22	0	2.51	0.58	0.79	0.56	52.8
20113	0.63	0.08	38.25	0.26	0.19	2.68	0.05	9.9	0	0	13.84	1.97	3.46	7.8	0
20115	0.14	0.01	0	0.11	0.03	0.58	0.05	7.98	0	0	0.11	0.02	0.03	0.04	0
20121	0.74	0.14	0	0.29	0.14	2.34	0.05	9.8	0	0	0.94	0.13	0.11	0.38	0
20127	1.51	0.29	212.8	0.14	0.14	2.14	0.13	16.8	0	0	0.88	0.13	0.1	0.36	0
20125	1.13	0.23	0	0.15	0.06	0.99	0.11	7	0	0	0.76	0.14	0.11	0.3	0
Herbs, spices, and condiments															
02001	0.02	0.01	10.26	0	0	0.05	0.01	0.68	0	0.74	0.17	0.05	0.01	0.04	0
02002	0.11	0.02	6.53	0.01	0.01	0.06	0.01	0.21	0	0.44	0.33	0.01	0.21	0.07	0
02003	0.08	0.02	131.25	0	0	0.1	0.02	3.84	0	0.86	0.06	0	0.01	0.03	0
02004	0.02	0	37.11	0	0	0.01	0.01	1.08	0	0.28	0.05	0.01	0.01	0.01	0
02005	0.12	0.02	7.62	0.01	0.01	0.08	0.01	0.21	0	0.44	0.31	0.01	0.15	0.07	0
02006	0.15	0.01	0	0	0	0.02	0	0	0	0.42	0.13	0.01	0.02	0.01	0
11935	0.03	0.03	152.4	0.01	0.01	0.21	0.03	2.25	0	2.27	0.05	0.01	0.01	0.01	0
02007	0.14	0.03	1.04	0.01	0.01	0.06	0.01	0.2	0	0.34	0.51	0.04	0.32	0.07	0
02008	0.05	0	35.1	0	0	0.03	0.01	1.64	0	0.3	0.02	0	0.01	0.01	0
02009	0.07	0.01	908.1	0.01	0.02	0.21	0.05	2.6	0	1.67	0.44	0.08	0.09	0.19	0
11615	0.01	0	136.6	0	0	0.01	0	0.22	0	1.32	0.01	0	0	0	0

NDB#	Description & Serving	Grams	Water	Calories	Protein	Carbohydrates	Fiber	Calcium	Phosphorus	Iron	Sodium	Potassium	Magnesium
			gm	kcal	gm	gm	gm	mg	mg	mg	mg	mg	mg
11156	**Chives, raw** 1 teaspoon, chopped	1	0.91	0.3	0.03	0.04	0.03	0.92	0.58	0.02	0.03	2.96	0.42
02010	**Cinnamon, ground** 1 teaspoon	2.3	0.22	6.01	0.09	1.84	1.25	28.25	1.41	0.88	0.61	11.5	1.28
02011	**Cloves, ground** 1 teaspoon	2.1	0.14	6.78	0.13	1.29	0.72	13.56	2.21	0.18	5.1	23.14	5.54
02012	**Coriander leaf, dried** 1 teaspoon	0.6	0.04	1.67	0.13	0.31	0.06	7.48	2.89	0.25	1.27	26.8	4.16
02013	**Coriander seed** 1 teaspoon	1.8	0.16	5.36	0.22	0.99	0.75	12.76	7.36	0.29	0.64	22.81	5.94
02014	**Cumin seed** 1 teaspoon	2.1	0.17	7.87	0.37	0.93	0.22	19.54	10.47	1.39	3.52	37.54	7.68
02015	**Curry powder** 1 teaspoon	2	0.19	6.5	0.25	1.16	0.66	9.56	6.98	0.59	1.04	30.86	5.08
02016	**Dill seed** 1 teaspoon	2.1	0.16	6.4	0.34	1.16	0.44	31.83	5.81	0.34	0.41	24.91	5.37
02017	**Dill weed, dried** 1 teaspoon	1	0.07	2.53	0.2	0.56	0.14	17.84	5.43	0.49	2.08	33.08	4.51
02045	**Dill weed, fresh** 5 sprigs	1	0.86	0.43	0.03	0.07	0.02	2.08	0.66	0.07	0.61	7.38	0.55
11957	**Fennel, bulb, raw** 1 cup, sliced	87	78.48	26.97	1.08	6.34	2.7	42.63	43.5	0.63	45.24	360.18	14.79
02018	**Fennel seed** 1 teaspoon	2	0.18	6.9	0.32	1.05	0.8	23.93	9.75	0.37	1.76	33.88	7.7
02019	**Fenugreek seed** 1 teaspoon	3.7	0.33	11.95	0.85	2.16	0.91	6.5	10.96	1.24	2.49	28.48	7.05
11215	**Garlic, raw** 1 teaspoon	2.8	1.64	4.17	0.18	0.93	0.06	5.07	4.28	0.05	0.48	11.23	0.7
02021	**Ginger, ground** 1 teaspoon	1.8	0.17	6.25	0.16	1.27	0.23	2.09	2.66	0.21	0.58	24.17	3.31
02022	**Mace, ground** 1 teaspoon	1.7	0.14	8.08	0.11	0.86	0.34	4.29	1.87	0.24	1.36	7.87	2.77
02023	**Marjoram, dried** 1 teaspoon	0.6	0.05	1.63	0.08	0.36	0.24	11.94	1.84	0.5	0.46	9.13	2.08
02024	**Mustard seed, yellow** 1 teaspoon	3.3	0.23	15.49	0.82	1.15	0.49	17.2	27.74	0.33	0.15	22.52	9.85
02025	**Nutmeg, ground** 1 teaspoon	2.2	0.14	11.54	0.13	1.08	0.46	4.06	4.68	0.07	0.36	7.69	4.03
02026	**Onion powder** 1 teaspoon	2.1	0.11	7.28	0.21	1.69	0.12	7.62	7.14	0.05	1.12	19.81	2.55
02027	**Oregano, ground** 1 teaspoon	1.5	0.11	4.59	0.17	0.97	0.64	23.64	3	0.66	0.22	25.03	4.05
02028	**Paprika** 1 teaspoon	2.1	0.2	6.07	0.31	1.17	0.44	3.72	7.24	0.5	0.71	49.23	3.88
02029	**Parsley, dried** 1 teaspoon	0.3	0.03	0.83	0.07	0.15	0.09	4.4	1.05	0.29	1.36	11.41	0.75
11297	**Parsley, raw** 1 tablespoon	3.8	3.33	1.37	0.11	0.24	0.13	5.24	2.2	0.24	2.13	21.05	1.9

NDB#	Zinc	Copper	Vitamin A	Thiamin	Riboflavin	Niacin	Vitamin B6	Folate	Vitamin B12	Vitamin C	Fat	Fat:Saturated	Fat:Monounsaturated	Fat:Polyunsaturated	Cholesterol
	mg	mg	IU	mg	mg	mg	mg	mcg	mcg	mg	gm	gm	gm	gm	mg
11156	0.01	0	43.53	0	0	0.01	0	1.05	0	0.58	0.01	0	0	0	0
02010	0.05	0.01	5.98	0	0	0.03	0.01	0.67	0	0.65	0.07	0.01	0.01	0.01	0
02011	0.02	0.01	11.13	0	0.01	0.03	0.03	1.95	0	1.7	0.42	0.11	0.03	0.15	0
02012	0.03	0.01	35.1	0.01	0.01	0.06	0.01	1.64	0	3.4	0.03	0	0.01	0	0
02013	0.08	0.02	0	0	0.01	0.04	0	0	0	0.38	0.32	0.02	0.24	0.03	0
02014	0.1	0.02	26.67	0.01	0.01	0.1	0.01	0.21	0	0.16	0.47	0.03	0.29	0.07	0
02015	0.08	0.02	19.72	0.01	0.01	0.07	0.01	3.08	0	0.23	0.28	0.04	0.11	0.05	0
02016	0.11	0.02	1.11	0.01	0.01	0.06	0.01	0.21	0	0.44	0.31	0.02	0.2	0.02	0
02017	0.03	0	58.5	0	0	0.03	0.01	0	0	0.5	0.04	0	0	0	0
02045	0.01	0	77.18	0	0	0.02	0	1.5	0	0.85	0.01	0	0.01	0	0
11957	0.17	0.06	116.58	0.01	0.03	0.56	0.04	23.49	0	10.44	0.17	0	0	0	0
02018	0.07	0.02	2.7	0.01	0.01	0.12	0	0	0	0.42	0.3	0.01	0.2	0.03	0
02019	0.09	0.04	2.22	0.01	0.01	0.06	0	2.11	0	0.11	0.24	0.05	0	0	0
11215	0.03	0.01	0	0.01	0	0.02	0.03	0.09	0	0.87	0.01	0	0	0.01	0
02021	0.08	0.01	2.65	0	0	0.09	0.02	0.7	0	0.13	0.11	0.03	0.02	0.02	0
02022	0.04	0.04	13.6	0.01	0.01	0.02	0.01	1.29	0	0.36	0.55	0.16	0.19	0.07	0
02023	0.02	0.01	48.41	0	0	0.02	0.01	1.64	0	0.31	0.04	0	0.01	0.03	0
02024	0.19	0.01	2.05	0.02	0.01	0.26	0.01	2.51	0	0.1	0.95	0.05	0.65	0.18	0
02025	0.05	0.02	2.24	0.01	0	0.03	0.01	1.67	0	0.07	0.8	0.57	0.07	0.01	0
02026	0.05	0	0	0.01	0	0.01	0.03	3.49	0	0.31	0.02	0	0	0.01	0
02027	0.07	0.01	103.55	0.01	0	0.09	0.02	4.11	0	0.75	0.15	0.04	0.01	0.08	0
02028	0.09	0.01	1272.68	0.01	0.04	0.32	0.04	2.23	0	1.49	0.27	0.04	0.03	0.17	0
02029	0.01	0	70.02	0	0	0.02	0	0.54	0	0.37	0.01	0	0.01	0	0
11297	0.04	0.01	197.6	0	0	0.05	0	5.78	0	5.05	0.03	0.01	0.01	0	0

NDB#	Description & Serving	Grams	Water	Calories	Protein	Carbohydrates	Fiber	Calcium	Phosphorus	Iron	Sodium	Potassium	Magnesium
			gm	kcal	gm	gm	gm	mg	mg	mg	mg	mg	mg
02030	Pepper, black 1 teaspoon	2.1	0.22	5.36	0.23	1.36	0.56	9.17	3.64	0.61	0.92	26.44	4.06
02031	Pepper, red or cayenne 1 teaspoon	1.8	0.14	5.72	0.22	1.02	0.49	2.67	5.28	0.14	0.54	36.25	2.74
02032	Pepper, white 1 teaspoon	2.4	0.27	7.1	0.25	1.65	0.63	6.37	4.22	0.34	0.12	1.74	2.16
11937	Pickles, cucumber, dill 1 cup (about 23 slices)	155	142.09	27.9	0.96	6.4	1.86	13.95	32.55	0.82	1987.1	179.8	17.05
11940	Pickle, cucumber, sweet 1 cup, sliced	170	110.94	198.9	0.63	54.08	1.87	6.8	20.4	1	1596.3	54.4	6.8
11941	Pickle, cucumber, sour 1 large (4" long)	135	127.01	14.85	0.45	3.04	1.62	0	18.9	0.54	1630.8	31.05	5.4
11945	Pickle relish, sweet 1 tablespoon	15	9.31	19.5	0.06	5.26	0.17	0.45	2.1	0.13	121.65	3.75	0.75
11943	Pimento, canned 1 tablespoon	12	11.17	2.76	0.13	0.61	0.23	0.72	2.04	0.2	1.68	18.96	0.72
02033	Poppy seed 1 teaspoon	2.8	0.19	14.93	0.51	0.66	0.28	40.56	23.76	0.26	0.59	19.59	9.28
02034	Poultry seasoning 1 teaspoon	1.5	0.14	4.61	0.14	0.98	0.17	14.94	2.57	0.53	0.41	10.26	3.36
02035	Pumpkin pie spice 1 teaspoon	1.7	0.14	5.81	0.1	1.18	0.25	11.59	2.01	0.34	0.88	11.27	2.31
02036	Rosemary, dried 1 teaspoon	1.2	0.11	3.98	0.06	0.77	0.51	15.36	0.84	0.35	0.59	11.46	2.64
02063	Rosemary, fresh 1 teaspoon	0.7	0.47	0.92	0.02	0.14	0.1	2.22	0.46	0.05	0.18	4.68	0.64
02037	Saffron 1 teaspoon	0.7	0.08	2.17	0.08	0.46	0.03	0.78	1.76	0.08	1.04	12.07	1.85
02038	Sage, ground 1 teaspoon	0.7	0.06	2.2	0.07	0.43	0.28	11.56	0.64	0.2	0.08	7.49	3
02047	Salt, table 1 tablespoon	18	0.04	0	0	0	0	4.32	0	0.06	6976.44	1.44	0.18
02039	Savory, ground 1 teaspoon	1.4	0.13	3.81	0.09	0.96	0.64	29.84	1.96	0.53	0.34	14.71	5.27
02066	Spearmint, dried 1 teaspoon	0.5	0.06	1.43	0.1	0.26	0.15	7.44	1.38	0.44	1.72	9.62	3.01
02041	Tarragon, ground 1 teaspoon	1.6	0.12	4.73	0.36	0.8	0.12	18.23	5.01	0.52	1	48.31	5.55
02049	Thyme, fresh 1 teaspoon	0.8	0.52	0.81	0.04	0.2	0.11	3.24	0.85	0.14	0.07	4.87	1.28
02042	Thyme, ground 1 teaspoon	1.4	0.11	3.87	0.13	0.9	0.52	26.45	2.81	1.73	0.77	11.4	3.09
02043	Turmeric, ground 1 teaspoon	2.2	0.25	7.79	0.17	1.43	0.46	4.02	5.89	0.91	0.83	55.55	4.25
02050	Vanilla extract 1 tablespoon	13	6.84	37.44	0.01	1.64	0	1.43	0.78	0.02	1.17	19.24	1.56
02048	Vinegar, cider 1 tablespoon	15	14.07	2.1	0	0.89	0	0.9	1.35	0.09	0.15	15	3.3

NDB#	Zinc	Copper	Vitamin A	Thiamin	Riboflavin	Niacin	Vitamin B6	Folate	Vitamin B12	Vitamin C	Fat	Fat:Saturated	Fat:Monounsaturated	Fat:Polyunsaturated	Cholesterol
	mg	mg	IU	mg	mg	mg	mg	mcg	mcg	mg	gm	gm	gm	gm	mg
02030	0.03	0.02	3.99	0	0.01	0.02	0.01	0.21	0	0.44	0.07	0.02	0.02	0.02	0
02031	0.04	0.01	748.98	0.01	0.02	0.16	0.04	1.91	0	1.38	0.31	0.06	0.05	0.15	0
02032	0.03	0.02	0	0	0	0.01	0.01	0.24	0	0.5	0.05	0.02	0.02	0.01	0
11937	0.22	0.12	509.95	0.02	0.04	0.09	0.02	1.55	0	2.95	0.29	0.07	0	0.12	0
11940	0.14	0.18	214.2	0.02	0.05	0.3	0.03	1.7	0	2.04	0.44	0.11	0.01	0.18	0
11941	0.03	0.11	195.75	0	0.01	0	0.01	0.96	0	1.35	0.27	0.07	0	0.11	0
11945	0.02	0.01	23.25	0	0	0.03	0	0.15	0	0.15	0.07	0.01	0.03	0.02	0
11943	0.02	0.01	318.6	0	0.01	0.07	0.03	0.72	0	10.19	0.04	0.01	0	0.02	0
02033	0.29	0.05	0	0.02	0	0.03	0.01	1.62	0	0.08	1.25	0.14	0.18	0.86	0
02034	0.05	0.01	39.48	0	0	0.04	0.01	2.07	0	0.18	0.11	0.05	0.02	0.03	0
02035	0.04	0.01	4.44	0	0	0.04	0.01	0.87	0	0.4	0.21	0.11	0.02	0.01	0
02036	0.04	0.01	37.54	0.01	0	0.01	0	0	0	0.73	0.18	0.1	0	0	0
02063	0.01	0	20.47	0	0	0.01	0	0.76	0	0.15	0.04	0.02	0.01	0.01	0
02037	0.01	0	3.71	0	0	0.01	0.01	0.65	0	0.57	0.04	0.01	0	0.01	0
02038	0.03	0.01	41.3	0.01	0	0.04	0.01	1.92	0	0.23	0.09	0.05	0.01	0.01	0
02047	0.02	0.01	0	0	0	0	0	0	0	0	0	0	0	0	0
02039	0.06	0.01	71.82	0.01	0	0.06	0	0	0	0.7	0.08	0.05	0	0	0
02066	0.01	0.01	52.9	0	0.01	0.03	0.01	2.65	0	0	0.03	0.01	0	0.02	0
02041	0.06	0.01	67.2	0	0.02	0.14	0.02	4.38	0	0.8	0.12	0.03	0.01	0.06	0
2049	0.01	0	38.02	0	0	0.01	0	0.36	0	1.28	0.01	0	0	0	0
02042	0.09	0.01	53.2	0.01	0.01	0.07	0.02	3.84	0	0.7	0.1	0.04	0.01	0.02	0
02043	0.1	0.01	0	0	0.01	0.11	0.04	0.86	0	0.57	0.22	0.07	0.04	0.05	0
02050	0.01	0.01	0	0	0.01	0.06	0	0	0	0	0.01	0	0	0	0
02048	0	0.01	0	0	0	0	0	0	0	0	0	0	0	0	0

NDB#	Description & Serving	Grams	Water	Calories	Protein	Carbohydrates	Fiber	Calcium	Phosphorus	Iron	Sodium	Potassium	Magnesium
		gm	gm	kcal	gm	gm	gm	mg	mg	mg	mg	mg	mg

Meat

Beef

NDB#	Description & Serving	Grams	Water	Calories	Protein	Carbohydrates	Fiber	Calcium	Phosphorus	Iron	Sodium	Potassium	Magnesium
13369	Brisket, flat half, lean & fat, 0" fat, braised 3 oz	85	49.08	182.75	25.91	0	0	4.25	210.8	2.34	52.7	245.65	20.4
13034	Chuck, arm pot rst, lean & fat, 1/4" fat, braised 3 oz	85	40.79	282.2	23.32	0	0	8.5	187	2.64	51	209.1	16.15
13073	Rib, whole (ribs 6-12), lean & fat, 1/4" fat, roasted 3 oz	85	40.37	304.3	19.13	0	0	9.35	148.75	1.99	53.55	255.85	17
13148	Shortribs, lean & fat, choice, braised 3 oz	85	30.36	400.35	18.33	0	0	10.2	137.7	1.96	42.5	190.4	12.75
13160	Bttm round, lean & fat, 1/4" fat, all grds, braised 3 oz	85	44.32	233.75	24.36	0	0	5.1	208.25	2.65	42.5	239.7	18.7
13176	Eye of round, lean & fat, 1/4" fat, roasted 3 oz	85	50.52	194.65	22.77	0	0	5.1	176.8	1.56	50.15	307.7	20.4
13184	Eye of round, lean, 1/4" fat, roasted 3 oz	85	55.25	142.8	24.64	0	0	4.25	192.1	1.66	52.7	335.75	22.95
13238	Tenderloin, lean & fat, 1/4" fat, broiled 3 oz	85	45.08	247.35	21.47	0	0	6.8	178.5	2.68	50.15	312.8	22.1
13298	Ground, extra lean, broiled, med 3 oz	85	48.67	217.6	21.59	0	0	5.95	136.85	2	59.5	266.05	17.85
13305	Ground, lean, broiled, med 3 oz	85	47.38	231.2	21.01	0	0	9.35	134.3	1.79	65.45	255.85	17.85
13312	Ground, reg, broiled, med 3 oz	85	55.25	142.8	24.64	0	0	4.25	192.1	1.66	52.7	335.75	22.95
13322	Heart, simmered 3 oz	85	54.47	148.75	24.47	0.36	0	5.1	212.5	6.38	53.55	198.05	21.25
13324	Kidneys, simmered 3 oz	85	58.51	122.4	21.66	0.82	0	14.45	260.1	6.21	113.9	152.15	15.3
13327	Liver, pan-fried 3 oz	85	47.33	184.45	22.71	6.67	0	9.35	391.85	5.34	90.1	309.4	19.55
13340	Tongue, simmered 3 oz	85	47.64	240.55	18.79	0.28	0	5.95	120.7	2.88	51	153	14.45
13347	Corned bf, brisket 3 oz	85	50.82	213.35	15.44	0.4	0	6.8	106.25	1.58	963.9	123.25	10.2

Lamb

NDB#	Description & Serving	Grams	Water	Calories	Protein	Carbohydrates	Fiber	Calcium	Phosphorus	Iron	Sodium	Potassium	Magnesium
17014	Dom, leg, whole (shk & sirl), lean, 1/4" fat, choice, roasted 3 oz	85	54.31	162.35	24.06	0	0	6.8	175.1	1.8	57.8	287.3	22.1
17025	Dom, loin, lean & fat, 1/4" fat, choice, roasted 3 oz	85	44.63	262.65	19.17	0	0	15.3	153	1.8	54.4	209.1	19.55
17060	Dom, cubed for stew (leg & shoulder), lean, 1/4" fat, braised 3 oz	85	47.8	189.55	28.64	0	0	12.75	174.25	2.38	59.5	221	23.8
17073	Nz, imp, frz, leg, whole (shk & sirl), lean & fat, roasted 3 oz	85	49.19	209.1	21.09	0	0	8.5	185.3	1.79	36.55	141.95	17
17075	Nz, imp, frz, leg, whole (shk & sirl), lean, roasted 3 oz	85	54.33	153.85	23.53	0	0	5.95	198.9	1.9	38.25	155.55	17.85

NDB#	Zinc	Copper	Vitamin A	Thiamin	Riboflavin	Niacin	Vitamin B6	Folate	Vitamin B12	Vitamin C	Fat	Fat: Saturated	Fat: Monounsaturated	Fat: Polyunsaturated	Cholesterol
	mg	mg	IU	mg	mg	mg	mg	mcg	mcg	mg	gm	gm	gm	gm	mg
Meat															
Beef															
13369	5.19	0.1	0	0.06	0.18	3.18	0.26	6.8	2.19	0	8	2.85	3.53	0.31	80.75
13034	5.81	0.11	0	0.06	0.2	2.7	0.24	7.65	2.51	0	20.24	7.97	8.68	0.77	84.15
13073	4.55	0.07	0	0.06	0.14	2.9	0.2	5.95	2.16	0	24.66	9.95	10.6	0.88	71.4
13148	4.15	0.08	0	0.04	0.13	2.08	0.19	4.25	2.23	0	35.68	15.13	16.05	1.3	79.9
13160	4.17	0.1	0	0.06	0.2	3.17	0.28	8.5	2	0	14.37	5.41	6.25	0.54	81.6
13176	3.69	0.08	0	0.07	0.14	2.97	0.3	5.95	1.79	0	10.84	4.23	4.66	0.39	61.2
13184	4.03	0.09	0	0.08	0.14	3.19	0.32	5.95	1.84	0	4.17	1.51	1.77	0.14	58.65
13238	4.15	0.13	0	0.09	0.22	2.99	0.33	5.1	2.05	0	17.22	6.76	7.06	0.65	73.1
13298	4.63	0.06	0	0.05	0.23	4.22	0.23	7.65	1.84	0	13.88	5.46	6.08	0.52	71.4
13305	4.56	0.06	0	0.04	0.18	4.39	0.22	7.65	2	0	15.69	6.16	6.87	0.59	73.95
13312	4.4	0.07	0	0.03	0.16	4.9	0.23	7.65	2.49	0	17.59	6.91	7.7	0.65	76.5
13322	2.66	0.63	0	0.12	1.31	3.46	0.18	1.7	12.16	1.28	4.78	1.43	1.06	1.16	164.05
13324	3.59	0.58	1054.85	0.16	3.45	5.12	0.44	83.3	43.61	0.68	2.92	0.93	0.63	0.63	328.95
13327	4.63	3.8	30689.25	0.18	3.52	12.27	1.22	187	95.03	19.55	6.8	2.27	1.38	1.45	409.7
13340	4.08	0.19	0	0.03	0.3	1.83	0.14	4.25	5.02	0.43	17.63	7.59	8.05	0.66	90.95
13347	3.89	0.13	0	0.02	0.14	2.58	0.2	5.1	1.39	0	16.13	5.39	7.84	0.57	83.3
Lamb															
17014	4.2	0.1	0	0.09	0.25	5.39	0.14	19.55	2.24	0	6.58	2.35	2.88	0.43	75.65
17025	2.9	0.1	0	0.09	0.2	6.04	0.09	16.15	1.88	0	20.05	8.7	8.23	1.59	80.75
17060	5.59	0.12	0	0.06	0.2	5.06	0.1	17.85	2.32	0	7.48	2.68	3.01	0.69	91.8
17073	3.04	0.09	0	0.1	0.38	6.45	0.11	0.85	2.21	0	13.23	6.47	5.11	0.64	85.85
17075	3.43	0.09	0	0.1	0.43	6.38	0.12	0	2.24	0	5.96	2.59	2.34	0.35	85

NDB#	Description & Serving	Grams	Water	Calories	Protein	Carbohydrates	Fiber	Calcium	Phosphorus	Iron	Sodium	Potassium	Magnesium
		gm	gm	kcal	gm	gm	gm	mg	mg	mg	mg	mg	mg
Veal													
17103	Leg, lean, roasted 3 oz	85	56.96	127.5	23.86	0	0	5.1	200.6	0.77	57.8	334.05	23.8
17109	Loin, lean, roasted 3 oz	85	54.9	148.75	22.37	0	0	17.85	188.7	0.72	81.6	289	22.1
17115	Rib, lean, roasted 3 oz	85	54.94	150.45	21.9	0	0	10.2	175.95	0.82	82.45	264.35	20.4
17143	Ground, broiled 3 oz	85	56.75	146.2	20.72	0	0	14.45	184.45	0.84	70.55	286.45	20.4
Pork													
10011	Frsh, (ham), whole, lean, roasted 3 oz	85	51.56	179.35	25	0	0	5.95	238.85	0.95	54.4	317.05	21.25
10019	Frsh, (ham), shank half, lean, roasted 3 oz	85	51.37	182.75	23.98	0	0	5.95	236.3	0.94	54.4	306	21.25
10027	Frsh, loin, whole, lean, roasted 3 oz	85	51.87	177.65	24.33	0	0	15.3	211.65	0.93	49.3	361.25	23.8
10042	Frsh, center loin (chops), bone-in, lean, broiled 3 oz	85	51.98	171.7	25.66	0	0	26.35	204.85	0.72	51	318.75	22.95
10050	Frsh, center rib (chops), bone-in, lean, broiled 3 oz	85	48.41	186.15	26.15	0	0	26.35	208.25	0.7	55.25	357	23.8
10059	Frsh, sirloin (roasts), bone-in, lean, roasted 3 oz	85	51.46	183.6	24.49	0	0	17	193.8	0.95	53.55	311.1	21.25
10079	Frsh, shoulder, arm picnic, lean, roasted 3 oz	85	51.23	193.8	22.68	0	0	7.65	209.95	1.21	68	298.35	17
10089	Frsh, spareribs, lean & fat, braised 3 oz	85	34.36	337.45	24.7	0	0	39.95	221.85	1.57	79.05	272	20.4
10124	Cured, bacon, broiled, pan-fried or roasted 3 medium slices packed 20/lb raw, after cooking	19	2.46	109.44	5.79	0.11	0	2.28	63.84	0.31	303.24	92.34	4.56
10131	Cured, canadian-style bacon, grilled 2 slices (6 per 6-oz pkg.)	46.5	28.69	86.03	11.27	0.63	0	4.65	137.64	0.38	718.89	181.35	9.77
10132	Cured, feet, pickled 1 lb	453.6	311.26	920.81	61.33	0.09	0	145.15	154.22	2.81	4186.73	1065.96	18.14
10134	Cured, ham, bnless, extra lean (approx 5% fat), roasted 3 oz	85	57.52	123.25	17.79	1.28	0	6.8	166.6	1.26	1022.55	243.95	11.9
10136	Cured, ham, bnless, reg (approx 11% fat), roasted 3 oz	85	54.86	151.3	19.23	0	0	6.8	238.85	1.14	1275	347.65	18.7
10153	Cured, ham, whole, lean, roasted 3 oz	85	55.91	133.45	21.29	0	0	5.95	192.95	0.8	1127.95	268.6	18.7
10169	Cured, shoulder, arm picnic, lean, roasted 3 oz	85	54.28	144.5	21.2	0	0	9.35	206.55	0.92	1046.35	248.2	13.6
Poultry: Chicken (broilers or fryers)													
05030	Light meat, meat & skin, fried, batter 1/2 chicken, bone removed	188	94.43	520.76	44.27	17.86	0	37.6	315.84	2.37	539.56	347.8	41.36
05031	Light meat, meat & skin, fried, flour 1/2 chicken, bone removed	130	71.06	319.8	39.59	2.37	0.13	20.8	276.9	1.57	100.1	310.7	35.1

NDB#	Zinc	Copper	Vitamin A	Thiamin	Riboflavin	Niacin	Vitamin B6	Folate	Vitamin B12	Vitamin C	Fat	Fat-Saturated	Fat-Monounsaturated	Fat-Polyunsaturated	Cholesterol
	mg	mg	IU	mg	mg	mg	mg	mcg	mcg	mg	gm	gm	gm	gm	mg
Veal															
17103	2.62	0.11	0	0.05	0.28	8.57	0.26	13.6	1	0	2.88	1.04	1.01	0.25	87.55
17109	2.75	0.1	0	0.05	0.26	8.04	0.31	13.6	1.11	0	5.9	2.19	2.12	0.48	90.1
17115	3.82	0.09	0	0.05	0.25	6.38	0.23	11.9	1.34	0	6.32	1.77	2.26	0.57	97.75
17143	3.29	0.09	0	0.06	0.23	6.83	0.33	9.35	1.08	0	6.43	2.58	2.41	0.47	87.55
Pork															
10011	2.77	0.09	7.65	0.59	0.3	4.19	0.38	10.2	0.61	0.34	8.02	2.81	3.78	0.72	79.9
10019	2.93	0.09	6.8	0.54	0.29	4.15	0.39	5.1	0.6	0.34	8.93	3.09	4.27	0.77	78.2
10027	2.15	0.05	6.8	0.86	0.28	5.01	0.47	5.95	0.62	0.51	8.19	2.98	3.67	0.65	68.85
10042	2.02	0.04	6.8	0.98	0.26	4.71	0.4	5.1	0.63	0.34	6.86	2.51	3.09	0.49	69.7
10050	2.02	0.06	5.1	0.95	0.28	5.24	0.4	2.55	0.65	0.26	8.28	2.94	3.78	0.53	68.85
10059	2.18	0.07	5.95	0.68	0.28	4.72	0.36	5.1	0.66	0.26	8.75	3.08	3.84	0.74	73.1
10079	3.46	0.11	5.95	0.49	0.3	3.67	0.35	4.25	0.66	0.26	10.73	3.66	5.08	1.02	80.75
10089	3.91	0.12	8.5	0.35	0.32	4.65	0.3	3.4	0.92	0	25.76	9.45	11.46	2.32	102.85
10124	0.62	0.03	0	0.13	0.05	1.39	0.05	0.95	0.33	0	9.36	3.31	4.5	1.1	16.15
10131	0.79	0.03	0	0.38	0.09	3.22	0.21	1.86	0.36	0	3.92	1.32	1.88	0.38	26.97
10132	5.62	0.23	0	0.03	0.19	1.66	1.72	18.14	2.81	0	73.21	25.27	34.34	7.94	417.31
10134	2.45	0.07	0	0.64	0.17	3.42	0.34	2.55	0.55	0	4.7	1.54	2.23	0.46	45.05
10136	2.1	0.12	0	0.62	0.28	5.23	0.26	2.55	0.6	0	7.67	2.65	3.77	1.2	50.15
10153	2.18	0.07	0	0.58	0.22	4.27	0.4	3.4	0.6	0	4.68	1.56	2.15	0.54	46.75
10169	2.5	0.11	0	0.62	0.19	4.08	0.31	3.4	0.94	0	5.98	2.01	2.75	0.69	40.8
Poultry: Chicken (broilers or fryers)															
05030	1.99	0.11	148.52	0.21	0.28	17.21	0.73	11.28	0.53	0	29.03	7.75	11.98	6.77	157.92
05031	1.64	0.08	88.4	0.1	0.17	15.65	0.7	5.2	0.43	0	15.72	4.32	6.24	3.5	113.1

NDB#	Description & Serving	Grams	Water	Calories	Protein	Carbohydrates	Fiber	Calcium	Phosphorus	Iron	Sodium	Potassium	Magnesium
		gm	*gm*	*kcal*	*gm*	*gm*	*gm*	*mg*	*mg*	*mg*	*mg*	*mg*	*mg*
05032	**Light meat, meat & skin, roasted** 1/2 chicken, bone removed	132	79.87	293.04	38.31	0	0	19.8	264	1.5	99	299.64	33
05033	**Light meat, meat & skin, stewed** 1/2 chicken, bone removed	150	97.7	301.5	39.21	0	0	19.5	219	1.47	94.5	250.5	30
05035	**Dark meat, meat & skin, fried, batter** 1/2 chicken, bone removed	278	135.72	828.44	60.74	26.08	0	58.38	403.1	4	820.1	514.3	55.6
05037	**Dark meat, meat & skin, roasted** 1/2 chicken, bone removed	167	97.91	422.51	43.37	0	0	25.05	280.56	2.27	145.29	367.4	36.74
05038	**Dark meat, meat & skin, stewed** 1/2 chicken, bone removed	184	115.9	428.72	43.24	0	0	25.76	244.72	2.41	128.8	305.44	33.12
05040	**Light meat, meat only, fried** 1 cup	140	84.2	268.8	45.95	0.59	0	22.4	323.4	1.6	113.4	368.2	40.6
05041	**Light meat, meat only, roasted** 1 cup, chopped or diced	140	90.66	242.2	43.27	0	0	21	302.4	1.48	107.8	345.8	37.8
05042	**Light meat, meat only, stewed** 1 cup, chopped or diced	140	95.23	222.6	40.43	0	0	18.2	222.6	1.3	91	252	30.8
05044	**Dark meat, meat only, fried** 1 cup	140	77.98	334.6	40.59	3.63	0	25.2	261.8	2.09	135.8	354.2	35
05045	**Dark meat, meat only, roasted** 1 cup, chopped or diced	140	88.28	287	38.32	0	0	21	250.6	1.86	130.2	336	32.2
05046	**Dark meat, meat only, stewed** 1 cup, chopped or diced	140	92.16	268.8	36.36	0	0	19.6	200.2	1.9	103.6	253.4	28
05028	**Chicken, liver, all classes, simmered** 1 cup, chopped or diced	140	95.63	219.8	34.1	1.23	0	19.6	436.8	11.86	71.4	196	29.4
05310	**Cornish game hens, meat only, roasted** 1/2 bird	110	79.09	147.4	25.63	0	0	14.3	163.9	0.85	69.3	275	20.9
	Poultry: Duck												
05140	**Duck, domesticated, meat & skin, roasted** 1 cup, chopped or diced	140	72.58	471.8	26.59	0	0	15.4	218.4	3.78	82.6	285.6	22.4
05142	**Duck, domesticated, meat only, roasted** 1 cup, chopped or diced	140	89.91	281.4	32.87	0	0	16.8	284.2	3.78	91	352.8	28
	Poultry: Goose												
05147	**Goose, domesticated, meat & skin, roasted** 1 cup, chopped or diced	140	72.73	427	35.22	0	0	18.2	378	3.96	98	460.6	30.8
05149	**Goose, domesticated, meat only, roasted** 1/2 goose	591	338.23	1406.58	171.21	0	0	82.74	1826.19	16.96	449.16	2293.08	147.75
	Poultry: Turkey												
05192	**Turkey, breast, meat & skin, roasted** 1/2 breast, bone removed	864	546.22	1632.96	248.05	0	0	181.44	1814.4	12.1	544.32	2488.32	233.28
05194	**Turkey, leg, meat & skin, roasted** 1 leg, bone removed	546	334.1	1135.68	152.17	0	0	174.72	1086.54	12.56	420.42	1528.8	125.58
	Luncheon meat												
07007	**Bologna, beef** 1 slice (4" dia x 1/8" thick)	23	12.72	71.76	2.81	0.18	0	2.76	20.24	0.38	225.63	36.11	2.76
07011	**Bologna, turkey** 2 slices	56.7	36.9	112.83	7.78	0.55	0	47.63	74.28	0.87	497.83	112.83	7.94

NDB#	Zinc	Copper	Vitamin A	Thiamin	Riboflavin	Niacin	Vitamin B6	Folate	Vitamin B12	Vitamin C	Fat	Fat:Saturated	Fat:Monounsaturated	Fat:Polyunsaturated	Cholesterol
	mg	mg	IU	mg	mg	mg	mg	mcg	mcg	mg	gm	gm	gm	gm	mg
05032	1.62	0.07	145.2	0.08	0.16	14.7	0.69	3.96	0.42	0	14.32	4.03	5.62	3.05	110.88
05033	1.71	0.07	144	0.06	0.17	10.4	0.41	4.5	0.3	0	14.96	4.2	5.88	3.18	111
05035	5.78	0.22	286.34	0.33	0.61	15.59	0.7	25.02	0.75	0	51.82	13.76	21.07	12.32	247.42
05037	4.16	0.13	335.67	0.11	0.35	10.62	0.52	11.69	0.48	0	26.35	7.3	10.34	5.83	151.97
05038	4.16	0.13	342.24	0.09	0.33	8.3	0.31	11.04	0.37	0	26.97	7.47	10.58	5.96	150.88
05040	1.78	0.08	42	0.1	0.18	18.71	0.88	5.6	0.5	0	7.76	2.13	2.76	1.76	126
05041	1.72	0.07	40.6	0.09	0.16	17.39	0.84	5.6	0.48	0	6.31	1.78	2.16	1.37	119
05042	1.67	0.06	37.8	0.06	0.16	10.91	0.46	4.2	0.32	0	5.59	1.57	1.89	1.22	107.8
05044	4.07	0.12	110.6	0.13	0.35	9.9	0.52	12.6	0.46	0	16.27	4.37	6.05	3.88	134.4
05045	3.92	0.11	100.8	0.1	0.32	9.17	0.5	11.2	0.45	0	13.62	3.72	4.98	3.16	130.2
05046	3.72	0.11	96.6	0.08	0.28	6.63	0.29	9.8	0.31	0	12.57	3.43	4.56	2.93	123.2
05028	6.08	0.52	22925	0.21	2.45	6.23	0.81	1078	27.15	22.12	7.63	2.58	1.88	1.26	883.4
05310	1.68	0.06	71.5	0.08	0.25	6.9	0.39	2.2	0.33	0.66	4.26	1.09	1.36	1.03	116.6
Poultry: Duck															
05140	2.6	0.32	294	0.24	0.38	6.76	0.25	8.4	0.42	0	39.69	13.54	18.06	5.11	117.6
05142	3.64	0.32	107.8	0.36	0.66	7.14	0.35	14	0.56	0	15.68	5.84	5.18	2	124.6
Poultry: Goose															
05147	3.67	0.37	98	0.11	0.45	5.84	0.52	2.8	0.57	0	30.69	9.62	14.35	3.53	127.4
05149	18.73	1.63	236.4	0.54	2.3	24.12	2.78	70.92	2.9	0	74.88	26.95	25.65	9.1	567.36
Poultry: Turkey															
05192	17.54	0.41	0	0.49	1.13	54.99	4.15	51.84	3.11	0	64.02	18.14	21.17	15.55	639.36
05194	23.31	0.84	0	0.33	1.32	19.44	1.8	49.14	1.97	0	53.62	16.71	15.67	14.85	464.1
Luncheon meat															
07007	0.5	0.01	0	0.01	0.03	0.55	0.03	1.15	0.33	0	6.56	2.78	3.17	0.25	13.34
07011	0.99	0.02	0	0.03	0.09	2	0.12	3.97	0.15	0	8.62	2.87	2.72	2.43	56.13

NDB#	Description & Serving	Grams	Water	Calories	Protein	Carbohydrates	Fiber	Calcium	Phosphorus	Iron	Sodium	Potassium	Magnesium
		gm	gm	kcal	gm	gm	gm	mg	mg	mg	mg	mg	mg
07017	Chicken roll, light meat 2 slices	56.7	38.9	90.15	11.07	1.39	0	24.38	89.02	0.55	331.13	129.28	10.77
07022	Frankfurter, beef 1 frankfurter (5 in long x 3/4 in dia, 10 per pound)	45	24.62	141.75	5.4	0.81	0	9	39.15	0.64	461.7	74.7	1.35
07024	Frankfurter, chicken 1 frankfurter	45	25.89	115.65	5.82	3.06	0	42.75	48.15	0.9	616.5	37.8	4.5
07025	Frankfurter, turkey 1 frankfurter	45	28.35	101.7	6.43	0.67	0	47.7	60.3	0.83	641.7	80.55	6.3
07028	Ham, sliced, extra lean (approx 5% fat) 1 slice (6-1/4" x 4" x 1/16")	28.35	19.99	37.14	5.49	0.27	0	1.98	61.8	0.22	405.12	99.23	4.82
07029	Ham, sliced, reg (approx 11% fat) 1 slice (6-1/4" x 4" x 1/16")	28.35	18.33	51.6	4.98	0.88	0	1.98	70.02	0.28	373.37	94.12	5.39
07069	Salami, bf & pork 1 slice (4" dia x 1/8" thick) (10 per 8 oz package)	23	13.89	57.5	3.2	0.52	0	2.99	26.45	0.61	244.95	45.54	3.45
07070	Salami, cooked, turkey 2 slices	56.7	37.34	111.13	9.28	0.31	0	11.34	60.1	0.91	569.27	138.35	8.51
07071	Salami, dry or hard, pork 1 slice (3-1/8" dia x 1/16" thick)	10	3.62	40.7	2.26	0.16	0	1.3	22.9	0.13	226	37.8	2.2
07079	Turkey breast meat 1 slice (3-1/2" square; 8 per 6 oz package)	21	15.09	23.1	4.73	0	0	1.47	48.09	0.08	300.51	58.38	4.2
07081	Turkey roll, light meat 2 slices	56.7	40.57	83.35	10.6	0.3	0	22.68	103.76	0.73	277.26	142.32	9.07
07082	Turkey roll, light & dark meat 2 slices	56.7	39.78	84.48	10.29	1.21	0	18.14	95.26	0.77	332.26	153.09	10.21
Nuts, seeds, and related products													
12061	Almonds, dried, unblanched 1 cup, sliced, unblanched	95	4.2	559.55	18.95	19.38	10.36	252.7	494	3.48	10.45	695.4	281.2
12063	Almonds, dry roasted, unblanched, wo/salt 1 cup whole kernels	138	4.14	810.06	22.54	33.35	18.91	389.16	756.24	5.24	15.18	1062.6	419.52
12065	Almonds, oil roasted, unblanched, wo/salt 1 cup whole kernels	157	4.84	970.26	32.01	24.93	17.58	367.38	858.79	6.01	15.7	1072.31	477.28
12071	Almond paste 1 oz	28.35	4	129.84	2.55	13.55	1.36	48.76	73.14	0.45	2.55	89.02	36.86
12078	Brazil nuts, dried, unblanched 1 cup, shelled (32 kernels)	140	4.68	918.4	20.08	17.92	7.56	246.4	840	4.76	2.8	840	315
12085	Cashew nuts, dry roasted, wo/salt 1 cup, halves and whole	137	2.33	786.38	20.97	44.79	4.11	61.65	671.3	8.22	21.92	774.05	356.2
12086	Cashew nuts, oil roasted, wo/salt 1 cup, halves and whole	130	5.08	748.8	21	37.08	4.94	53.3	553.8	5.33	22.1	689	331.5
12095	Chestnuts, chinese, roasted 1 oz	28.35	11.4	67.76	1.27	14.84	0	5.39	28.92	0.43	1.13	135.23	25.52
12104	Coconut meat, raw 1 cup, shredded	80	37.59	283.2	2.66	12.18	7.2	11.2	90.4	1.94	16	284.8	25.6
12108	Coconut meat, dried (desiccated), not swtnd 1 oz	28.35	0.85	187.11	1.95	6.92	4.62	7.37	58.4	0.94	10.49	153.94	25.52

NDB#	Zinc	Copper	Vitamin A	Thiamin	Riboflavin	Niacin	Vitamin B6	Folate	Vitamin B12	Vitamin C	Fat	Fat-Saturated	Fat-Monounsaturated	Fat-Polyunsaturated	Cholesterol
	mg	mg	IU	mg	mg	mg	mg	mcg	mcg	mg	gm	gm	gm	gm	mg
07017	0.41	0.02	46.49	0.04	0.07	3	0.12	1.13	0.09	0	4.18	1.15	1.68	0.91	28.35
07022	0.98	0.03	0	0.02	0.05	1.09	0.05	1.8	0.69	0	12.83	5.42	6.13	0.62	27.45
07024	0.47	0.02	58.5	0.03	0.05	1.39	0.14	1.8	0.11	0	8.77	2.49	3.82	1.82	45.45
07025	1.4	0.05	0	0.02	0.08	1.86	0.1	3.6	0.13	0	7.97	2.65	2.51	2.25	48.15
07028	0.55	0.02	0	0.26	0.06	1.37	0.13	1.13	0.21	0	1.41	0.46	0.67	0.14	13.32
07029	0.61	0.03	0	0.24	0.07	1.49	0.1	0.85	0.24	0	3	0.96	1.4	0.34	16.16
07069	0.49	0.05	0	0.05	0.09	0.82	0.05	0.46	0.84	0	4.63	1.86	2.11	0.46	14.95
07070	1.03	0.03	0	0.04	0.1	2	0.14	2.27	0.12	0	7.82	2.28	2.58	2	46.49
07071	0.42	0.02	0	0.09	0.03	0.56	0.06	0.2	0.28	0	3.37	1.19	1.6	0.37	7.9
07079	0.24	0.01	0	0.01	0.02	1.75	0.08	0.84	0.42	0	0.33	0.1	0.09	0.06	8.61
07081	0.88	0.02	0	0.05	0.13	3.97	0.18	2.27	0.14	0	4.09	1.15	1.42	0.99	24.38
07082	1.13	0.04	0	0.05	0.16	2.72	0.15	2.84	0.13	0	3.96	1.16	1.3	1.01	31.19

Nuts, seeds, and related products

NDB#	Zinc	Copper	Vitamin A	Thiamin	Riboflavin	Niacin	Vitamin B6	Folate	Vitamin B12	Vitamin C	Fat	Fat-Saturated	Fat-Monounsaturated	Fat-Polyunsaturated	Cholesterol
12061	2.77	0.89	0	0.2	0.74	3.19	0.11	55.77	0	0.57	49.6	4.7	32.21	10.41	0
12063	6.76	1.69	0	0.18	0.83	3.89	0.1	88.04	0	0.97	71.21	6.75	46.24	14.94	0
12065	7.69	1.92	0	0.2	1.55	5.5	0.13	100.17	0	1.1	90.54	8.58	58.79	19	0
12071	0.42	0.13	0	0.02	0.12	0.4	0.01	20.7	0	0.14	7.85	0.74	5.1	1.65	0
12078	6.43	2.48	0	1.4	0.17	2.27	0.35	5.6	0	0.98	92.71	22.62	32.22	33.78	0
12085	7.67	3.04	0	0.27	0.27	1.92	0.35	94.8	0	0	63.5	12.55	37.42	10.74	0
12086	6.18	2.82	0	0.55	0.23	2.34	0.33	88.01	0	0	62.67	12.38	36.94	10.6	0
12095	0.17	0.07	39.12	0.03	0.03	0.16	0.08	13.15	0	7	0.22	0.03	0.11	0.06	0
12104	0.88	0.35	0	0.05	0.02	0.43	0.04	21.12	0	2.64	26.79	23.76	1.14	0.29	0
12108	0.57	0.23	0	0.02	0.03	0.17	0.09	2.55	0	0.43	18.29	16.22	0.78	0.2	0

NDB#	Description & Serving	Grams	Water	Calories	Protein	Carbohydrates	Fiber	Calcium	Phosphorus	Iron	Sodium	Potassium	Magnesium
		gm	gm	kcal	gm	gm	gm	mg	mg	mg	mg	mg	mg
12115	Coconut cream, raw (liquid expressed from grated meat) 1 tablespoon	15	8.09	49.5	0.54	1	0.33	1.65	18.3	0.34	0.6	48.75	4.2
12121	Filberts or hazelnuts, dried, blanched 1 oz	28.35	0.54	190.51	3.61	4.53	1.81	55.28	91.57	0.96	0.85	130.98	83.92
12122	Filberts or hazelnuts, dry roasted, unblanched, wo/salt 1 oz	28.35	0.54	187.68	2.84	5.07	2.04	55.28	91.57	0.96	0.85	130.98	83.92
12123	Filberts or hazelnuts, oil roasted, unblanched, wo/salt 1 oz	28.35	0.34	187.11	4.04	5.43	1.81	55.57	92.42	0.97	0.85	131.83	84.48
12131	Macadamia nuts, dried 1 oz (11 whole kernels)	28.35	0.82	199.02	2.35	3.89	2.64	19.85	38.56	0.68	1.42	104.33	32.89
12133	Macadamia nuts, oil roasted, wo/salt 1 cup, whole or halves	134	2.24	962.12	9.73	17.29	12.46	60.3	268	2.41	9.38	440.86	156.78
12143	Pecans, dry roasted, wo/salt 1 oz	28.35	0.31	186.83	2.26	6.33	2.64	9.92	86.18	0.62	0.28	104.9	37.71
12144	Pecans, oil roasted, wo/salt 1 oz (15 halves)	28.35	1.19	194.2	1.97	4.55	1.9	9.64	83.35	0.6	0.28	101.78	36.57
12152	Pistachio nuts, dry roasted, wo/salt 1 cup	128	2.68	775.68	19.11	35.24	13.82	89.6	609.28	4.06	7.68	1241.6	166.4
12166	Sesame butter, tahini, from roasted & toasted kernels (most common type) 1 tablespoon	15	0.46	89.25	2.55	3.18	1.4	63.9	109.8	1.34	17.25	62.1	14.25
12537	Sunflower seed kernels, dry roasted, w/salt 1 cup	128	1.54	744.96	24.74	30.81	11.52	89.6	1478.4	4.86	998.4	1088	165.12
12023	Sesame seeds, whole, dried 1 tablespoon	9	0.42	51.57	1.6	2.11	1.06	87.75	56.61	1.31	0.99	42.12	31.59
12036	Sunflower seed kernels, dried 1 cup, with hulls, edible yield	46	2.47	262.2	10.48	8.63	4.83	53.36	324.3	3.11	1.38	316.94	162.84
12154	Walnuts, black, dried 1 cup, chopped	125	5.45	758.75	30.44	15.13	6.25	72.5	580	3.84	1.25	655	252.5

Seafood

Fish

NDB#	Description & Serving	Grams	Water	Calories	Protein	Carbohydrates	Fiber	Calcium	Phosphorus	Iron	Sodium	Potassium	Magnesium
15187	Bass, freshwater, mxd sp, cooked, dry heat 3 oz	85	58.47	124.1	20.55	0	0	87.55	217.6	1.62	76.5	387.6	32.3
15188	Bass, striped, cooked, dry heat 3 oz	85	62.36	105.4	19.32	0	0	16.15	215.9	0.92	74.8	278.8	43.35
15189	Bluefish, cooked, dry heat 3 oz	85	53.24	135.15	21.84	0	0	7.65	247.35	0.53	65.45	405.45	35.7
15009	Carp, cooked, dry heat 3 oz	85	59.19	137.7	19.43	0	0	44.2	451.35	1.35	53.55	362.95	32.3
15235	Catfish, channel, farmed, cooked, dry heat 3 oz	85	60.84	129.2	15.91	0	0	7.65	208.25	0.7	68	272.85	22.1
15012	Caviar, black & red, granular 1 tablespoon	16	7.6	40.32	3.94	0.64	0	44	56.96	1.9	240	28.96	48
15016	Cod, Atlantic, cooked, dry heat 3 oz	85	64.53	89.25	19.41	0	0	11.9	117.3	0.42	66.3	207.4	35.7
15192	Cod, Pacific, cooked, dry heat 3 oz	85	64.6	89.25	19.51	0	0	7.65	189.55	0.28	77.35	439.45	26.35

NDB#	Zinc	Copper	Vitamin A	Thiamin	Riboflavin	Niacin	Vitamin B6	Folate	Vitamin B12	Vitamin C	Fat	Fat:Saturated	Fat:Monounsaturated	Fat:Polyunsaturated	Cholesterol
	mg	mg	IU	mg	mg	mg	mg	mcg	mcg	mg	gm	gm	gm	gm	mg
12115	0.14	0.06	0	0	0	0.13	0.01	3.45	0	0.42	5.2	4.61	0.22	0.06	0
12121	0.71	0.44	19.56	0.15	0.03	0.33	0.18	21.12	0	0.28	19.08	1.4	14.95	1.83	0
12122	0.71	0.44	19.56	0.06	0.06	0.79	0.18	21.12	0	0.28	18.8	1.38	14.73	1.8	0
12123	0.71	0.45	19.85	0.06	0.06	0.79	0.18	21.29	0	0.28	18.03	1.33	14.13	1.73	0
12131	0.48	0.08	0	0.1	0.03	0.61	0.06	4.45	0	0	20.9	3.13	16.49	0.36	0
12133	1.47	0.4	12.06	0.29	0.15	2.71	0.27	21.31	0	0	102.54	15.35	80.91	1.77	0
12143	1.61	0.35	37.71	0.09	0.03	0.26	0.06	11.54	0	0.57	18.31	1.47	11.42	4.53	0
12144	1.56	0.34	36.57	0.09	0.03	0.25	0.05	11.17	0	0.57	20.19	1.62	12.58	5	0
12152	1.74	1.55	304.64	0.54	0.31	1.8	0.33	75.65	0	9.34	67.61	8.56	45.64	10.22	0
12166	0.69	0.24	10.05	0.18	0.07	0.82	0.02	14.66	0	0	8.06	1.13	3.05	3.53	0
12537	6.77	2.34	0	0.14	0.31	9.01	1.03	303.87	0	1.79	63.74	6.68	12.17	42.09	0
12023	0.7	0.37	0.81	0.07	0.02	0.41	0.07	8.7	0	0	4.47	0.63	1.69	1.96	0
12036	2.33	0.81	23	1.05	0.12	2.07	0.35	104.6	0	0.64	22.8	2.39	4.35	15.06	0
12154	4.28	1.28	370	0.27	0.14	0.86	0.69	81.88	0	4	70.73	4.54	15.91	46.87	0

Seafood
Fish

NDB#	Zinc	Copper	Vitamin A	Thiamin	Riboflavin	Niacin	Vitamin B6	Folate	Vitamin B12	Vitamin C	Fat	Fat:Saturated	Fat:Monounsaturated	Fat:Polyunsaturated	Cholesterol
15187	0.71	0.1	97.75	0.07	0.08	1.29	0.12	14.45	1.96	1.79	4.02	0.85	1.56	1.16	73.95
15188	0.43	0.03	88.4	0.1	0.03	2.17	0.29	8.5	3.75	0	2.54	0.55	0.72	0.85	87.55
15189	0.88	0.06	390.15	0.06	0.08	6.16	0.39	1.7	5.29	0	4.62	1	1.95	1.15	64.6
15009	1.62	0.06	27.2	0.12	0.06	1.79	0.19	14.71	1.25	1.36	6.09	1.18	2.54	1.56	71.4
15235	0.89	0.1	42.5	0.36	0.06	2.14	0.14	5.95	2.38	0.68	6.82	1.52	3.53	1.18	54.4
15012	0.15	0.02	298.88	0.03	0.1	0.02	0.05	8	3.2	0	2.86	0.65	0.74	1.18	94.08
15016	0.49	0.03	39.1	0.07	0.07	2.14	0.24	6.89	0.89	0.85	0.73	0.14	0.11	0.25	46.75
15192	0.43	0.03	27.2	0.02	0.04	2.11	0.39	6.8	0.88	2.55	0.69	0.09	0.09	0.27	39.95

NDB#	Description & Serving	Grams	Water	Calories	Protein	Carbohydrates	Fiber	Calcium	Phosphorus	Iron	Sodium	Potassium	Magnesium
		gm	gm	kcal	gm	gm	gm	mg	mg	mg	mg	mg	mg
15229	Cuttlefish, mxd sp, cooked, moist heat 3 oz	85	51.95	134.3	27.61	1.39	0	153	493	9.21	632.4	541.45	51
15194	Dolphinfish, cooked, dry heat 3 oz	85	60.54	92.65	20.16	0	0	16.15	155.55	1.23	96.05	453.05	32.3
15195	Drum, freshwater, cooked, dry heat 3 oz	85	60.3	130.05	19.12	0	0	65.45	196.35	0.98	81.6	300.05	32.3
15026	Eel, mxd sp, cooked, dry heat 1 oz, boneless	28.35	16.81	66.91	6.7	0	0	7.37	78.53	0.18	18.43	98.94	7.37
15029	Flatfish (flounder & sole sp), cooked, dry heat 3 oz	85	62.19	99.45	20.54	0	0	15.3	245.65	0.29	89.25	292.4	49.3
15032	Grouper, mxd sp, cooked, dry heat 3 oz	85	62.36	100.3	21.11	0	0	17.85	121.55	0.97	45.05	403.75	31.45
15034	Haddock, cooked, dry heat 3 oz	85	63.11	95.2	20.6	0	0	35.7	204.85	1.15	73.95	339.15	42.5
15035	Haddock, smoked 1 oz, boneless	28.35	20.26	32.89	7.15	0	0	13.89	71.16	0.4	216.31	117.65	15.31
15037	Halibut, Atlantic & Pacific, cooked, dry heat 3 oz	85	60.94	119	22.69	0	0	51	242.25	0.91	58.65	489.6	90.95
15041	Herring, Atlantic, pickled 1 oz, boneless	28.35	15.65	74.28	4.02	2.73	0	21.83	25.23	0.35	246.65	19.56	2.27
15042	Herring, Atlantic, kippered 1 oz, boneless	28.35	16.92	61.52	6.97	0	0	23.81	92.14	0.43	260.25	126.72	13.04
15047	Mackerel, Atlantic, cooked, dry heat 3 oz	85	45.28	222.7	20.27	0	0	12.75	236.3	1.33	70.55	340.85	82.45
15201	Mackerel, Pacific & jack, mxd sp, cooked, dry heat 1 oz, boneless	28.35	17.5	56.98	7.29	0	0	8.22	45.36	0.42	31.19	147.7	10.21
15203	Monkfish, cooked, dry heat 3 oz	85	66.73	82.45	15.78	0	0	8.5	217.6	0.35	19.55	436.05	22.95
15056	Mullet, striped, cooked, dry heat 3 oz	85	59.94	127.5	21.09	0	0	26.35	207.4	1.2	60.35	389.3	28.05
15061	Perch, mxd sp, cooked, dry heat 3 oz	85	62.26	99.45	21.13	0	0	86.7	218.45	0.99	67.15	292.4	32.3
15063	Pike, northern, cooked, dry heat 3 oz	85	62.02	96.05	20.99	0	0	62.05	239.7	0.6	41.65	281.35	34
15204	Pike, walleye, cooked, dry heat 3 oz	85	62.45	101.15	20.86	0	0	119.85	228.65	1.42	55.25	424.15	32.3
15205	Pollock, Atlantic, cooked, dry heat 3 oz	85	61.23	100.3	21.18	0	0	65.45	240.55	0.5	93.5	387.6	73.1
15067	Pollock, walleye, cooked, dry heat 3 oz	85	62.95	96.05	19.98	0	0	5.1	409.7	0.24	98.6	328.95	62.05
15069	Pompano, Florida, cooked, dry heat 3 oz	85	53.52	179.35	20.14	0	0	36.55	289.85	0.57	64.6	540.6	26.35
15207	Roe, mxd sp, cooked, dry heat 1 oz	28.35	16.62	57.83	8.11	0.54	0	7.94	146	0.22	33.17	80.23	7.37
15232	Roughy, orange, cooked, dry heat 3 oz	85	58.74	75.65	16.02	0	0	32.3	217.6	0.2	68.85	327.25	32.3
15075	Sablefish, smoked 3 oz	85	51.12	218.45	15	0	0	42.5	188.7	1.44	626.45	400.35	62.9

NDB#	Zinc	Copper	Vitamin A	Thiamin	Riboflavin	Niacin	Vitamin B6	Folate	Vitamin B12	Vitamin C	Fat	Fat: Saturated	Fat: Monounsaturated	Fat: Polyunsaturated	Cholesterol
	mg	mg	IU	mg	mg	mg	mg	mcg	mcg	mg	gm	gm	gm	gm	mg
15229	2.94	0.85	573.75	0.01	1.47	1.86	0.23	20.4	4.59	7.23	1.19	0.2	0.14	0.23	190.4
15194	0.5	0.05	176.8	0.02	0.07	6.31	0.39	5.1	0.59	0	0.77	0.2	0.13	0.18	79.9
15195	0.72	0.25	166.6	0.07	0.18	2.43	0.29	14.45	1.96	0.85	5.37	1.22	2.39	1.26	69.7
15026	0.59	0.01	1073.61	0.05	0.01	1.27	0.02	4.9	0.82	0.51	4.24	0.86	2.61	0.34	45.64
15029	0.54	0.02	32.3	0.07	0.1	1.85	0.2	7.82	2.13	0	1.3	0.31	0.2	0.55	57.8
15032	0.43	0.04	140.25	0.07	0.01	0.32	0.3	8.67	0.59	0	1.11	0.25	0.23	0.34	39.95
15034	0.41	0.03	53.55	0.03	0.04	3.94	0.29	11.31	1.18	0	0.79	0.14	0.13	0.26	62.9
15035	0.14	0.01	20.7	0.01	0.01	1.44	0.11	4.34	0.45	0	0.27	0.05	0.04	0.09	21.83
15037	0.45	0.03	152.15	0.06	0.08	6.05	0.34	11.73	1.16	0	2.5	0.35	0.82	0.8	34.85
15041	0.15	0.03	244.09	0.01	0.04	0.94	0.05	0.68	1.21	0	5.1	0.68	3.39	0.48	3.69
15042	0.39	0.04	36.29	0.04	0.09	1.25	0.12	3.88	5.3	0.28	3.51	0.79	1.45	0.83	23.25
15047	0.8	0.08	153	0.14	0.35	5.82	0.39	1.28	16.15	0.34	15.14	3.55	5.96	3.66	63.75
15201	0.24	0.03	13.32	0.04	0.15	3.02	0.11	0.57	1.2	0.6	2.87	0.82	0.96	0.71	17.01
15203	0.45	0.03	39.1	0.02	0.06	2.17	0.24	6.8	0.88	0.85	1.66	0	0	0	27.2
15056	0.75	0.12	119.85	0.09	0.09	5.36	0.42	8.33	0.21	1.02	4.13	1.22	1.17	0.78	53.55
15061	1.22	0.16	27.2	0.07	0.1	1.62	0.12	4.93	1.87	1.45	1	0.2	0.17	0.4	97.75
15063	0.73	0.06	68.85	0.06	0.07	2.38	0.11	14.71	1.96	3.23	0.75	0.13	0.17	0.22	42.5
15204	0.67	0.19	68.85	0.27	0.17	2.38	0.12	14.45	1.96	0	1.33	0.27	0.32	0.49	93.5
15205	0.51	0.05	34	0.05	0.19	3.39	0.28	2.55	3.13	0	1.07	0.14	0.12	0.53	77.35
15067	0.51	0.05	64.6	0.06	0.06	1.4	0.06	3.06	3.57	0	0.95	0.2	0.15	0.45	81.6
15069	0.59	0.07	102	0.58	0.13	3.23	0.2	14.71	1.02	0	10.32	3.82	2.82	1.24	54.4
15207	0.36	0.04	85.9	0.08	0.27	0.62	0.05	26.08	3.27	4.65	2.33	0.53	0.6	0.97	135.8
15232	0.82	0.15	68.85	0.1	0.16	3.11	0.29	6.8	1.96	0	0.77	0.02	0.52	0.01	22.1
15075	0.37	0.03	346.8	0.11	0.1	4.51	0.33	16.75	1.7	0	17.12	3.58	9.01	2.28	54.4

NDB#	Description & Serving	Grams	Water	Calories	Protein	Carbohydrates	Fiber	Calcium	Phosphorus	Iron	Sodium	Potassium	Magnesium
		gm	gm	kcal	gm	gm	gm	mg	mg	mg	mg	mg	mg
15179	Salmon, chinook, smoked (lox), reg 3 oz	85	61.2	99.45	15.54	0	0	9.35	139.4	0.72	1700	148.75	15.3
15209	Salmon, Atlantic, wild, cooked, dry heat 3 oz	85	50.68	154.7	21.62	0	0	12.75	217.6	0.88	47.6	533.8	31.45
15210	Salmon, chinook, cooked, dry heat 3 oz	85	55.76	196.35	21.86	0	0	23.8	315.35	0.77	51	429.25	103.7
15211	Salmon, chum, cooked, dry heat 3 oz	85	58.17	130.9	21.95	0	0	11.9	308.55	0.6	54.4	467.5	23.8
15212	Salmon, pink, cooked, dry heat 3 oz	85	59.23	126.65	21.73	0	0	14.45	250.75	0.84	73.1	351.9	28.05
15086	Salmon, sockeye, cooked, dry heat 3 oz	85	52.56	183.6	23.21	0	0	5.95	234.6	0.47	56.1	318.75	26.35
15088	Sardine, Atlantic, canned in oil, drained sol w/bone 1 oz	28.35	16.9	58.97	6.98	0	0	108.3	138.92	0.83	143.17	112.55	11.06
15092	Sea bass, mxd sp, cooked, dry heat 3 oz	85	61.32	105.4	20.09	0	0	11.05	210.8	0.31	73.95	278.8	45.05
15215	Shad, American, cooked, dry heat 3 oz	85	50.34	214.2	18.45	0	0	51	296.65	1.05	55.25	418.2	32.3
15100	Smelt, rainbow, cooked, dry heat 3 oz	85	61.87	105.4	19.21	0	0	65.45	250.75	0.98	65.45	316.2	32.3
15102	Snapper, mxd sp, cooked, dry heat 3 oz	85	59.8	108.8	22.36	0	0	34	170.85	0.2	48.45	443.7	31.45
15106	Sturgeon, mxd sp, smoked 3 oz	85	53.13	147.05	26.52	0	0	14.45	238.85	0.79	628.15	322.15	39.95
15109	Surimi 3 oz	85	64.89	84.15	12.9	5.82	0	7.65	239.7	0.22	121.55	95.2	36.55
15111	Swordfish, cooked, dry heat 3 oz	85	58.44	131.75	21.58	0	0	5.1	286.45	0.88	97.75	313.65	28.9
15116	Trout, rainbow, wild, cooked, dry heat 3 oz	85	59.93	127.5	19.48	0	0	73.1	228.65	0.32	47.6	380.8	26.35
15118	Tuna, fresh, bluefin, cooked, dry heat 3 oz	85	50.23	156.4	25.42	0	0	8.5	277.1	1.11	42.5	274.55	54.4
15221	Tuna, yellowfin, fresh, cooked, dry heat 3 oz	85	53.39	118.15	25.47	0	0	17.85	208.25	0.8	39.95	483.65	54.4
15222	Turbot, European, cooked, dry heat 3 oz	85	59.88	103.7	17.49	0	0	19.55	140.25	0.39	163.2	259.25	55.25
15131	Whitefish, mxd sp, smoked 1 oz, boneless	28.35	20.08	30.62	6.63	0	0	5.1	37.42	0.14	288.89	119.92	6.52
	Shellfish												
15156	Abalone, mxd sp, cooked, fried 3 oz	85	51.09	160.65	16.69	9.39	0	31.45	184.45	3.23	502.35	241.4	47.6
15159	Clam, mxd sp, cooked, moist heat 20 small clams	190	120.92	281.2	48.55	9.75	0	174.8	642.2	53.12	212.8	1193.2	34.2
15137	Crab, Alaska king, cooked, moist heat 1 leg	134	103.92	129.98	25.93	0	0	79.06	375.2	1.02	1436.48	351.08	84.42
15140	Crab, blue, cooked, moist heat 1 cup (not packed)	135	104.53	137.7	27.27	0	0	140.4	278.1	1.23	376.65	437.4	44.55

NDB#	Zinc	Copper	Vitamin A	Thiamin	Riboflavin	Niacin	Vitamin B6	Folate	Vitamin B12	Vitamin C	Fat	Fat: Saturated	Fat: Monounsaturated	Fat: Polyunsaturated	Cholesterol
	mg	mg	IU	mg	mg	mg	mg	mcg	mcg	mg	gm	gm	gm	gm	mg
15179	0.26	0.2	74.8	0.02	0.09	4.01	0.24	1.62	2.77	0	3.67	0.79	1.72	0.85	19.55
15209	0.7	0.27	37.4	0.23	0.41	8.57	0.8	24.65	2.59	0	6.91	1.07	2.29	2.77	60.35
15210	0.48	0.05	421.6	0.04	0.13	8.54	0.39	29.75	2.44	3.49	11.37	2.73	4.88	2.26	72.25
15211	0.51	0.06	96.9	0.08	0.19	7.25	0.39	4.25	2.94	0	4.11	0.92	1.68	0.98	80.75
15212	0.6	0.08	115.6	0.17	0.06	7.25	0.2	4.25	2.94	0	3.76	0.61	1.02	1.47	56.95
15086	0.43	0.06	177.65	0.18	0.15	5.67	0.19	4.25	4.93	0	9.32	1.63	4.5	2.05	73.95
15088	0.37	0.05	63.5	0.02	0.06	1.49	0.05	3.35	2.53	0	3.25	0.43	1.1	1.46	40.26
15092	0.44	0.02	181.05	0.11	0.13	1.62	0.39	4.93	0.26	0	2.18	0.56	0.46	0.81	45.05
15215	0.4	0.07	102	0.16	0.26	9.15	0.39	14.45	0.12	0	15	0	0	0	81.6
15100	1.8	0.15	49.3	0.01	0.12	1.5	0.14	3.91	3.37	0	2.64	0.49	0.7	0.96	76.5
15102	0.37	0.04	97.75	0.05	0	0.29	0.39	4.93	2.98	1.36	1.46	0.31	0.27	0.5	39.95
15106	0.48	0.04	793.05	0.08	0.08	9.44	0.23	17	2.47	0	3.74	0.88	2	0.37	68
15109	0.28	0.03	56.1	0.02	0.02	0.19	0.03	1.36	1.36	0	0.77	0.15	0.12	0.39	25.5
15111	1.25	0.14	116.45	0.04	0.1	10.02	0.32	1.96	1.72	0.94	4.37	1.2	1.68	1	42.5
15116	0.43	0.05	42.5	0.13	0.08	4.9	0.29	16.15	5.36	1.7	4.95	1.38	1.48	1.56	58.65
15118	0.65	0.09	2142	0.24	0.26	8.96	0.45	1.87	9.25	0	5.34	1.37	1.75	1.57	41.65
15221	0.57	0.07	57.8	0.43	0.05	10.15	0.88	1.7	0.51	0.85	1.04	0.26	0.17	0.31	49.3
15222	0.24	0.04	34	0.06	0.08	2.28	0.21	7.65	2.16	1.45	3.21	0	0	0	52.7
15131	0.14	0.09	53.87	0.01	0.03	0.68	0.11	2.07	0.92	0	0.26	0.06	0.08	0.08	9.36
Shellfish															
15156	0.81	0.19	4.25	0.19	0.11	1.62	0.13	4.59	0.59	1.53	5.76	1.4	2.33	1.42	79.9
15159	5.19	1.31	1083	0.29	0.81	6.37	0.21	54.72	187.89	41.99	3.71	0.36	0.33	1.05	127.3
15137	10.21	1.58	38.86	0.07	0.07	1.8	0.24	68.34	15.41	10.18	2.06	0.18	0.25	0.72	71.02
15140	5.7	0.87	8.1	0.14	0.07	4.46	0.24	68.58	9.86	4.46	2.39	0.31	0.38	0.92	135

NDB#	Description & Serving	Grams	Water gm	Calories kcal	Protein gm	Carbohydrates gm	Fiber gm	Calcium mg	Phosphorus mg	Iron mg	Sodium mg	Potassium mg	Magnesium mg
15226	Crab, dungeness, cooked, moist heat 1 crab	127	93.1	139.7	28.35	1.21	0	74.93	222.25	0.55	480.06	518.16	73.66
15227	Crab, queen, cooked, moist heat 3 oz	85	63.84	97.75	20.16	0	0	28.05	108.8	2.45	587.35	170	53.55
15243	Crayfish, mxd sp, farmed, cooked, moist heat 3 oz	85	68.68	73.95	14.89	0	0	43.35	204.85	0.94	82.45	202.3	28.05
15148	Lobster, northern, cooked, moist heat 3 oz	85	64.63	83.3	17.43	1.09	0	51.85	157.25	0.33	323	299.2	29.75
15165	Mussel, blue, cooked, moist heat 3 oz	85	51.98	146.2	20.23	6.28	0	28.05	242.25	5.71	313.65	227.8	31.45
15167	Oyster, eastern, wild, raw 6 medium	84	71.53	57.12	5.92	3.28	0	37.8	113.4	5.59	177.24	131.04	39.48
15169	Oyster, eastern, wild, cooked, moist heat 6 medium	42	29.53	57.54	5.92	3.28	0	37.8	85.26	5.04	177.24	118.02	39.9
15244	Oyster, eastern, wild, cooked, dry heat 6 medium	59	49.15	42.48	4.87	2.83	0	26.55	80.24	2.55	143.96	99.12	27.14
15171	Oyster, Pacific, raw 3 oz	85	69.75	68.85	8.03	4.21	0	6.8	137.7	4.34	90.1	142.8	18.7
15231	Oyster, Pacific, cooked, moist heat 3 oz	85	54.5	138.55	16.07	8.42	0	13.6	206.55	7.82	180.2	256.7	37.4
15173	Scallop, mxd sp, cooked, breaded & fried 2 large scallops	31	18.12	66.65	5.6	3.14	0	13.02	73.16	0.25	143.84	103.23	18.29
15151	Shrimp, mxd sp, cooked, moist heat 4 large	22	17	21.78	4.6	0	0	8.58	30.14	0.68	49.28	40.04	7.48
15176	Squid, mxd sp, cooked, fried 3 oz	85	54.86	148.75	15.25	6.62	0	33.15	213.35	0.86	260.1	237.15	32.3

Vegetables and vegetable juices

NDB#	Description & Serving	Grams	Water	Calories	Protein	Carb	Fiber	Calcium	Phosphorus	Iron	Sodium	Potassium	Magnesium
11008	Artichokes (globe or French), cooked, boiled, drained, wo/salt 1 medium artichoke	120	100.76	60	4.18	13.42	6.48	54	103.2	1.55	114	424.8	72
11011	Asparagus, raw 1 small spear (5" long or less)	12	11.09	2.76	0.27	0.54	0.25	2.52	6.72	0.1	0.24	32.76	2.16
11027	Bamboo shoots, cooked, boiled, drained, wo/salt 1 cup (1/2" slices)	120	115.1	14.4	1.84	2.3	1.2	14.4	24	0.29	4.8	639.6	3.6
11053	Beans, snap, green, cooked, boiled, drained, wo/salt 1 cup	125	111.53	43.75	2.36	9.86	4	57.5	48.75	1.6	3.75	373.75	31.25
11081	Beets, cooked, boiled, drained 1/2 cup slices	85	74	37.4	1.43	8.47	1.7	13.6	32.3	0.67	65.45	259.25	19.55
11090	Broccoli, raw 1 cup, flowerets	71	64.39	19.88	2.12	3.72	2.13	34.08	46.86	0.62	19.17	230.75	17.75
11099	Brussels sprouts, cooked, boiled, drained, wo/salt 1/2 cup	78	68.11	30.42	1.99	6.76	2.03	28.08	43.68	0.94	16.38	247.26	15.6
11109	Cabbage, raw 1 cup, shredded	70	64.51	17.5	1.01	3.8	1.61	32.9	16.1	0.41	12.6	172.2	10.5
11110	Cabbage, cooked, boiled, drained, wo/salt 1/2 cup shredded	75	70.2	16.5	0.77	3.35	1.73	23.25	11.25	0.13	6	72.75	6
11112	Cabbage, red, raw 1 cup, shredded	70	64.09	18.9	0.97	4.28	1.4	35.7	29.4	0.34	7.7	144.2	10.5

NDB#	Zinc	Copper	Vitamin A	Thiamin	Riboflavin	Niacin	Vitamin B6	Folate	Vitamin B12	Vitamin C	Fat	Fat-Saturated	Fat-Monounsaturated	Fat-Polyunsaturated	Cholesterol
	mg	mg	IU	mg	mg	mg	mg	mcg	mcg	mg	gm	gm	gm	gm	mg
15226	6.95	0.93	132.08	0.07	0.26	4.6	0.22	53.34	13.18	4.57	1.57	0.21	0.27	0.52	96.52
15227	3.05	0.53	147.05	0.08	0.21	2.45	0.15	35.7	8.82	6.12	1.28	0.16	0.28	0.46	60.35
15243	1.26	0.49	42.5	0.04	0.07	1.42	0.11	9.35	2.64	0.43	1.11	0.18	0.21	0.35	116.45
15148	2.48	1.65	73.95	0.01	0.06	0.91	0.07	9.44	2.64	0	0.5	0.09	0.14	0.08	61.2
15165	2.27	0.13	258.4	0.26	0.36	2.55	0.09	64.26	20.4	11.56	3.81	0.72	0.86	1.03	47.6
15167	76.28	3.74	84	0.08	0.08	1.16	0.05	8.4	16.35	3.11	2.07	0.65	0.26	0.81	44.52
15169	76.28	3.18	75.6	0.08	0.08	1.04	0.05	5.88	14.71	2.52	2.06	0.65	0.26	0.81	44.1
15244	43.42	2.04	0	0.05	0.05	0.99	0.06	10.62	16.4	2.42	1.12	0.32	0.14	0.48	28.91
15171	14.13	1.34	229.5	0.06	0.2	1.71	0.04	8.5	13.6	6.8	1.96	0.43	0.3	0.76	42.5
15231	28.25	2.28	413.1	0.11	0.38	3.08	0.08	12.75	24.48	10.88	3.91	0.87	0.61	1.52	85
15173	0.33	0.02	23.25	0.01	0.03	0.47	0.04	5.64	0.41	0.71	3.39	0.83	1.39	0.89	18.91
15151	0.34	0.04	48.18	0.01	0.01	0.57	0.03	0.77	0.33	0.48	0.24	0.06	0.04	0.1	42.9
15176	1.48	1.8	29.75	0.05	0.39	2.21	0.05	4.51	1.04	3.57	6.36	1.6	2.34	1.82	221
Vegetables and vegetable juices															
11008	0.59	0.28	212.4	0.08	0.08	1.2	0.13	61.2	0	12	0.19	0.04	0.01	0.08	0
11011	0.06	0.02	69.96	0.02	0.02	0.14	0.02	15.36	0	1.58	0.02	0.01	0	0.01	0
11027	0.56	0.1	0	0.02	0.06	0.36	0.12	2.76	0	0	0.26	0.06	0.01	0.12	0
11053	0.45	0.13	832.5	0.09	0.12	0.77	0.07	41.63	0	12.13	0.35	0.08	0.01	0.18	0
11081	0.3	0.06	29.75	0.02	0.03	0.28	0.06	68	0	3.06	0.15	0.02	0.03	0.05	0
11090	0.28	0.03	1094.82	0.05	0.08	0.45	0.11	50.41	0	66.17	0.25	0.04	0.02	0.12	0
11099	0.26	0.06	560.82	0.08	0.06	0.47	0.14	46.8	0	48.36	0.4	0.08	0.03	0.2	0
11109	0.13	0.02	93.1	0.04	0.03	0.21	0.07	30.1	0	22.54	0.19	0.02	0.01	0.09	0
11110	0.07	0.01	99	0.04	0.04	0.21	0.08	15	0	15.08	0.32	0.04	0.02	0.15	0
11112	0.15	0.07	28	0.04	0.02	0.21	0.15	14.49	0	39.9	0.18	0.02	0.01	0.09	0

NDB#	Description & Serving	Grams	Water	Calories	Protein	Carbohydrates	Fiber	Calcium	Phosphorus	Iron	Sodium	Potassium	Magnesium
			gm	kcal	gm	gm	gm	mg	mg	mg	mg	mg	mg
11113	Cabbage, red, cooked, boiled, drained, wo/salt 1/2 cup shredded	75	70.2	15.75	0.79	3.48	1.5	27.75	21.75	0.26	6	105	8.25
11115	Cabbage, savoy, cooked, boiled, drained, wo/salt 1 cup, shredded	145	133.4	34.8	2.61	7.84	4.06	43.5	47.85	0.55	34.8	266.8	34.8
11117	Cabbage, Chinese (pak-choi), cooked, boiled, drained, wo/salt 1 cup, shredded	170	162.44	20.4	2.65	3.03	2.72	158.1	49.3	1.77	57.8	630.7	18.7
11124	Carrots, raw 1 cup, grated	110	96.57	47.3	1.13	11.15	3.3	29.7	48.4	0.55	38.5	355.3	16.5
11960	Carrots, baby, raw 1 medium	10	8.98	3.8	0.08	0.82	0.18	2.3	3.8	0.08	3.5	27.9	1.2
11125	Carrots, cooked, boiled, drained, wo/salt 1/2 cup slices	78	68.16	35.1	0.85	8.17	2.57	24.18	23.4	0.48	51.48	177.06	10.14
11135	Cauliflower, raw 1 cup	100	91.91	25	1.98	5.2	2.5	22	44	0.44	30	303	15
11136	Cauliflower, cooked, boiled, drained, wo/salt 1/2 cup (1" pieces)	62	57.66	14.26	1.14	2.55	1.67	9.92	19.84	0.2	9.3	88.04	5.58
11965	Cauliflower, green, raw 1 cup	64	57.47	19.84	1.89	3.9	2.05	21.12	39.68	0.47	14.72	192	12.8
11967	Cauliflower, green, cooked, no salt 1/5 head	90	80.52	28.8	2.74	5.65	2.97	28.8	51.3	0.65	20.7	250.2	17.1
11143	Celery, raw 1 cup, diced	120	113.57	19.2	0.9	4.38	2.04	48	30	0.48	104.4	344.4	13.2
11148	Chard, swiss, cooked, boiled, drained, wo/salt 1 cup, chopped	175	162.14	35	3.29	7.25	3.68	101.5	57.75	3.96	313.25	960.75	150.5
11151	Chicory, witloof, raw 1/2 cup	45	42.53	7.65	0.41	1.8	1.4	8.55	11.7	0.11	0.9	94.95	4.5
11162	Collards, cooked, boiled, drained, wo/salt 1 cup, chopped	190	174.53	51.3	2.57	11.65	5.32	43.7	15.2	0.3	30.4	248.9	13.3
11168	Corn, swt, yellow, cooked, boiled, drained, wo/salt 1 baby ear	8	5.57	8.64	0.27	2.01	0.22	0.16	8.24	0.05	1.36	19.92	2.56
11203	Cress, garden, raw 1 cup	50	44.7	16	1.3	2.75	0.55	40.5	38	0.65	7	303	19
11205	Cucumber, with peel, raw 1/2 cup slices	52	49.93	6.76	0.36	1.44	0.42	7.28	10.4	0.14	1.04	74.88	5.72
11210	Eggplant, cooked, boiled, drained, wo/salt 1 cup (1" cubes)	99	90.85	27.72	0.82	6.57	2.48	5.94	21.78	0.35	2.97	245.52	12.87
11213	Endive, raw 1/2 cup, chopped	25	23.45	4.25	0.31	0.84	0.78	13	7	0.21	5.5	78.5	3.75
11234	Kale, cooked, boiled, drained, wo/salt 1 cup, chopped	130	118.56	41.6	2.47	7.32	2.6	93.6	36.4	1.17	29.9	296.4	23.4
11242	Kohlrabi, cooked, boiled, drained, wo/salt 1 cup, sliced	165	149	47.85	2.97	11.04	1.82	41.25	74.25	0.66	34.65	561	31.35
11247	Leeks (bulb & lower leaf-portion), cooked, boiled, drained, wo/salt 1/4 cup chopped or diced	26	23.61	8.06	0.21	1.98	0.26	7.8	4.42	0.29	2.6	22.62	3.64
11250	Lettuce, butterhead (incl Boston & bibb types), raw 1 cup, shredded or chopped	55	52.57	7.15	0.71	1.28	0.55	17.6	12.65	0.17	2.75	141.35	7.15
11251	Lettuce, cos or romaine, raw 1/2 cup shredded	28	26.57	4.48	0.45	0.66	0.48	10.08	12.6	0.31	2.24	81.2	1.68

NDB#	Zinc	Copper	Vitamin A	Thiamin	Riboflavin	Niacin	Vitamin B6	Folate	Vitamin B12	Vitamin C	Fat	Fat: Saturated	Fat: Monounsaturated	Fat: Polyunsaturated	Cholesterol
	mg	mg	IU	mg	mg	mg	mg	mcg	mcg	mg	gm	gm	gm	gm	mg
11113	0.11	0.05	20.25	0.03	0.02	0.15	0.11	9.45	0	25.8	0.15	0.02	0.01	0.07	0
11115	0.33	0.08	1289.05	0.07	0.03	0.03	0.22	67.14	0	24.65	0.13	0.02	0.01	0.06	0
11117	0.29	0.03	4365.6	0.05	0.11	0.73	0.28	69.02	0	44.2	0.27	0.04	0.02	0.13	0
11124	0.22	0.05	30941.9	0.11	0.06	1.02	0.16	15.4	0	10.23	0.21	0.03	0.01	0.08	0
11960	0.02	0	197.2	0	0.01	0.09	0.01	3.3	0	0.84	0.05	0.01	0	0.03	0
11125	0.23	0.1	19152.12	0.03	0.04	0.39	0.19	10.84	0	1.79	0.14	0.03	0.01	0.07	0
11135	0.28	0.04	19	0.06	0.06	0.53	0.22	57	0	46.4	0.21	0.03	0.01	0.1	0
11136	0.11	0.02	10.54	0.03	0.03	0.25	0.11	27.28	0	27.47	0.28	0.04	0.02	0.13	0
11965	0.41	0.03	97.28	0.05	0.07	0.47	0.14	36.48	0	56.38	0.19	0.03	0.02	0.09	0
11967	0.57	0.04	126.9	0.06	0.09	0.61	0.19	36.9	0	65.34	0.28	0.04	0.03	0.12	0
11143	0.16	0.04	160.8	0.06	0.05	0.39	0.1	33.6	0	8.4	0.17	0.04	0.03	0.08	0
11148	0.58	0.29	5493.25	0.06	0.15	0.63	0.15	15.05	0	31.5	0.14	0.02	0.03	0.05	0
11151	0.07	0.02	13.05	0.03	0.01	0.07	0.02	16.65	0	1.26	0.05	0.01	0	0.02	0
11162	0.21	0.06	5181.3	0.04	0.1	0.55	0.1	11.4	0	22.99	0.36	0.05	0.03	0.17	0
11168	0.04	0	17.36	0.02	0.01	0.13	0	3.71	0	0.5	0.1	0.02	0.03	0.05	0
11203	0.12	0.09	4650	0.04	0.13	0.5	0.12	40.2	0	34.5	0.35	0.01	0.12	0.11	0
11205	0.1	0.02	111.8	0.01	0.01	0.11	0.02	6.76	0	2.76	0.07	0.02	0	0.03	0
11210	0.15	0.11	63.36	0.08	0.02	0.59	0.09	14.26	0	1.29	0.23	0.04	0.02	0.09	0
11213	0.2	0.02	512.5	0.02	0.02	0.1	0.01	35.5	0	1.63	0.05	0.01	0	0.02	0
11234	0.31	0.2	9620	0.07	0.09	0.65	0.18	17.29	0	53.3	0.52	0.07	0.04	0.25	0
11242	0.51	0.22	57.75	0.07	0.03	0.64	0.25	19.97	0	89.1	0.18	0.02	0.01	0.09	0
11247	0.02	0.02	11.96	0.01	0.01	0.05	0.03	6.32	0	1.09	0.05	0.01	0	0.03	0
11250	0.09	0.01	533.5	0.03	0.03	0.17	0.03	40.32	0	4.4	0.12	0.02	0	0.06	0
11251	0.07	0.01	728	0.03	0.03	0.14	0.01	38	0	6.72	0.06	0.01	0	0.03	0

NDB#	Description & Serving	Grams	Water	Calories	Protein	Carbohydrates	Fiber	Calcium	Phosphorus	Iron	Sodium	Potassium	Magnesium
		gm	gm	kcal	gm	gm	gm	mg	mg	mg	mg	mg	mg
11252	**Lettuce, iceberg (incl crisphead types), raw** 1 cup, shredded or chopped	55	52.74	6.6	0.56	1.15	0.77	10.45	11	0.28	4.95	86.9	4.95
11253	**Lettuce, looseleaf, raw** 1/2 cup shredded	28	26.32	5.04	0.36	0.98	0.53	19.04	7	0.39	2.52	73.92	3.08
11260	**Mushrooms, raw** 1 cup, whole	96	88.14	24	2.01	4.46	1.15	4.8	99.84	1.19	3.84	355.2	9.6
11950	**Mushrooms, enoki, raw** 1 large	5	4.47	1.7	0.12	0.35	0.13	0.05	5.65	0.04	0.15	19.05	0.8
11268	**Mushrooms, shiitake, dried** 1 mushroom	3.6	0.34	10.66	0.34	2.71	0.41	0.4	10.58	0.06	0.47	55.22	4.75
11269	**Mushrooms, shiitake, cooked, wo/salt** 1 cup (pieces)	145	121.05	79.75	2.26	20.71	3.05	4.35	42.05	0.64	5.8	169.65	20.3
11279	**Okra, cooked, boiled, drained, wo/salt** 8 pods (3" long)	85	76.42	27.2	1.59	6.13	2.13	53.55	47.6	0.38	4.25	273.7	48.45
11282	**Onions, raw** 1 cup, chopped	160	143.49	60.8	1.86	13.81	2.88	32	52.8	0.35	4.8	251.2	16
11283	**Onions, cooked, boiled, drained, wo/salt** 1 cup	210	184.51	92.4	2.86	21.32	2.94	46.2	73.5	0.5	6.3	348.6	23.1
11291	**Onions, spring (incl tops & bulb), raw** 1 tablespoon, chopped	6	5.39	1.92	0.11	0.44	0.16	4.32	2.22	0.09	0.96	16.56	1.2
11297	**Parsley, raw** 1 cup	60	52.63	21.6	1.78	3.8	1.98	82.8	34.8	3.72	33.6	332.4	30
11299	**Parsnips, cooked, boiled, drained, wo/salt** 1/2 cup slices	78	60.62	63.18	1.03	15.23	3.12	28.86	53.82	0.45	7.8	286.26	22.62
11305	**Peas, green, cooked, boiled, drained, wo/salt** 1 cup	160	124.59	134.4	8.58	25.02	8.8	43.2	187.2	2.46	4.8	433.6	62.4
11333	**Peppers, sweet, green, raw** 1 cup, chopped	149	137.36	40.23	1.33	9.58	2.68	13.41	28.31	0.69	2.98	263.73	14.9
11951	**Peppers, sweet, yellow, raw** 10 strips	52	47.85	14.04	0.52	3.29	0.47	5.72	12.48	0.24	1.04	110.24	6.24
11363	**Potatoes, baked, flesh, wo/salt** 1 potato (2-1/3" x 4-3/4")	156	117.66	145.08	3.06	33.63	2.34	7.8	78	0.55	7.8	609.96	39
11364	**Potatoes, baked, skin, wo/salt** 1 potato skin	58	27.44	114.84	2.49	26.72	4.58	19.72	58.58	4.08	12.18	332.34	24.94
11365	**Potatoes, boiled, cooked in skin, flesh, wo/salt** 1 potato (2-1/2" dia, sphere)	136	104.69	118.32	2.54	27.38	2.45	6.8	59.84	0.42	5.44	515.44	29.92
11423	**Pumpkin, cooked, boiled, drained, wo/salt** 1 cup, mashed	245	229.54	49	1.76	11.98	2.7	36.75	73.5	1.4	2.45	563.5	22.05
11952	**Radicchio, raw** 1 cup, shredded	40	37.26	9.2	0.57	1.79	0.36	7.6	16	0.23	8.8	120.8	5.2
11429	**Radishes, raw** 1 cup, slices	116	110.01	19.72	0.7	4.16	1.86	24.36	20.88	0.34	27.84	269.12	10.44
11436	**Rutabagas, cooked, boiled, drained, wo/salt** 1 cup, mashed	240	213.31	93.6	3.1	20.98	4.32	115.2	134.4	1.27	48	782.4	55.2
11458	**Spinach, cooked, boiled, drained, wo/salt** 1 cup	180	164.18	41.4	5.35	6.75	4.32	244.8	100.8	6.43	126	838.8	156.6
11477	**Squash, summer, zucchini, incl skin, raw** 1 cup, sliced	113	107.67	15.82	1.31	3.28	1.36	16.95	36.16	0.47	3.39	280.24	24.86

NDB #	Zinc	Copper	Vitamin A	Thiamin	Riboflavin	Niacin	Vitamin B6	Folate	Vitamin B12	Vitamin C	Fat	Fat-Saturated	Fat-Monounsaturated	Fat-Polyunsaturated	Cholesterol
	mg	mg	IU	mg	mg	mg	mg	mcg	mcg	mg	gm	gm	gm	gm	mg
11252	0.12	0.02	181.5	0.03	0.02	0.1	0.02	30.8	0	2.15	0.1	0.01	0	0.06	0
11253	0.08	0.01	532	0.01	0.02	0.11	0.02	13.94	0	5.04	0.08	0.01	0	0.04	0
11260	0.7	0.47	0	0.1	0.43	3.95	0.09	20.26	0	3.36	0.4	0.05	0.01	0.16	0
11950	0.03	0	0.35	0	0.01	0.18	0	1.5	0	0.6	0.02	0	0	0.01	0
11268	0.28	0.19	0	0.01	0.05	0.51	0.03	5.88	0	0.13	0.04	0.01	0.01	0.01	0
11269	1.93	1.3	0	0.05	0.25	2.18	0.23	30.31	0	0.44	0.32	0.08	0.1	0.04	0
11279	0.47	0.07	488.75	0.11	0.05	0.74	0.16	38.85	0	13.86	0.14	0.04	0.02	0.04	0
11282	0.3	0.1	0	0.07	0.03	0.24	0.19	30.4	0	10.24	0.26	0.04	0.04	0.1	0
11283	0.44	0.14	0	0.09	0.05	0.35	0.27	31.5	0	10.92	0.4	0.07	0.06	0.15	0
11291	0.02	0	23.1	0	0	0.03	0	3.84	0	1.13	0.01	0	0	0	0
11297	0.64	0.09	3120	0.05	0.06	0.79	0.05	91.2	0	79.8	0.47	0.08	0.18	0.07	0
11299	0.2	0.11	0	0.06	0.04	0.56	0.07	45.4	0	10.14	0.23	0.04	0.09	0.04	0
11305	1.9	0.28	955.2	0.41	0.24	3.23	0.35	101.28	0	22.72	0.35	0.06	0.03	0.16	0
11333	0.18	0.1	941.68	0.1	0.04	0.76	0.37	32.78	0	133.06	0.28	0.04	0.02	0.15	0
11951	0.09	0.06	123.76	0.01	0.01	0.46	0.09	13.52	0	95.42	0.11	0	0	0	0
11363	0.45	0.34	0	0.16	0.03	2.18	0.47	14.2	0	19.97	0.16	0.04	0	0.07	0
11364	0.28	0.47	0	0.07	0.06	1.78	0.36	12.53	0	7.83	0.06	0.02	0	0.02	0
11365	0.41	0.26	0	0.14	0.03	1.96	0.41	13.6	0	17.68	0.14	0.04	0	0.06	0
11423	0.56	0.22	2650.9	0.08	0.19	1.01	0.11	20.83	0	11.52	0.17	0.09	0.02	0.01	0
11952	0.25	0.14	10.8	0.01	0.01	0.1	0.02	24	0	3.2	0.1	0.02	0	0.04	0
11429	0.35	0.05	9.28	0.01	0.05	0.35	0.08	31.32	0	26.45	0.63	0.03	0.02	0.05	0
11436	0.84	0.1	1346.4	0.2	0.1	1.72	0.24	36	0	45.12	0.53	0.07	0.06	0.23	0
11458	1.37	0.31	14742	0.17	0.42	0.88	0.44	262.44	0	17.64	0.47	0.08	0.01	0.19	0
11477	0.23	0.06	384.2	0.08	0.03	0.45	0.1	24.97	0	10.17	0.16	0.03	0.01	0.07	0

NDB#	Description & Serving	Grams	Water	Calories	Protein	Carbohydrates	Fiber	Calcium	Phosphorus	Iron	Sodium	Potassium	Magnesium
		gm	gm	kcal	gm	gm	gm	mg	mg	mg	mg	mg	mg
11480	Squash, summer, zucchini, incl skin, frz, cooked, boiled, drained, wo/salt												
	1 cup	223	211.27	37.91	2.56	7.94	2.9	37.91	55.75	1.07	4.46	432.62	28.99
11483	Squash, winter, acorn, cooked, baked, wo/salt												
	1 cup, cubes	205	169.95	114.8	2.3	29.89	9.02	90.2	92.25	1.91	8.2	895.85	88.15
11486	Squash, winter, butternut, cooked, baked, wo/salt												
	1 cup, cubes	205	179.99	82	1.85	21.5	0	84.05	55.35	1.23	8.2	582.2	59.45
11490	Squash, winter, hubbard, cooked, baked, wo/salt												
	1 cup, cubes	205	174.46	102.5	5.08	22.16	0	34.85	47.15	0.96	16.4	733.9	45.1
11493	Squash, winter, spaghetti, cooked, boiled, drained, or baked, wo/salt												
	1 cup	155	143.07	44.95	1.02	10.01	2.17	32.55	21.7	0.53	27.9	181.35	17.05
11496	Succotash (corn & limas), cooked, boiled, drained, wo/salt												
	1 cup	192	131.27	220.8	9.73	46.81	8.64	32.64	224.64	2.92	32.64	787.2	101.76
11508	Sweetpotato, cooked, baked in skin, wo/salt												
	1 large	180	131.13	185.4	3.1	43.69	5.4	50.4	99	0.81	18	626.4	36
11510	Sweetpotato, cooked, boiled, wo/skin, wo/salt												
	1 medium	151	109.99	158.55	2.49	36.66	2.72	31.71	40.77	0.85	19.63	277.84	15.1
11529	Tomatoes, red, ripe, raw, year round average												
	1 cup, chopped or sliced	180	168.77	37.8	1.53	8.35	1.98	9	43.2	0.81	16.2	399.6	19.8
11530	Tomatoes, red, ripe, cooked, boiled, wo/salt												
	2 medium	246	226.71	66.42	2.63	14.34	2.46	14.76	76.26	1.38	27.06	686.34	34.44
11565	Turnips, cooked, boiled, drained, wo/salt												
	1 cup, mashed	230	215.28	41.4	1.63	11.27	4.6	50.6	43.7	0.51	115	310.5	18.4
11591	Watercress, raw												
	1 cup, chopped	34	32.34	3.74	0.78	0.44	0.51	40.8	20.4	0.07	13.94	112.2	7.14

NDB#	Zinc	Copper	Vitamin A	Thiamin	Riboflavin	Niacin	Vitamin B6	Folate	Vitamin B12	Vitamin C	Fat	Fat Saturated	Fat Monounsaturated	Fat Polyunsaturated	Cholesterol
	mg	mg	IU	mg	mg	mg	mg	mcg	mcg	mg	gm	gm	gm	gm	mg
11480	0.45	0.1	963.36	0.09	0.09	0.86	0.1	17.39	0	8.25	0.29	0.06	0.02	0.12	0
11483	0.35	0.18	877.4	0.34	0.03	1.81	0.4	38.34	0	22.14	0.29	0.06	0.02	0.12	0
11486	0.27	0.13	14352.05	0.15	0.03	1.99	0.25	39.36	0	30.96	0.18	0.04	0.01	0.08	0
11490	0.31	0.09	12371.75	0.15	0.1	1.14	0.35	33.21	0	19.48	1.27	0.26	0.09	0.53	0
11493	0.31	0.05	170.5	0.06	0.03	1.26	0.15	12.4	0	5.43	0.4	0.1	0.03	0.2	0
11496	1.21	0.34	564.48	0.32	0.18	2.55	0.22	62.98	0	15.74	1.54	0.28	0.3	0.73	0
11508	0.52	0.37	39279.6	0.13	0.23	1.09	0.43	40.68	0	44.28	0.2	0.04	0.01	0.09	0
11510	0.41	0.24	25751.54	0.08	0.21	0.97	0.37	16.76	0	25.82	0.45	0.1	0.02	0.2	0
11529	0.16	0.13	1121.4	0.11	0.09	1.13	0.14	27	0	34.38	0.59	0.08	0.09	0.24	0
11530	0.27	0.23	1827.78	0.17	0.14	1.84	0.23	31.98	0	56.09	1.01	0.14	0.15	0.42	0
11565	0.46	0.15	0	0.06	0.05	0.69	0.15	21.16	0	26.68	0.18	0.02	0.01	0.1	0
11591	0.04	0.03	1598	0.03	0.04	0.07	0.04	3.13	0	14.62	0.03	0.01	0	0.01	0

Appendix B

Diet and Nutrition Help Lines

• •

*A*s you thumb through this book, you'll see phone numbers, FAX numbers, and Web site addresses for groups, businesses, and organizations offering information and assistance with one or more aspects of weight loss and weight control.

To make it easier for you to find a particular number in a hurry, I've collected them all in one spot, right here in this appendix. Consult it whenever you feel the need for online exploration, 800-number chats, or just plain browsing.

You can add your own numbers to this list, or you can tear out these pages and pin them up on the front of the fridge or next to your PC.

Yes, I know Ms. Jones taught you way back in first grade that it's a sin to write in a book. As for tearing out pages, well, that would probably have given her the vapors. But as an avid collector of facts and odd bits of information, not to mention a certified book lover, I say, go ahead. Right now! While nobody's watching!

If you feel guilty, buy another copy of this book and give it to your local library in honor of Ms. Jones. She'd love that!

Help Lines

American Anorexia and Bulimia Association, Inc.: Offers: Information about eating disorders, support for patients and families, links to other sites. Telephone: (212) 575-6200. Web site: www.aabainc.org

American College of Sports Medicine: Offers: Information about specialists and the medical effects of exercise. Telephone: (317) 637-9200. Web site: www.acsm.org

American Diabetes Association: Offers: Medical and nutritional guidance, support, publications. Telephone: (800) DIABETES, (800) 342-2382. Web site: www.diabetes.org

American Dietetic Association: Offers: The skinny on nutrition and health, everything from calorie charts to diet recommendations, publications, referrals to dietitians, links to other sites. Telephone: (800) 366-1655 (Find a dietitian). Web site: www.eatright.org

American Heart Association: Offers: Medical and dietary advice for a healthy heart. Telephone: (800) 242-8721. Web site: www.americanheart.org

American Society of Bariatric Physicians (ASBP): Offers: Responsible weight loss guidance plus assistance in locating an obesity specialist. Telephone: (303) 779-4833. Web site: www.asbp.org

American Society of Clinical Nutrition: Offers: Authoritative information about nutrition. Telephone: (301) 530-7110. Web site: www.faseb.org

Anorexia Nervosa and Related Eating Disorders, Inc.: Offers: Information about eating disorders, support for patients and families, links to other sites. Web site: www.anred.com

Arby's: Offers: Restaurant locations, nutrition charts. Web site: www.arbys.com

Atkins Diet Center: Offers: Information and products for low-carb weight loss. Telephone: (212) 758-2110. Web site: www.atkinscenter.com

Au Bon Pain: Offers: Restaurant locations, nutrition charts. Web site: www.aubonpain.com

Burger King: Offers: Restaurant locations, nutrition charts. Web site: www.burgerking.com

Calorie Control Council: Offers: Information about foods that reduce calorie consumption, nutrition news and publications. Telephone: (404) 252-3663. Web site: www.caloriecontrol.org

The Carbohydrate Addict's Diet: Offers: Information and products for low-carb weight loss. Web site: www.carbohydrateaddicts.com

Center for Science in the Public Interest: Offers: Health tips, nutrition info, newsletter (with membership), publications, links to other sites. FAX: (202) 265-4954. Web site: www.cspinet.org

Consumer's Union: Offers: Consumer product evaluations (including diet products), publications including Consumer Reports. Telephone: (914) 378-2000. Web site: www.consumersunion.org

Council on Size & Weight Discrimination: Offers: Advocacy support to counter bias against large persons. Web site: www.cswd.org

CyberDiet: Offers: Online weight loss information, evaluations of weight loss diets and links to related sites. Web site: www.CyberDiet.com

Dunkin' Donuts: Offers: Restaurant locations and nutrition charts. Web site: www.dunkindonuts.com

Eating Disorder Referral & Information Center: Offers: Assistance in dealing with eating disorders, plus referrals to specialists and support groups. Telephone: (858) 792-7463. Web site: www.edreferral.com

EDiets: Offers: Online nutrition information and diet evaluations. Web site: www.ediets.com

Federal Trade Commission: Offers: Help line, information on product recalls, complaint forms. Telephone: (887) FTC-HELP. Web site: www.ftc.gov, www.ftc.gov/ftc/complaint.htm (complaint forms)

Food and Drug Administration: Offers: Enough nutrition information to satisfy even the hungriest data junkie:charts, regulations, legal information, nutrition news, and on and on and on. . . .Telephone: (301) 443-3170, (consumer affairs) (202) 205-4561 (nutrition and food sciences). Web site: www.fda.gov

Institute of Food Technologists (IFT): Offers: Expert information on food processing and nutrients. Telephone: (312) 782-8424. Web site: www.ift.org

International Food Information Council: Offers: Expert information on food and nutrition. Telephone: (202) 296-6540. Web site: ificinfo.health.org

iVillage: Offers: Online nutrition and diet advice. Web site: www.ivillage.com

Jenny Craig: Offers: Diet information and products. Telephone: (800) 597-5366. Web site: www.jennycraig.com

Mayo Clinic Health Oasis: Offers: A broad variety of Online health and diet news, reports, evaluations, publications (including the Mayo Clinic Health Letter). Web site: www.mayohealth.org

McDonald's Nutrition Information Center: Offers: Restaurant locations and nutrition charts. Web site: www.mcdonalds.com

National Association to Advance Fat Acceptance (NAAFA): Offers: Advocacy and support, legal and health issue positions.Web site: www.naafa.org

National Heart, Lung, and Blood Institute (NHLBI): Offers: Nutrition and health information, publications, help lines, links to related sites. Telephone: (301) 951-3260. Web site: www.nhlbi.nih.gov

National Institute for Diabetes, Digestive and Kidney Disease (NIDDK): Offers: Nutrition and health information, publications, help lines, links to related sites. Web site: www.niddk/nih.gov

Nutrisystem: Offers: Online, sometimes interactive, information and support plus product sales. Web site: www.nutrisystem.com

Overeaters Anonymous: Offers: Information and support. Web site: www.overeatersanonymous.org

Pizza Hut: Offers: Restaurant locations and nutrition charts. Web site: www.pizzahut.com

President's Council on Physical Fitness and Sports: Offers: Authoritative information on the virtues of fitness for every age group. Telephone: (202) 690-9000. Web site: www.fitness.gov

Pritikin Diet: Offers: Targeted information for lowfat weight loss. Telephone: Web site: www.pritikin.com

Subway: Offers: Restaurant locations and nutrition charts. Web site: www.subway.com

SugarBusters!: Offers: Targeted information and products for low-carb weight loss. Web site: www.sugarbusters.com

TOPS (Take Off Pounds Sensibly): Offers: Support group, assistance with weight loss and maintenance. Telephone: (800) 932-8777. Web site: www.tops.org

Tufts University Nutrition Navigator: Offers: Authoritative evaluation of nutrition and diet Web sites. Web site: navigator.tufts.edu

1-800-Therapist Network: Offers: Referral source for patient with eating disorders. Telephone: (800) 843-7274. Web site: www.1-800-therapist.com

U.S. Department of Agriculture Nutrient Database: Offers: The world's most complete nutrition chart. Web site: www.nal.usda.gov/fnic/cgi-bin/nut_search.pl

Weight Control Information Network (WIN): Offers: Authoritative information on obesity and weight control. Telephone: (202) 828-1025, (877) 946-4627. Web site: www.niddk.nih.gov/health/nutrit/win.htm

Weight Watchers: Offers: Weight loss support, products. Telephone: (800) 651-6000. Web site: www.weight_watchers.org

Wendy's International Inc.: Offers: Restaurant locations and nutrition charts. Web site: www.wendys.com

World Health Organization (WHO) Washington, D.C., Office: Offers: International statistics and information on health including weight. Telephone: (202) 861-3200. Web site: www.who.int/

The Zone: Offers: Targeted information and products for carb-based weight loss. Web site: www.zoneperfect.com

Appendix C

About the CD

● ●

*W*riting the CD-ROM for *Weight Loss Kit For Dummies* was a blast because it let me create "print out" charts that give you tools to make taking off pounds easier. And I get to include some statements and data from Big Name sources such as the American Dietetic Association that just wouldn't fit into the pages of this book.

System Requirements

Make sure that your computer meets the minimum system requirements that follow. If your computer doesn't match up to most of these requirements, you may have problems using the contents of the CD.

- ✔ A PC with a Pentium or faster processor, or a Mac OS computer with a 68040 or faster processor.
- ✔ Microsoft Windows 95 or later, or Mac OS system software 7.55 or later.
- ✔ At least 16MB of total RAM installed on your computer. For best performance, we recommend at least 32MB of RAM installed.
- ✔ A CD-ROM drive — double-speed (2x) or faster.
- ✔ A sound card for PCs. (Mac OS computers have built-in sound support.)
- ✔ A monitor capable of displaying at least 256 colors or grayscale.
- ✔ A modem with a speed of at least 14,400 bps.

If you need more information on the basics, check out *PCs For Dummies,* 7th Edition, by Dan Gookin; *Macs For Dummies,* 6th Edition, by David Pogue; *iMac For Dummies,* by David Pogue; *Windows 98 For Dummies, or Windows 95 For Dummies,* 2nd Edition, all by Andy Rathbone (all published by Hungry Minds, Inc.).

Using the CD with Microsoft Windows

To install the items from the CD to your hard drive, follow these steps:

1. **Insert the CD into your computer's CD-ROM drive.**

2. **Open your browser.**

   If you do not have a browser, I have included Microsoft Internet Explorer as well as Netscape Communicator. You can find them in the Programs folders at the root of the CD.

3. **Click Start⇨Run.**

4. **In the dialog box that appears, type D:\START.HTM**

   Replace *D* with the proper drive letter if your CD-ROM drive uses a different letter. (If you don't know the letter, see how your CD-ROM drive is listed under My Computer.)

5. **Read through the license agreement, nod your head, and then click the Accept button if you want to use the CD — after you click Accept, you'll jump to the Main Menu.**

   This action displays the file that will walk you through the content of the CD.

6. **To navigate within the interface, simply click on any topic of interest to take you to an explanation of the files on the CD and how to use or install them.**

7. **To install the software from the CD, simply click on the software name.**

   You'll see two options — the option to run or open the file from the current location or the option to save the file to your hard drive. Choose to run or open the file from its current location and the installation procedure will continue. After you are done with the interface, simply close your browser as usual.

To run some of the programs, you may need to keep the CD inside your CD-ROM drive. This is a Good Thing. Otherwise, the installed program would have required you to install a very large chunk of the program to your hard drive space, which would have kept you from installing other software.

How to use the CD using the Mac OS

To install the items from the CD to your hard drive, follow these steps:

1. **Insert the CD into your computer's CD-ROM drive.**

   In a moment, an icon representing the CD you just inserted appears on your Mac desktop. Chances are, the icon looks like a CD-ROM.

2. **Double-click the CD icon to show the CD's contents.**

3. **Double-click the Read Me First icon.**

   This text file contains information about the CD's programs and any last-minute instructions you need to know about installing the programs on the CD that I don't cover in this appendix.

4. **Open your browser.**

   If you don't have a browser, I have included the two most popular ones for your convenience — Microsoft Internet Explorer and Netscape Communicator.

5. **Click on File⇨Open and select the CD.**

6. **Click on the Links.htm file to see an explanation of all files and folders included on the CD.**

7. **Some programs come with installer programs — with those you simply open the program's folder on the CD and double-click the icon with the words "Install" or "Installer."**

   Once you have installed the programs that you want, you can eject the CD. Carefully place it back in the plastic jacket of the book for safekeeping.

What You'll Find Here

I've organized this "index" to the CD-ROM by chapters to make it easier for you to key the data on disc to what you're reading. So first up is, Ta! Ta! Chapter 1.

Chapter 1: Why Weight Matters

Your best guide to your own risk of weight-related health problems is your family history. The Family Fat Tree enables you to set up an easily viewable family album. If your family is fat but fit, fine. If your relatives are skinny and fit, that's fine, too. But if you see a pattern of weight-related illness, that's a warning. So check it out with your doctor, okay?

The American Dietetic Association statement on weight control is a perfect introduction not only to the state of your weight (as well as that of your friends and relatives), it's also a great introduction to what you'll find in this book. So click up and take a look.

Chapter 2: How to Tell Who's Fat

The Body Mass Index gives you a handle on whether your weight is within reasonable bounds or edging up toward trouble. Chapter 2 shows you how to calculate your own BMI. This guide (BMIs) does it for you. And for most other people on this planet, I might add.

Chapter 3: How to Tell If You're Losing Weight

One way to tell if your losing weight is to watch what happens to your clothing sizes. Going up? Booo! Going down? Hooray! But what exactly does a clothing size measure? As you can read in Chapter 3, men's clothing sizes are standard to a fault. But women's clothing sizes are a guessing game. DOC Body Measurements for the Sizing of Women's Patterns and Apparel shows early size measurements drawn up by the Department of Commerce. ASTM Standard Tables of Body Measurements for Adult Female Misses Figure Type, Sizes 2-20 is a more recent compilation that's replaced the DOC figures. As it says in the text for this chapter, comparing the two is an interesting game.

Whichever size you turn out to be, Tracking Your Weight is a printable chart that enables you to keep track of the results of your weigh-ins.

Chapter 4: Healthful Rules for Healthy Weight Loss Programs

Before you choose a weight loss program, you need to know if you're ready to take on the challenge of taking off the pounds. Are You ready to Lose Weight? is a simple questionnaire that can help you decide.

Fad Versus Fit: Does Your Weight Loss Plan Measure Up? is a printable, fill-in chart that rates your proposed diet plan.

Chapter 5: Calories Count

After you've read the first part of Chapter 5 and know how many calories your body requires each day to work in tiptop form, click on to Counting Your Personal Calories. The printable chart shows you how to set up one week's worth of calorie consumption. Neat.

Chapter 6: Playing with Carbs

The carbohydrate-based diet is endorsed by a slew of nutrition gurus. To win your heart and make it easy as (lowfat) pie for you to set up your own carb-based weight loss plan, I've created three printable charts: One Week's Carb-Based Weight Loss Diet 1,200 calories, One Week's Carb-Based Weight Loss Diet 1,500 calories, and One Week's Carb-Based Weight Loss Diet 1,800 calories. These charts show serving allowances based on the USDA/HHS Food Guide Pyramid. Pick a chart, print it, and go!

Chapter 7: Praising Protein

Yes, low-carb, high-protein diets do take off weight, at least temporarily. But USDA still prefers carb-based plans. An Executive Summary of the agency's January 2000 Report tells why.

Chapter 8: Fiddling with Fats

Fats come in so many different varieties that just contemplating them can make your head spin. Chapter 8 unravels the mysteries. Tracking the Fat shows you how to keep track of the fats in your food (and on your plate).

Chapter 10: Nutrition for Dieters

When it comes to counting nutrients, what would we do without the Recommended Dietary Allowances (RDA) from the National Academy of Sciences? Frankly, I have no idea, so the first chart I planned for the CD-ROM was, you guessed it, RDAs for Adults. ESADDIs for Adults is a second guide to essential nutrients. Click! Click!

Chapter 11: Shopping for Weight Loss Meals

You can't build weight loss meals if you don't purchase the right foods. The Food Guide Pyramid Shopping List isn't just a pretty picture. It's a useful fill-in chart that shows you how to plan a shopping list that creates a healthful diet.

Chapter 14: Weight Loss Pills and Potions

Diet drugs can be valuable when used with medical supervision. Ingredients in Weight Loss Products Not Approved is a list of ingredients the Food and Drug Administration banned or questioned when the agency reviewed weight loss products several years ago.

Chapter 16: Gadgets and Gimmicks

Trade Advertising Cases Involving Weight Loss Products and Services, 1927lowfat1997 is a super guide to dubious products. The Partnership lists members in a private/public group designed to keep weight loss products healthful. The FTC Complaint Form shows you how to complain when things go wrong.

Chapter 17: Changing Your Food Attitudes

Changing your mind about food can help change your body. A food trigger tracker enables you to keep track of the "triggers" that send you in search of food so that you can plan strategies to avoid eating when you're not hungry.

Chapter 18: Exercise: The Essential Extra

Oh, boy, what can I say about the virtues of exercise that hasn't already been said, including by me, in Chapter 18? Not much! But you may want to read USDA's recommendations for a new guideline (on exercise) and use A Daily Exercise Chart to let you figure out what works for you. Then do it!

And more!

Shareware programs are fully functional, free trial versions of copyrighted programs. If you like particular programs, register with their authors for a nominal fee and receive licenses, enhanced versions, and technical support. *Freeware programs* are free, copyrighted games, applications, and utilities. You can copy them to as many PCs as you like — free — but they have no technical support. GNU software is governed by its own license, which is included inside the folder of the GNU software. There are no restrictions on distribution of this software. See the GNU license for more details. Trial, demo, or evaluation versions are usually limited either by time or functionality (such as being unable to save projects).

And just so that you have everything you need, I've also included a few more bonus items on the CD, including:

- ✔ All Web site links in the book so that you don't have to type them yourself
- ✔ An evaluation version of Acrobat Reader, from Adobe Systems, Inc.
- ✔ A commercial version of MindSpring Internet Access, from MindSpring
- ✔ A commercial version of Netscape Communicator 4.7, from Netscape
- ✔ A commercial version of Internet Explorer 5.5, from Microsoft

Happy surfing!

If You've Got Problems (Of the CD Kind)

I tried my best to compile programs that work on most computers with the minimum system requirements. Alas, your computer may differ, and some programs may not work properly for some reason.

The two likeliest problems are that you don't have enough memory (RAM) for the programs you want to use, or you have other programs running that are affecting installation or running of a program. If you get error messages like Not enough memory or Setup cannot continue, try one or more of these methods and then try using the software again:

- ✔ **Turn off any antivirus software that you have on your computer.** Installers sometimes mimic virus activity and may make your computer incorrectly believe that it is being infected by a virus.

- ✔ **Close all running programs.** The more programs you're running, the less memory is available to other programs. Installers also typically update files and programs. So if you keep other programs running, installation may not work properly.

- ✔ **Have your local computer store add more RAM to your computer.** This is, admittedly, a drastic and somewhat expensive step. However, if you have a Windows 95 PC or a Mac OS computer with a PowerPC chip, adding more memory can really help the speed of your computer and allow more programs to run at the same time. This may include closing the CD interface and running a product's installation program from Windows Explorer.

If you still have trouble with installing the items from the CD, please call the Hungry Minds Customer Service phone number: 800-762-2974 (outside the U.S.: 317-572-3993).

Index

• E •

• F •

• O •

• *Y* •

• *Z* •

Notes

Hungry Minds, Inc., End-User License Agreement

READ THIS. You should carefully read these terms and conditions before opening the software packet(s) included with this book ("Book"). This is a license agreement ("Agreement") between you and Hungry Minds, Inc. ("HMI"). By opening the accompanying software packet(s), you acknowledge that you have read and accept the following terms and conditions. If you do not agree and do not want to be bound by such terms and conditions, promptly return the Book and the unopened software packet(s) to the place you obtained them for a full refund.

1. **License Grant.** HMI grants to you (either an individual or entity) a nonexclusive license to use one copy of the enclosed software program(s) (collectively, the "Software") solely for your own personal or business purposes on a single computer (whether a standard computer or a workstation component of a multiuser network). The Software is in use on a computer when it is loaded into temporary memory (RAM) or installed into permanent memory (hard disk, CD-ROM, or other storage device). HMI reserves all rights not expressly granted herein.

2. **Ownership.** HMI is the owner of all right, title, and interest, including copyright, in and to the compilation of the Software recorded on the disk(s) or CD-ROM ("Software Media"). Copyright to the individual programs recorded on the Software Media is owned by the author or other authorized copyright owner of each program. Ownership of the Software and all proprietary rights relating thereto remain with HMI and its licensers.

3. **Restrictions on Use and Transfer.**

   (a) You may only (i) make one copy of the Software for backup or archival purposes, or (ii) transfer the Software to a single hard disk, provided that you keep the original for backup or archival purposes. You may not (i) rent or lease the Software, (ii) copy or reproduce the Software through a LAN or other network system or through any computer subscriber system or bulletin-board system, or (iii) modify, adapt, or create derivative works based on the Software.

   (b) You may not reverse engineer, decompile, or disassemble the Software. You may transfer the Software and user documentation on a permanent basis, provided that the transferee agrees to accept the terms and conditions of this Agreement and you retain no copies. If the Software is an update or has been updated, any transfer must include the most recent update and all prior versions.

4. **Restrictions on Use of Individual Programs.** You must follow the individual requirements and restrictions detailed for each individual program in Appendix C of this Book. These limitations are also contained in the individual license agreements recorded on the Software Media. These limitations may include a requirement that after using the program for a specified period of time, the user must pay a registration fee or discontinue use. By opening the Software packet(s), you will be agreeing to abide by the licenses and restrictions for these individual programs that are detailed in Appendix C and on the Software Media. None of the material on this Software Media or listed in this Book may ever be redistributed, in original or modified form, for commercial purposes.

Installation Instructions

The *Weight Loss Kit For Dummies* CD offers valuable information that you won't want to miss. To install the items from the CD to your hard drive, follow these steps.

1. **Insert the CD into your computer's CD-ROM drive.**

   In a moment, an icon representing the CD you just inserted appears on your Mac desktop. Chances are, the icon looks like a CD-ROM.

2. **Double-click the CD icon to show the CD's contents.**

3. **Double-click the Read Me First icon.**

   The Read Me First text file contains information about the CD's programs and any last-minute instructions you may need in order to correctly install them.

4. **To install most programs, just drag the program's folder from the CD window and drop it on your hard drive icon.**

5. **Other programs come with installer programs — with these, you simply open the program's folder on the CD and then double-click the icon with the words "Install" or "Installer."**

   Sometimes the installers are actually self extracting archives, which just means that the program files have been bundled up into an archive, and this self extractor unbundles the files and places them on your hard drive. This kind of program is often called an .sea. Double-click anything with .sea in the title, and it will run just like an installer.

   After you have installed the programs you want, you can eject the CD. Carefully place it back in the plastic jacket of the book for safekeeping.

For more information, see Appendix C.

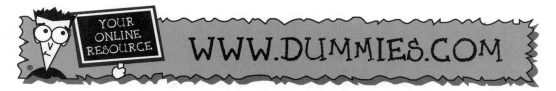

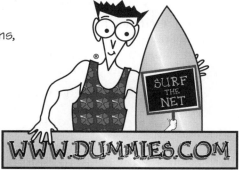

FOR DUMMIES
BOOK REGISTRATION

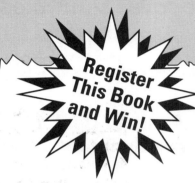

Register This Book and Win!

We want to hear from you!

Visit **dummies.com** to register this book and tell us how you liked it!

✔ Get entered in our monthly prize giveaway.

✔ Give us feedback about this book — tell us what you like best, what you like least, or maybe what you'd like to ask the author and us to change!

✔ Let us know any other *For Dummies* topics that interest you.

Your feedback helps us determine what books to publish, tells us what coverage to add as we revise our books, and lets us know whether we're meeting your needs as a *For Dummies* reader. You're our most valuable resource, and what you have to say is important to us!

Not on the Web yet? It's easy to get started with *Dummies 101: The Internet For Windows 98* or *The Internet For Dummies* at local retailers everywhere.

Or let us know what you think by sending us a letter at the following address:

For Dummies Book Registration
Dummies Press
10475 Crosspoint Blvd.
Indianapolis, IN 46256

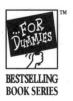

...FOR DUMMIES™

BESTSELLING
BOOK SERIES